INTERNATIONAL FALK WORKSHOP

Vanishing Bile Duct Syndrome – Pathophysiology and Treatment

EDITED BY

D. Alvaro

II Cattedra di Gastroenterologia
Dipartimento di Medicina Clinica,
Università di Roma "La Sapienza"
Viale dell'Università, 37
I-00185 Roma
Italy

A. Benedetti

Clinica di Gastroenterologia
Ospedale Torrette
I-60026 Ancona
Italy

M. Strazzabosco

Istituto d Medicina Interna
Università degli Studi di Padova
Via Giustiniani, 2
I-35128 Padova
Italy

Proceedings of the International Falk Workshop held in Spoleto (Perugia), Italy, May 30–June 1, 1996

KLUWER ACADEMIC PUBLISHERS
DORDRECHT / BOSTON / LONDON

Distributors

for the United States and Canada: Kluwer Academic Publishers, PO Box 358, Accord Station, Hingham, MA 02018-0358, USA

for all other countries: Kluwer Academic Publishers Group, Distribution Center, PO Box 322, 3300 AH Dordrecht, The Netherlands

A catalogue record for this book is available from the British Library

ISBN 0–7923–8721–X

Copyright

Published in the United Kingdom by Kluwer Academic Publishers, PO Box 55, Lancaster, UK.

Kluwer Academic Publishers BV incorporates the publishing programmes of D. Reidel, Martinus Nijhoff, Dr W. Junk and MTP Press.

Typeset by EXPO Holdings, Malaysia

Printed and bound in Great Britain by Hartnolls Ltd., Bodmin, Cornwall.

Contents

List of principal contributors

G. Alpini
Texas A & M University
Health Science Center
College of Medicine, Building 147
Olin E. Teague Veterans' Center
1901 South 1st Street
Temple
TX 76504
USA

D. Alvaro
Il Cattedra di Gastroenterologia
Dipartimento di Medicina Clinica
Università di Roma 'La Sapienza'
Viale dell'Università, 37
I-00185 Roma
Italy

A. Benedetti
Clinica di Gastroenterologia
Ospedale Torrette C.P. 38
Università di Ancona
I-60020 Ancona
Italy

U. Beuers
Department of Internal Medicine
Klinikum Grosshadern
University of Munich
D-81377 Munich
Germany

J. L. Boyer
Liver Center/Section of Digestive Diseases
Yale University School of Medicine
333 Cedar Street
New Haven
CT 06520-8019
USA

Y. Calmus
Hôpital Cochin
27 rue Faubourg Saint-Jacques
F-75014 Paris
France

L. Capocaccia
Il Cattedra di Gastroenterologia
Dipartimento di Medicina Clinica
Università di Roma 'La Sapienza'
Viale dell'Università, 37
I-00185 Roma
Italy

C. Clerici
Istituto di Gastroenterologia e Endoscopia Digestiva
Clinica Medica I
Policlinico Monteluce
Via Brunamonti, 51
I-06122 Perugia
Italy

A. J. Demetris
Division of Transplantation Pathology
Department of Pathology
University of Pittsburgh School of Medicine
E1548 Biomedical Science Tower
Pittsburgh
PA 15261
USA

V. J. Desmet
Universitaire Ziekenhuizen Sint Rafael
Lab voor Histochemie en Cytochemie
Minderbroedersstraat 12
B-3000 Leuven
Belgium

LIST OF PRINCIPAL CONTRIBUTORS

J. G. Fitz
Duke University Medical Center
Box 3671
Room 307 Sands Building
Durham
NC 27710
USA

M. E. Gershwin
Division of Rheumatology,
Allergy and Clinical Immunology
TB 192
University of California
Davis
CA 95616
USA

A. F. Hofmann
Division of Gastroenterology
Department of Medicine (0813)
University of California
San Diego
La Jolla
CA 92093-0813
USA

A. M. Jezequel
Istituto di Patologia Sperimentale
C.P. 38
Università di Ancona
I-60020 Torrette (Ancona)
Italy

R. Joplin
The Liver Research Laboratories
Queen Elizabeth Hospital
Edgbaston
Birmingham
B15 2TH
UK

S. A. Levine
Division of Gastroenterology
Mayo Clinic
Mayo Medical School
200 First St. SW
Rochester
MN 55905-0001
USA

U. Leuschner
Universitätsklinik
Medizinische Klinik II
Theodor-Stern-Kai 7
D-60590 Frankfurt am Main
Germany

P. J. Meier-Abt
Abteilung für Klinische Pharmakologie
Departement Innere Medizin
Universitätsspital
Rämistr. 100
CH-8091 Zurich
Switzerland

J. M. Neuberger
The Liver Unit
The Queen Elizabeth Hospital
Queen Elizabeth Medical Centre
Edgbaston
Birmingham B15 2TH
UK

R. P. J. Oude Elferink
Division Gastrointestinal and Liver Diseases
Academic Medical Center
University of Amsterdam
Meibergdreef 9
1105 AZ Amsterdam
The Netherlands

M. Podda
Division of Internal Medicine
School of Medicine San Paolo
University of Milan
Via di Rudiní 8
I-20142 Milano
Italy

M. Strazzabosco
Istituto di Medicina Interna
Università degli Studi di Padova
Via Giustiniani, 2
I-35100 Padova
Italy

J. M. Vierling
Center for Liver Diseases and Transplantation
Cedars-Sinai Medical Center
8635 West Third Street, 590W
Los Angeles
CA 90048-1865
USA

Preface

This book contains the contributions to the International Falk Workshop held in Spoleto, Italy, May 30–June 1, 1996. The focus of this meeting was on the physiological, pathological and clinical aspects of vanishing bile duct syndrome.

This syndrome comprises a number of chronic cholestatic diseases caused by primary immunological and functional damage to the biliary epithelium. Many of these chronic cholestatic disorders are genetic or developmental, while many others, such as primary biliary cirrhosis, primary sclerosing cholangitis and chronic rejection of liver transplant, are acquired. Although representing an important cause of morbidity and mortality, and a major indication for liver transplantation, until recently little was known regarding the pathogenesis of this group of disorders, mainly because of the lack of experimental models allowing the study of the biliary epithelium at a cellular and molecular level. Important advances have recently been made in the biology, physiology and treatment of vanishing bile duct syndrome. In particular, progress in the biology and physiology of the intrahepatic biliary epithelium has added considerably to the current understanding of the pathophysiology of this syndrome. This Workshop brought together the vast experience of investigators and clinicians actively working on the various aspects of this syndrome, from basic science to clinical practice.

The first section of the book deals with the anatomy and ultrastructure of bile duct epithelium, as well as the experimental models recently developed for the investigation of cholangiocyte functions. In addition, this section covers the physiology of cholangiocytes, with particular emphasis on transport processes and hormonal regulation.

The second section of the book is devoted to the pathophysiology of cholangiocytes, with particular focus on the cellular and molecular aspects of cholangiocyte injury and recent progress in the immunology of primary biliary cirrhosis and primary sclerosing cholangitis.

The final section deals with the clinical and therapeutic aspects of vanishing bile duct syndrome, with special emphasis on the medical treatment of early-stage primary biliary cirrhosis and primary sclerosing cholangitis and the indication for transplantation when the disease reaches an advanced stage.

As presidents of the Workshop, we are grateful to the scientific organizers, whose friendship and close collaboration were the inspiration behind this meeting. A special thanks goes to the speakers and the audience for the outstanding level of the presentations and the lively discussion.

A very special mention must also be given to the city of Spoleto whose historic atmosphere and cultural wealth made this event one to be remembered.

Our warmest gratitude to Dr. Falk, his Foundation and to Nordmark Spa without whose collaboration none of this would have been possible. Finally, thanks to O.I.C., Florence, and to Kluwer Academic Publishers whose efficiency and organization were essential.

L. Capocaccia
A. Morelli
L. Okolicsanyi
F. Orlandi

Rome: foundation and mysteries

L. CAPOCACCIA

By request of many of the participants we publish here an abridged version of the address delivered by Prof. Livio Capocaccia during the Symposium on the Vanishing Bile Duct Syndrome, held in Spoleto, 31 May – 1 June 1996. Prof. Capocaccia is not only an eminent hepatologist, but also a renowned amateur archaeologist, as well as a member of many national and international archaeological societies.

PROLOGUE

The history of the foundation of Rome clearly combines two distinct traditions: the Greek and Latin. As early as the seventh century BC (lines 1012–1017 from *Theogony*, by Esiodus) Greek folklore tells of the love affair between the Achaean, Ulysses, and the enchantress, Circe, giving birth to Latinos, obviously the root of Latium. At the beginning of the fifth century BC Greek legend celebrates the arrival of Aeneas in Latium, who together with his father and son were fleeing from the flames of Troy. Aeneas was then to marry Lavinia, and later founded the city of Lavinium. During this time the Greek colonies were in full expansion in southern Italy and we have proof that the ancient port along the Tiber was a calling ground for foreign merchants, many of whom were certainly Greek.

Roman literary tradition was the domain of certain groups of priests or scholars and was based on facts which were not part of the Greek world. First of all the name of Rome is not Greek but archaic Latin; secondly, the necessity to somehow include the city of Alba Longa (centre of the Latin League and traditionally considered as the mother-city of Rome) as part of the history of Rome; and, last of all, a chronology based on oral tales and annals of various pontifical and noble families, consistently dating the birth of Rome to around the eighth century BC. Greek tradition filled in the 400-year vacuum between the flames of Troy (twelfth to eleventh century BC) and local legend dating the foundation of Rome to the eighth century BC by inserting the dynasty of the kings of Alba Longa. The last king of Alba Longa, Numitor, was the father of Rhea Silvia, who was raped by the god Mars and bore the twin boys Romulus and Remus. Legend has it that they were breast-fed by the she-wolf, who was to become the symbol of Rome, and founded the walls of the city of Rome in 753 BC. Thus the two traditions were suitably wed, the Greeks being able to lay claim to the origins of the emerging city and the Romans glad that their status was acknowledged by the prevailing culture.

WHAT IS AUTHENTIC IN THE ANCIENT LEGENDS?

In the mid-eighteenth century historic research became imbued with the reigning positivist climate which was to last until the beginning of the following century, and whereby all traditional lore was regarded with enormous scepticism and criticism. However, with time the credibility of the tales told by classical writers was restored, and attempts were made to link these to a historical reconstruction of past events, inspired by tradition and backed up by known facts from the world of the Etruscans and Latins, not to mention linguistic developments and archaeological discoveries.

WHEN WAS ROME FOUNDED?

In 1948 Romanelli and Romagnosi, while excavating in an area to the west of the Germalo-Palatine, found traces of the foundations of a number of dwellings dating to the eighth century BC, exactly on the same site on which the ancient Romans preserved and venerated the 'House of Romulus' (*casa romuli*, in Latin). Remains dating to before the ninth century BC, of Greek and Etruscan origin (as well as Latin), were found near S. Omobono, where the Temples of Fortuna and Mater Matuta were excavated. This shows the existence of an already thriving commercial life in Rome by the ninth to eighth centuries BC (Figure 1).

The site of Rome lay near the mouth of the river Tiber, where its wide marshes narrowed, and where the firm banks allowed for easy crossing by people, herds and goods. Large salt deposits, a precious substance for ancient peoples, were also to be found. Therefore, it is not surprising that the hills which were to comprise the city were occupied way back in time by communities who were in a position to control the movement of people and goods inevitably converging on this point. This landscape itself must have greatly appealed to the early settlers. The marshy valleys and steep hills were a natural protection in themselves. Initially, the hill-tops were decked with the first villages, separated from each other by deep ravines. Gradually, as their population increased (eighth century BC), the settlements began to spread down the hillsides, soon invading the valley between the Capitol and Palatine. Around the seventh century, with the construction of the *Cloaca Maxima* (the Great Sewer) the valley, destined to be the site of the Roman Forum, was soon drained. The different communities (the Latins on the Palatine, the Sabines on the Quirinal and Capitol, the Etruscans on the Esquiline hill, and other groups on the Aventine) did not remain isolated for long, but soon began to assimilate. This can be seen in celebrations for the ancient festival of Septimontium, celebrated every year on 11 December, the day on which each of the communities offered sacrifice in honour of the hill on which they lived; proof that the different villages were beginning to feel a sense of unity. With time, alternating chiefs of important families or villages took up leading positions and later, in keeping with the habits and culture of the time, became kings, which explains the existence of Sabine, Latin and Etruscan kings.

These institutional events occurred around the end of the eighth century, coinciding with Roman tales dating the foundation of Rome to 753 BC. This is not necessarily in support of the legend of Romulus or even the very concept of 'foundation'. That the birth of the city was an act of will, taking place at a precise moment, was instinctive to the thinking of classical authors and had its origins in the story of the creation of the Greek colonies. Modern historians prefer a more gradual development, from being an isolated village to an urban aggregate, with some form of institutional structure or rituals in common.

DID THE KINGS OF ROME REALLY EXIST?

Excavations and the reconstruction of the site indicated by tradition as the 'Palace of the King', and the discovery of the fragment of a vase bearing the inscription REX found under this site, plus a number of rites maintained unchanged throughout the historical period of Rome, leave no doubts about this issue. Traditionally there were seven kings of Rome, Romulus (Latin), Numa Pompilius (Sabine), Tullius Hostilius (Latin), Ancus Marcius (Latin), Tarquinius Priscus (Tarquin I) (Etruscan), Servius Tullius (Etruscan), and Tarquinius Superbus (Etruscan), spanning a period from 753 to 509 BC.

According to legend the reign of each of the kings lasted more or less a single generation, which is almost an impossibility. The logical conclusion is that these were a necessary personalization of events and deeds of several royal successors, later restricted to a few individuals.

Apart from Romulus (clearly the eponym of Rome: *Rom-ulus* = an inhabitant of Rome), another obvious deduction may be made: among the various 'clans' and villages located in and around the hills Latins and Sabines tended to dominate, later followed by the Etruscans. On the other hand, the original three tribes of Rome were Tities (Sabines), Ramnes (Latins) and Luceres (Etruscans). These three ethnic components were maintained in the social and ritual structure of the city throughout the entire millennium when Rome ruled the world.

REGAL ROME: TRADITION AND INTERPRETATION

Of the first three kings of Rome (Latin–Sabine period), the possible historical genuineness of the alleged event refers only to Numa Pompilius, as the root of his name comes from the Sabine number 5; it is difficult to accept that this was an invention, particularly as Gens (family) Pomponia has left important traces in the life of Rome. Interpretation regarding the three Etruscan kings is easier, as legend and facts become more concrete. It suffices to state that the kings were not descendants of gods, heroes or former kings, but were in fact very human. Tarquin was the son of a merchant and Servius son of a slave, or anyway of humble parents (Servius = *servus* = servant). The story goes that Luxumo (Etruscan word for official), a rich merchant in Tarxuna (Tarquinia as we know it today) moved to Rome with his followers and all his wealth, where he gained power and sympathy. He was later adopted by the Latin king Ancus Marcius and changed his Etruscan name to the Latin Tarquinius Priscus. After the death of Ancus Marcius he became the king of Rome. He was later killed by the former king's son and his place was taken by an obscure son-in-law, Servius Tullius, in turn killed some years later by the sons of Tarquinius Priscus.

What lies behind this tale? First of all the dynasty of Tarquinius Priscus is a historical reality. It could also be hazarded that the monarchy of Tarquin is the human representation of trade links and other forms of traffic between the Etruscans and Romans, giving birth to a new order, political also, in the city, so that their economic potential prevailed over Sabine–Latin local oligarchies, finally substituting these with a true and proper monarchy, inspired by Greek and Etruscan models, and founding a dynasty. Moreover, paintings discovered by Francois in an old Etruscan tomb cast new light on the Etruscan monarchy of Tarquins. This tomb, dating back to the fifth century BC, depicts Maxstarna from the retinue of Avile Vipiennas, freeing Caile Vipiennas (Avile's brother), and then a series of warriors killing their enemies. The last warrior killed was called Cneve Tarxunies Rumax, i.e. Gneo Tarquinio Romano (Figure 2).

With regard to the intriguing figure of king Servius Tullius, today, we know enough to say that Servius can be equated with the Etruscan Maxstarna. This is clearly stated by the Emperor Claudius, who claimed to have access to Etruscan sources. His speech, delivered in AD 48, to the Senate, still survives, as it is engraved on a bronze plate found in Lyon, France (Lugdunium in Latin), the birthplace of the Emperor. The name *Maxstarna* comes from the Etruscan *Maxtr* (= chief) and *-na* (genitive or possessive case), i.e. belonging to the chief, who is easily identified as Caile Vipiennas, brother of Aville Vipiennas, whose name has also been found engraved on the fragment of a vase from the sixth century.

In light of all these considerations (the excessive duration of the reign of the legendary kings, the major public works and military deeds which could not be the work of just three kings alone, the existence of other Tarquins and the dynasty of Vipiennas, etc.) would lead us to believe in the existence of other Etruscan kings, although memory going back in time has focused only on the first and last of the Tarquins and on the outstanding personality, Maxstarna = Servius Tulius, who by force seized the leadership of Rome, perhaps the result of some form of plebeian pressure. He was killed on the return of the Tarquins, and perhaps Tarquinius Superbus was the grandson and not son of the previous Tarquinius Priscus.

Apart from these crude deeds what appears indisputable today is that at the end of the Etruscan monarchy Rome was already a great city (Figure 3). The built-up area spread over 300 hectares (the biggest Etruscan cities covered about 150 hectares), the population was between 50 000 and 100 000, the walls 13 kilometres long, and the hills at that time were about 50–60 metres high. The Rome of the Tarquins lies about 8–20 metres below present levels.

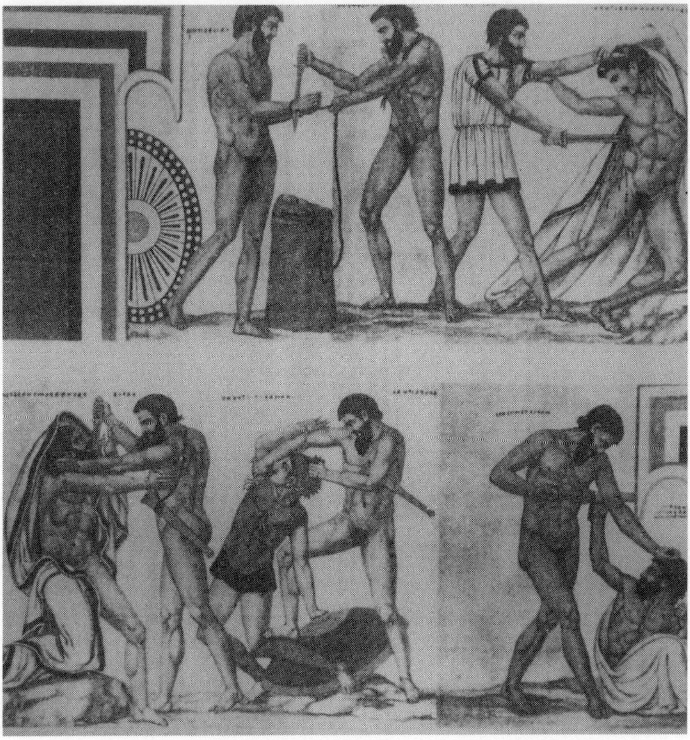

Figure 2 Etruscan tomb paintings, fifth century BC, depicting Maxstarna freeing Caile Vipiennas and a series of warriors killing their enemies

THE DECLINE OF THE MONARCHY AND THE BEGINNING OF THE REPUBLIC OF ROME?

Legend dates the end of the monarchy to 509 BC and attributes to this date the birth of 'Romana Libertas', the inauguration of the Temple of Jove on the Capitol, the beginning of the official year count marked each year by adding another nail to the Temple and, finally, the listing of the Higher Magistrates in the Consular Fasti. This list of names is today thought to be quite reliable, leaving aside their placing or pairing. The first names are plebeian, many of Etruscan ascendancy (Tarquin Collatin, Giunius Brutus) or Sabine (Publius Valerius Publicola), while from 485 BC the names of Etruscans disappear and are replaced by those of Latins. This is clear proof of the real existence of an Etruscan aristocracy, substituted by a plebeian–popular movement. A leading name in this movement was Publius Valerius Publicola (from the Latin, 'Friend of the people'), whose real existence is documented by the incision of his name above an arch in Satricum, his Sabine place of origin, dated to 480 BC (Figure 4).

The conclusion once again bears out the legend that in the early fifth century BC the Etruscan aristocracy was replaced by other Etruscan, Latin or Sabine personalities of plebeian origin, in keeping with known population movements in the Mediterranean region.

THE NAME OF ROME

Strangely enough, little is known about the origin of the name of Rome. The ancients believed that it derived from the mythical founder Romulus, which is instead an eponym (*Rom = ulus*, an inhabitant of Rome in old Latin).

According to Greek legend the word had a Greek root: ῥωμη = strength. Archaic Latin tradition has it that the name is derived from the Etruscan *rumn* = she-wolf or from the Latin *rumis* = breast, referring to the legend that the twins, Romulus and Remus, were breast fed by a she-wolf. However, as the ancients usually liked to give topographical or descriptive names to their cities, it may be that the root of Rome comes from *rumon*, i.e. river. This is further borne out by the existence of a gate to the city, *Romanula*, which led to the river.

The city also had another secret name, only used during arcane, mysterious ceremonies: this was unknown even to the most learned, the reason for the secrecy being the fear that it would be evoked by the enemy and used against the city. Thus once again we have the concept, as with the legend of Parsifal, where the name contains the essence and the force of the 'thing'. In other words the name of the city is totally identified with the city itself, and therefore the enemy should not be allowed to get hold of the secret name of the city and thus of the city itself.

There are numerous allusions regarding the existence of a secret name for Rome. One of these of Latin origin goes as follows: '*Feriae divae Angeronae Angeronalia appellantur. Huius deae simulacrum ... praenexo obsignatoque ne collocatum ... ut moneret ne quis nomen occultum urbis enuntiaret* (Plinium, *Fast. Prae., a.d. XII KAL.IAN*)', which could be translated as: 'Festivals of the Goddess Angerona are named Angeronalia. Her statue has its mouth gagged ... as if to warn everyone not to pronounce the secret name of the city.'

Secondly, as I already said, the Latins, like other ancient peoples, ritually personalized every single aspect of nature and human behaviour and, so as to be sure to be always on the right side, the Romans venerated not only these aspects but also their contrary. For example, the God Ianus, protector of the gates of Rome, from in to out and vice-versa, Aius Lucutius, personification of the 'spoken word', Tacita Muta, personification of 'silence'.

All these cults, either solar or cthonius, real or symbol-like, simple or double, have a confusing, but in some way or another a real, meaning, and were located along the Sacra Via or in the surroundings: however, within the circle of the old walls (Figure 5).

Dear friends, I know you are not enemies of Rome: thus in what I have said today I have given you the coordinates to discover the secret name of Rome. Should you come to discover it please do not say it aloud, at least only to people who already share the secret. By betraying the secret you could cause the fall of Rome and, as you know, if Rome falls the world falls with her.

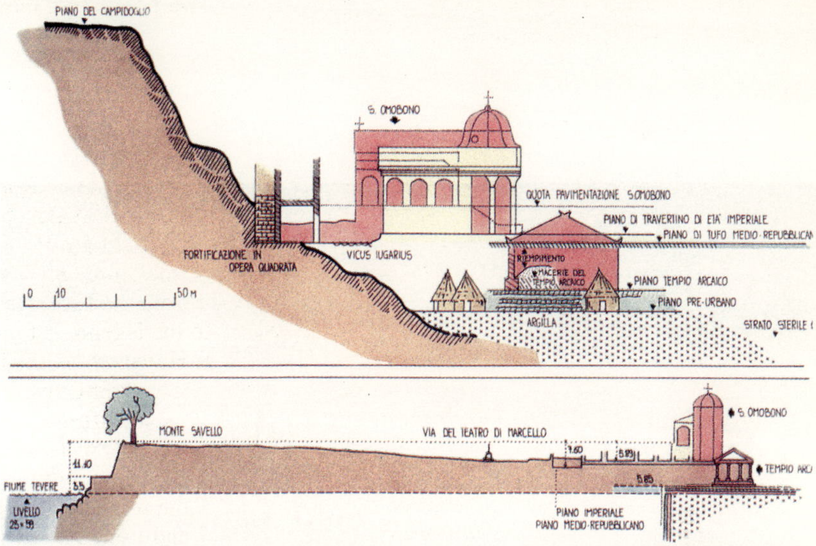

Figure 1 Cross-sectional view of the site near S. Omobono where remains dating back to before the ninth century BC were found

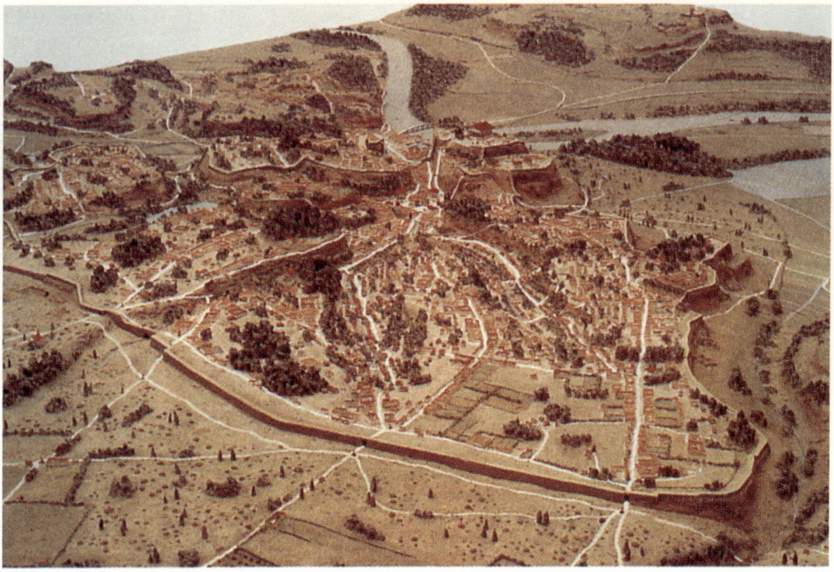

Figure 3 Reconstruction of an aerial view of Rome at the end of the Etruscan monarchy

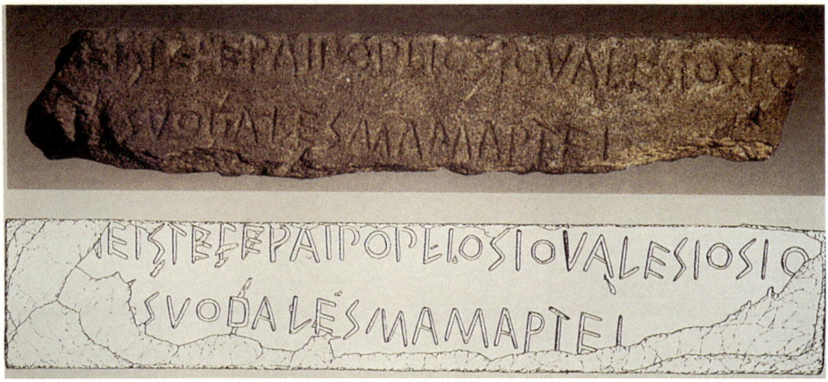

Figure 4 Incision above an arch in Satricum showing the name of Publius Valerius Publicola, 480 BC

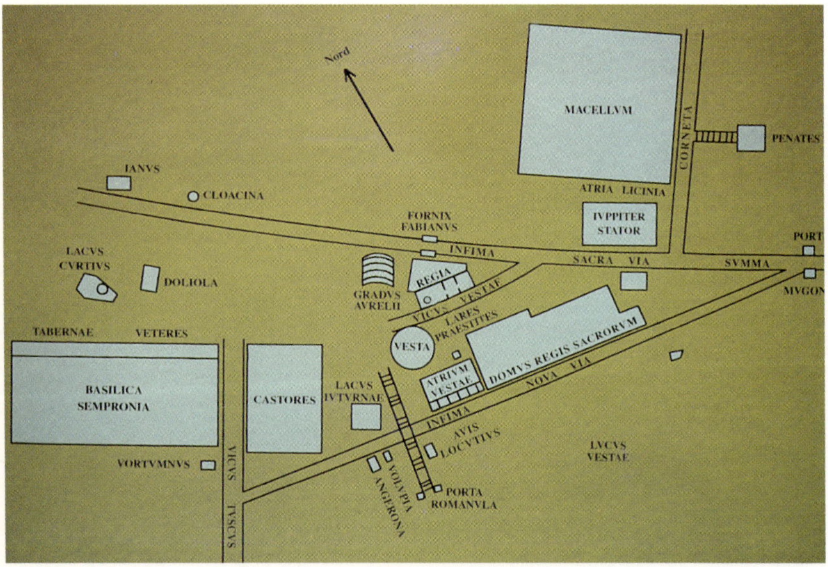

Figure 5 Sacra Via and surroundings

Section I
Basic sciences

1
Opening lecture: Vanishing bile duct syndrome – pathophysiology and treatment

J. L. BOYER

Professor Capocaccia and Co-members of the Steering Committee, Professors Morelli, Okolicsanyi and Orlandi; Distinguished Scientific Organizers, Drs Alvaro, Benedetti and Strazzabosco; ladies and gentlemen.

It is my honour and privilege to add my welcome to that of Professor Capocaccia to introduce and outline the goals of this International Falk Workshop, the Vanishing Bile Duct Syndrome – Pathophysiology and Treatment, here in Spoleto this 30 May–1 June 1996. In the next day and a half we will focus on the physiology and pathophysiology of the bile duct epithelium which, although representing only 2–5% of the total liver cell mass, occupies a strategic anatomical location where it is a collector and modifier of primary hepatocyte bile, and whose structures, when altered, may lead to chronic and even fatal cholestatic liver disorders. This audience needs no introduction to the importance of the bile duct epithelium, since the thought has long since been abandoned that it simply serves as a 'sewage pipe' for the delivery of bile from the liver to the intestine. In recent years many transport systems have been identified and characterized on this epithelium, and it is now well recognized that this is an important side of both secretory and absorptive transport functions that greatly modify primary bile constituents. Though not the focus of this meeting, the bile duct epithelium has enormous capacity for proliferation, and during obstructive cholestasis may assume as much as 30–40% of the total liver cell mass. It is, of course, a primary target for the development of chronic cholestatic liver diseases particularly primary biliary cirrhosis and sclerosing cholangitis.

From a historical viewpoint, early students of bile secretory physiology, particularly Paton Rous and P. D. McMaster, recognized that the bile duct epithelium was a distinct and separate source of secretion, from hepatocytes[1]. Rous studied the effects of common duct obstruction in several animal models in the cat and dog in the 1920s, and recognized that long-term obstruction was associated with 'white bile' previously described by surgeons. Despite this early interest, knowledge concerning the properties of the bile duct epithelium remained in its infancy. By 1965, when the first symposium of the 'NATO Advanced Study Institute, 1965' was first organized on work related to the biliary system, there was only a single page reference to bile ducts in the entire 700-page symposium. In this work there is an article by Professor W. H. H. Andrews, who said only 'I am still rash enough to consider that the biliary tract may have a function other than that of being of mere conductor of bile'[2]. Ten years later, when the second NATO Symposium on the Hepatobiliary System was held in 1975, a full chapter was devoted to bile duct function, by J. Chenderovitch. Here again he emphasizes 'For a long time the only site of bile secretion was located at the canalicular level and all the proposed mechanisms were devoted to the activity of the hepatocytes'[3]. However, as new techniques were developed for the isolation of bile duct epithelial cells, in the 1980s and 1990s, information rapidly increased, leading to the first scientific meeting devoted entirely to bile duct epithelial function in Ancona in 1992, entitled 'Basic science in gastroenterology: a seminar on biliary epithelial morphologic expression and physiology'. Two years later the AASLD sponsored a single-topic symposium on 'The pathophysiology of biliary epithelium' at Arlie House in Virginia on 23–26 June 1994, reflecting the Society's recognition of the growing importance of this topic. This meeting that we are about to begin will review the rapid progress made in only the past 2 years. This November the AASLD's postgraduate course will be devoted entirely to 'Diseases of the bile duct, pathogenesis and pathophysiology'.

Our symposium today and tomorrow is divided into three sessions: (1) Basic sciences, (2) Pathophysiology and (3) Clinical aspects and therapy. The session will begin with discussions on the anatomy and ultrastructure of the bile duct epithelium, reflecting increased knowledge of the structural heterogeneity of this epithelium. A great deal of work will be presented on transport systems for both secretion and absorptive functions. A session on pathophysiology will deal with our increasing understanding of the molecular biology of cholestasis, including translations of basic studies of defects in membrane transport systems to clinical liver disorders, as well as with defects in biliary lipid excretion and basic mechanisms in immunological disturbances that lead to the vanishing bile duct syndrome. The symposium will conclude with a session on therapeutic approaches, including transplantation, graft rejection, and medical treatment, and including studies on the mechanisms of action of ursodeoxycholic acid. The overall goal will be to review the basic science in this field and to assess its application to clinical disorders that comprise the vanishing bile duct syndromes. I look forward, with you, to the coming presentations.

References

1. Rous P, McMaster PD. Physiologic causes of stasis bile. J Exp Med. 1921;34:75–95.
2. Andrews WHH. Hepatic circulation with special reference to the relationship of the bile duct and the lymphatic system. In: Taylor W, editor. The biliary system. Oxford: Blackwell Scientific Publications; 1965:79–87.
3. Chenderovitch J. Bile duct function in biliary secretion. In: Taylor W, editor. The hepatobiliary system: fundamental and pathological mechanisms. London: Plenum Press; 1976:267–85.

2
Anatomy, development and pathology of the biliary tree

V. J. DESMET

ANATOMY OF THE BILIARY TREE

The biliary tree represents the tubular system which drains bile from inside the liver towards the duodenum. It comprises the extrahepatic and intrahepatic bile ducts. The extrahepatic part of the biliary tree is composed of the right and left hepatic ducts, which join together to form the common hepatic duct; the latter further descends in the lesser omentum and, after junction with the cystic duct from the gallbladder, forms the common bile duct. The latter continues downwards in the hepatoduodenal fold of peritoneum, passes behind the first part of the duodenum and the pancreas, then bends to the right to enter the second part of the duodenum at the papilla of Vater.

The intrahepatic part of the biliary tree comprises a system of ducts with 12 generations of branching[1]. From the hilum of the liver towards the periphery, one distinguishes with steadily decreasing diameter: the right and left hepatic ducts, the segmental ducts, the area ducts, the septal ducts, the interlobular ducts, the ductules or cholangioles, and canals of Hering (Table 1).

Table 1 Intrahepatic bile ducts terminology

Generation of branching	*Diameter* (μm)	*Terminology*
Large intrahepatic bile ducts: grossly recognizable		
First generation	> 800	Left and right hepatic duct
Second generation	400–800	Segmental ducts
Third generation	± 300–400	Area ducts
Small intrahepatic bile ducts: not grossly recognizable		
—	> 100	Septal ducts
—	15–100	Interlobular ducts
	15–40	small
	40–100	medium-sized
Twelfth generation	< 15	Ductules (cholangioles)
		Canal of Hering

'Large intrahepatic bile ducts' correspond to the branches which are grossly recognizable (hepatic, segmental and area ducts).

'Small intrahepatic bile ducts' is a collective term which refers to the part of the duct system which is not grossly recognizable, and needs study by microscopic techniques (septal and interlobular ducts, ductules and canals of Hering).

Larger ducts are lined by columnar cells, whereas smaller ducts are lined by less tall cells, gradually decreasing in size as the diameter of the ducts decreases; the ductules are lined by small cuboidal cells.

All bile duct lining cells rest on a basement membrane, and are vascularized by a peribiliary vascular plexus fed by branches from the hepatic artery[2]. Large intrahepatic ducts are provided with periductal or peribiliary glands[3,4].

Distinction can be made between intramural glands, which are sparse and represent simple epithelial evaginations into the periductal fibrous wall, and extramural glands. The latter correspond to arborizing tubulo-alveolar glands which are connected with the bile duct through a secretory duct[3].

The tubulo-alveolar gland clusters are surrounded by a layer of denser collagenized mesenchyme. They contain mucous and predominantly serous acini. The glands have been shown to secrete mucin glycoproteins (neutral, carboxylated, and sulphated mucins), serous fluid, lysozyme, lactoferrin, immunoglobulin A, secretory component, and pancreatic alpha-amylase, lipase and trypsin[5]. Some interspersed neuroendocrine cells occur between the mucous and serous glandular cells, showing immunoreactivity for somatostatin[6].

The extramural glands are mostly located on opposite sides of a duct, in a plane parallel to the orientation of the limiting parenchymal plate surrounding the portal tract[4,7].

The smallest intrahepatic ducts (ductules or cholangioles) measure less than 15 μm in diameter, and are lined by three or four cuboidal bile duct epithelial cells. Bile ductules appear to be the site of hepatic progenitor cells[8]. The canals of Hering can be viewed as the finest ramifications of the intrahepatic biliary tree, which establish connections with the intercellular canaliculi of the liver cell plates in the parenchyma. The canal of Hering is lined partly by bile ductular cells, partly by hepatic parenchymal cells. The areas lined by bile duct epithelial cells are surrounded by a basement membrane[1].

DEVELOPMENT OF THE BILIARY TREE

The biliary tree develops together with the liver from the liver bud, a thickening of the endoblastic epithelium in the ventral wall of the foregut near the origin of the yolk sac in the 18-day human embryo[9,10]. The liver bud develops into the hepatic diverticulum that protrudes into the septum transversum; the latter is a transverse sheet of mesodermal cells that separates the pericardial from the peritoneal cavity. In the 5 mm human embryo the hepatic diverticulum comprises two parts: a cranial pars hepatica and a caudal pars cystica. The latter one develops into the gallbladder, whereas the extrahepatic bile ducts derive from a prolongation of the caudal part of the hepatic diverticulum. From the beginning, and throughout their development, these structures are provided with a central lumen[10].

During the fifth week after conception the biliary channel above the junction of the cystic duct with the common bile duct becomes the site of some remodelling: it transforms into a funnel-like structure, in which endoblastic proliferation creates several folds giving rise to several channels. From these develop the left and right hepatic ducts, with considerable variability in the morphology of the Y-shaped junction between the hepatic ducts and the common bile duct[10].

The intrahepatic part of the biliary tree develops, like the liver, from the cranial pars hepatica of the hepatic diverticulum. The latter gives off irregular outgrowths of cells (hepatoblasts) that invade the septum transversum. This liver primordium is composed of a uniform population of bipotential progenitor cells that will give rise to both liver parenchymal cells and biliary epithelial cells[9,11]. During the first 7 weeks of embryonic life the primitive liver primordium does not comprise any intrahepatic bile ducts. The latter develop in close association with the portal vein branches, starting at the hilum of the liver, and gradually extending throughout the organ as it develops further during the whole foetal period.

The development of intrahepatic bile ducts is characterized by the formation of 'ductal plates', i.e. (partly) duplicated layers of hepatoblasts with altered phenotype surrounding the portal vein branches.

Three-dimensionally, the ductal plate corresponds to a double-walled epithelial cylinder ensheathing the portal vein branch with its layer of surrounding mesenchyme[12–14]. Gradually, tubular dilatations appear along the perimeter of the ductal plate. These tubular formations become incorporated into the mesenchyme surrounding the portal vein branches (future portal tracts), whereas the remaining non-dilated parts of the ductal plate gradually disappear. This remodelling process of the ductal plate results in the creation of tubular ducts, located within the portal mesenchyme, and connected through thin epithelial channels (future ductules) with the periportal parenchyma.

Formation of ductal plates and their remodelling occurs throughout the full period of foetal development, resulting in the presence of intrahepatic bile ducts in various stages of development at any given point in time: more mature ducts near the hilum, more immature types of structures towards the periphery.

At 40 weeks some of the smallest, most peripheral ramifications of the portal vein are still surrounded by immature ductal plates, indicating that the development of the intrahepatic biliary tree is not yet fully terminated at the time of birth[15,16].

The switch in phenotype from hepatoblasts into bile duct type cells is accompanied by changes in the expression of a number of molecules: decrease in α_1-antitrypsin and α-fetoprotein, increased expression of cytokeratins 19 and 7 and of carcinoembryonic antigen (CEA), and changed expression of surface carbohydrate chain structures[16].

Factors that regulate the differentiation of progenitor cells into biliary type epithelium appear to include matrix components, e.g. collagen type IV, laminin and tenascin[16]. The development of ductal plates and their remodelling involves production and deletion of considerable numbers of epithelial cells; the proliferation appears controlled by growth factors (TGFα) and their receptors, and differentiation factors such as parathyroid-hormone related peptide[16], while epithelial deletion, as expected, seems to involve the universal process of apoptosis[17].

Heterogeneity along the biliary tree is already apparent during foetal development. Larger, but not smaller, intrahepatic bile ducts express pancreatic enzymes

(α-amylase, trypsinogen, lipase) throughout development, and require expression of tenascin in the surrounding biomatrix[16], whereas the extrahepatic portion of the biliary tree expresses a 40 kDa epithelial antigen shared by the gut and the skin[18].

The peribiliary glands of the larger intrahepatic bile ducts develop as evaginations of the ductal plates or of the tubular structures in a somewhat more advanced stage of bile duct formation[16].

The peribiliary capillary or vascular plexus develops *pari-passu* with the emergence and maturation of the intrahepatic ducts, from primitive angioblasts through immature and premature stages, into the final mature stage of a double peribiliary plexus[19].

PATHOLOGY OF THE BILIARY TREE

The biliary tree may be the site of several pathological processes, of which only some pertaining to the intrahepatic bile ducts will be briefly considered. Besides infections, parasitic infestations and tumours, the intrahepatic bile ducts may be the seat of a number of disease processes which have been topics of considerable interest in recent years, and which can be categorized under two broad headings: congenital diseases of intrahepatic bile ducts and vanishing bile duct disorders.

Congenital diseases of intrahepatic bile ducts

A fundamental disturbance in bile duct development consists in a partial or complete lack of the remodelling of ductal plates. This results in the persistence throughout later (foetal, infantile, adult) stages of the primitive, embryonic patterns of bile ducts with excess epithelial structures in ductal plate configuration. This lesion is termed 'ductal plate malformation' (DPM), and is usually associated with an abnormality in the branching pattern of the portal vein characterized by too many, too small and too closely spaced branches: the 'pollard willow' pattern of branching[13].

DPM is a basic morphological component in most, if not all, congenital diseases of intrahepatic bile ducts: the latter can be categorized into 'atretic' and 'fibrocystic' varieties. The atretic diseases comprise extrahepatic bile duct atresia (EHBDA) and paucity of interlobular bile ducts (PILBD).

In a variable percentage of patients (20–60%) with EHBDA, the intrahepatic bile ducts display DPM[20,21]. This finding suggests an early, antenatal start of the disease, explaining the advanced degree of fibrosis at a very young age, and justifying the term 'early, severe EHBDA' for this subgroup of cases. Successful hepatic portoenterostomy in such patients often results over several years in a picture indistinguishable from that of congenital hepatic fibrosis (CHF)[20,22]. DPM has not yet been reported in syndromic or non-syndromic forms of PILBD, but seems to occur sporadically[1].

The fibrocystic group of congenital diseases of intrahepatic bile ducts represents a heterogeneous group of conditions, which have in common the morphological hallmark of DPM.

The liver lesion in autosomal recessive polycystic kidney disease corresponds to DPM of interlobular ducts[12]. Congenital hepatic fibrosis can be interpreted as

DPM of interlobular ducts, modulated by a slowly progressive, destructive cholangitis resulting in progressive biliary fibrosis[22].

Caroli's disease corresponds to DPM of larger intrahepatic bile ducts, whereas Caroli's syndrome combines the lesions of Caroli's disease and congenital hepatic fibrosis[13]. Von Meyenburg complexes represent DPM of smaller interlobular ducts; their progressive dilatation is at the origin of liver cysts in autosomal dominant polycystic kidney disease[23,24].

DPM at all levels of the intrahepatic biliary tree results in a combination of the various anatomical–clinical entities of fibrocystic diseases[13,25].

Although DPM may be recognized as a basic morphological component in virtually all congenital diseases of intrahepatic bile ducts, further studies are indicated into the genetic or other abnormalities responsible for total or partial lack of remodelling of ductal plates in these various anatomical–clinical entities[26].

Vanishing bile duct disorders

A number of diseases of the intrahepatic bile ducts are associated with progressive destruction and disappearance of particular segments of the intrahepatic biliary tree; constituting a group of 'vanishing bile duct disorders'[27].

The morphological types of cholangitis leading to destruction and disappearance of segments of the intrahepatic bile ducts have been categorized as lymphocytic, pleomorphic, granulomatous and fibro-obliterative cholangitis[28].

The putative mechanisms causing injury and destruction of bile ducts in diseases resulting in ductopenia can be classified as: developmental and genetic, neoplastic, immunological, toxic, infectious, ischaemic, and unclassified[29].

Developmental and genetic diseases

Extrahepatic bile duct atresia (EHBDA) results from the progressive destruction of extrahepatic and intrahepatic segments of the biliary tract by a necro-inflammatory process of unknown aetiology[20].

Paucity of interlobular bile ducts (PILBD) of the syndromic variety (Alagille's syndrome) is inherited as an autosomal dominant trait with variable penetrance. The non-syndromic varieties occur sporadically without apparent genetic transmission[30].

The basic histopathology in both the syndromic and non-syndromic forms of PILBD consists in a destructive, necro-inflammatory cholangitis[31].

Other genetic diseases associated with ductopenia include cystic fibrosis, α_1-antitrypsin deficiency, trihydroxycoprostanic acidaemia, trisomies 17, 18, 21 and Byler's disease[29].

Neoplastic disorders

Histiocytosis X, or Langerhans' cell histiocytosis, is a rare disorder occurring predominantly in childhood with rapidly progressive multisystem involvement and characterized by proliferation of dendritic Langerhans histiocytes. Histiocytic proliferation in the portal and periportal areas results in periductal fibrosis with cholangiographic features resembling sclerosing cholangitis, duct destruction, and ultimately biliary cirrhosis[32].

Hodgkin's disease may also be associated with destruction of intrahepatic bile ducts, even without lymphomatous portal tract infiltration, suggesting a possible role for cytokines released by lymphoma cells in bile duct destruction[33].

Immunological mechanisms

A primary immune pathogenesis appears to be responsible for destruction of bile ducts of different sizes in several diseases: primary biliary cirrhosis (PBC), immune cholangitis, primary sclerosing cholangitis (PSC), sarcoidosis, chronic graft versus host disease (CGVHD) and hepatic allograft rejection.

Discussions of immunological mechanisms involved can be found in several recent reviews[27,29,34–36] (and Vierling J, Gershwin E, Joplin R in this Symposium).

Infectious causes

Ascending cholangitis due to enteric organisms may result in focal ductopenia due to acute inflammatory destruction of bile duct epithelia in purulent cholangitis[29].

Several viral infections have been incriminated as causes of ductopenia: reovirus type 3, cytomegalovirus and hepatitis C virus, but the subject remains controversial at present. Infections with cryptosporidia may cause lesions resembling PSC in patients with AIDS[37].

Toxins, drugs and iatrogenic causes

Paraquat toxicity includes injury to intrahepatic bile ducts[38]. Several medications cause a cholestatic injury associated with an acute, destructive cholangitis, followed by a chronic cholestatic period with progressive ductopenia[39]. Iatrogenic bile duct lesions resembling primary sclerosing cholangitis may be caused by instillation of scolicidal solutions into echinococcal cysts, following intra-arterial injection of floxuridine for treatment of hepatic metastases, and after chemoembolization for treatment of hepatocellular carcinoma[29].

Ischaemic causes

Survival of bile duct epithelium is dependent upon an adequate arterial blood supply through the peribiliary vascular plexus fed by hepatic artery branches. Any interference with this arterial supply may cause ischaemic necrosis of bile duct segments, resulting in varying degrees of ductopenia at different levels of the biliary tree[29].

Unclassified causes

'Idiopathic adulthood ductopenia' is an entity described in 1988, which by definition occurs in adults, and is characterized by progressive destruction of intrahepatic bile ducts resulting in ductopenia. The aetiology and pathogenesis are unknown[40].

References

1. Desmet VJ, Roskams T, De Vos R. Gallbladder and bile ducts: normal anatomy. In: Feldman M, editor. Gastroenterology and hepatology: the comprehensive visual reference. Volume 'Gallbladder and bile ducts', La Russo N, editor. Philadelphia: Current Medicine, (In press).
2. Ohtani O. The peribiliary portal system in the rabbit liver. Arch Histol Jpn. 1979;42:153–67.
3. Terada T, Nakanuma Y, Ohta G. Glandular elements around the intrahepatic bile ducts in man: their morphology and distribution in normal livers. Liver. 1987;7:1–8.
4. Ishida F, Terada T, Nakanuma Y. Histologic and scanning electron microscopic observations of intrahepatic peribiliary glands in normal human livers. Lab Invest. 1989;60:260–5.
5. Terada T, Morita T, Hoso M, Nakanuma Y. Pancreatic enzymes in the epithelium of intrahepatic large bile ducts and in hepatic bile in patients with extrahepatic bile duct obstruction. J Clin Pathol. 1994;47:924–7.
6. Kurumaya H, Ohta G, Nakanuma Y. Endocrine cells in the intrahepatic biliary tree in normal livers and hepatolithiasis. Arch Pathol Lab Med. 1989;113:143–7.
7. Terada T, Nakanuma Y. Development of human intrahepatic peribiliary glands. Histological, keratin immunohistochemical, and mucus histochemical studies. Lab Invest. 1993;68:261–9.
8. Desmet V, Roskams T, Van Eyken P. Ductular reaction in the liver. Path Res Pract. 1995;191:513–24.
9. Desmet VJ. Embryogenèse des voies biliaires. Méd Thérapeut. 1995;1:227–35.
10. Tan CEL, Moscoso GJ. The developing human biliary system at the porta hepatis level between 29 days and 8 weeks of gestation: a way to understanding biliary atresia. Part 1. Pathol Int. 1994;44:587–99.
11. Desmet VJ. Embryology of the liver and intrahepatic biliary tract, and an overview of malformations of the bile duct. In: McIntyre N, Benhamou JP, Bircher J, Rizzetto M, Rodes J, editors. The Oxford textbook of clinical hepatology, Vol. 1. Oxford: Oxford University Press; 1991:497–519.
12. Jørgensen MJ. The ductal plate malformation. A study of the intrahepatic bile duct lesion in infantile polycystic disease and congenital hepatic fibrosis. Acta Pathol Microbiol Scand (Suppl.), 1977;257:1–88.
13. Desmet VJ. Congenital diseases of intrahepatic bile ducts: variations on the theme 'ductal plate malformation'. Hepatology. 1992;16:1069–83.
14. Desmet VJ. Intrahepatic bile ducts under the lens. J Hepatol. 1985;1:545–59.
15. Van Eyken P, Sciot R, Callea F, Van der Steen K, Moerman P, Desmet VJ. The development of the intrahepatic bile ducts in man: a keratin–immunohistochemical study. Hepatology. 1988;8:1586–95.
16. Van Eyken P, Desmet VJ. Embryology of the liver and bile ducts. In: Balistreri WF, Ohi R, Todani T, Tsuchida Y, editors. Hepato-biliary, pancreatic and splenic disease in children: medical and surgical management. Amsterdam: Elsevier (In press).
17. Terada T, Nakanuma Y. Detection of apoptosis and expression of apoptosis-related proteins during human intrahepatic bile duct development. Am J Pathol. 1995;146:67–74.
18. Das KM, Squillante L, Chitayet D, Kalousek DK. Simultaneous appearance of a unique common epitope in fetal colon, skin and biliary epithelial cells. A possible link for extracolonic manifestations in ulcerative colitis. J Clin Gastroenterol. 1992;15:311–16.
19. Terada T, Nakanuma Y. Development of human peribiliary capillary plexus: a lectin–histochemical and immunohistochemical study. Hepatology. 1993;18:529–36.
20. Desmet VJ, Callea F. Cholestatic syndromes of infancy and childhood. In: Zakim D, Boyer TD, editors. Hepatology: a textbook of liver disease, 2nd edn, vol. 2. Philadelphia: WB Saunders; 1990:1355–95.
21. Terracciano LM, Cathomas G, Vecchione R, Tornillo L, Gudat F, Bianchi L. Extrahepatic bile duct atresia associated with hyperplasia of the intrahepatic bile ducts ('early severe form'): high incidence in a south-italian population. Pathol Res Pract. 1995;191:192.
22. Desmet VJ. What is congenital hepatic fibrosis? Histopathology. 1992;20:465–77.
23. Melnick PJ. Polycystic liver. Analysis of seventy cases. Arch Pathol. 1955;59:162–72.
24. Karhunen PJ. Adult polycystic liver disease and biliary microhamartomas (Von Meyenburg's complexes). Acta Pathol Microbiol Immunol Scand. [A], 1986;94:397–400.
25. Desmet V. Pathogenesis of ductal plate abnormalities. Mayo Clin Proc. 1996 (In press).
26. D'Agata IDA, Jonas MM, Perez-Atayde AR, Guay-Woodford LM. Combined cystic disease of the liver and kidney. Semin Liver Dis. 1994;14:215–28.

27. Desmet VJ. Vanishing bile duct disorders. In: Boyer JL, Ockner RK, editors. Progress in liver diseases, vol. X. Philadelphia: WB Saunders; 1992:89–121.
28. Ludwig J. New concepts in biliary cirrhosis. Semin Liver Dis. 1987;7:293–301.
29. Woolf GM, Vierling JM. Disappearing intrahepatic bile ducts: the syndromes and their mechanisms. Semin Liver Dis. 1993;13:261–75.
30. Kahn E. Paucity of interlobular bile ducts. Arteriohepatic dysplasia and nonsyndromic duct paucity. In: Abramowsky CR, Bernstein J, Rosenberg HS, editors. Perspectives in pediatric pathology. Transplantation pathology – hepatic morphogenesis, vol. 14. Basel: Karger; 1991:168–215.
31. Desmet VJ. The cholangiopathies. In: Suchy FJ, editor. Liver disease in children. St Louis: Mosby; 1994:145–65.
32. Thompson PP, Pitt HA, Lewin KJ, Longmire JRWP. Sclerosing cholangitis and histiocytosis X. Gut. 1984;25:526–30.
33. Hubscher SG, Lumley MA, Elias E. Vanishing bile duct syndrome: a possible mechanism for intrahepatic cholestasis in Hodgkin's lymphoma. Hepatology. 1993;17:70–7.
34. Vierling JM. Primary biliary cirrhosis. In: Zakim D, Boyer TD, editors. Hepatology: a textbook of liver disease, 2nd edn. vol. 2. Philadelphia: WB Saunders; 1990:1158–205.
35. Nakanuma Y, Tsuneyama K, Gershwin ME, Yasoshima M. Pathology and immunopathology of primary biliary cirrhosis with emphasis on bile duct lesions: recent progress. Semin Liver Dis. 1995;15:313–28.
36. Vierling JM, Hu K-Q. immunologic mechanisms of hepatobiliary injury. In: Kaplowitz N, editor. Liver and biliary diseases. Baltimore: Williams & Wilkins; 1992:48–69.
37. Sherlock S. Pathogenesis of sclerosing cholangitis: the role of nonimmune factors. Semin Liver Dis. 1991;11:5–10.
38. Mullick FG, Ishak KG, Mahabir R, Stromeyer FW. Hepatic injury associated with paraquat toxicity in humans. Liver. 1981;1:209–21.
39. Degott C, Feldmann G, Larrey D *et al.* Drug-induced prolonged cholestasis in adults: a histological semiquantitative study demonstrating progressive ductopenia. Hepatology. 1992;15:244–51.
40. Ludwig J, Wiesner RH, La Russo NF. Idiopathic adulthood ductopenia. A cause of chronic cholestatic liver disease and biliary cirrhosis. J Hepatol. 1988;7:193–9.

3
Subcellular features of the biliary epithelium in health and disease

A. M. JEZEQUEL, A. BENEDETTI, C. BASSOTTI, K. RAPINO and F. ORLANDI

INTRODUCTION

The knowledge we currently have of the fine morphology of the intrahepatic biliary tree has been gradually and very slowly acquired. Hepatic lobules were identified by Malpighi in 1666[1]. Mascagni in 1819[2] recognized their grape-like configuration and Kiernan in 1833[3] further developed the concept of the hepatic lobule. In 1853 it was said that the liver tissue is composed of 'biliary cells, blood vessels and biliary canals'[4], but 'biliary cells' in this context was actually referring to hepatocytes. Although the presence of bile ducts in the portal spaces was recognized, nothing was known about the configuration of bile canaliculi or the transition between the liver cells and the biliary epithelium. Progress in the techniques of tissue processing, and in the resolution of optical microscopes, has produced additional information in this area, but not until 1960 did the development of techniques for processing and examination of biological samples for electron microscopy allow identification of the smallest branches of the intrahepatic biliary tree, up to the smallest components and the transitional areas[5]. A new impulse has been present in recent years, with the development of techniques for isolation of the intrahepatic biliary tree, fragments of ducts or isolated biliary cells[6–8], together with immunohistochemical techniques[9]. This has permitted investigations on preparations enriched in biliary cells, and has led to a remarkable expansion of knowledge concerning the pathophysiology of the biliary epithelium. Special attention has been devoted to the intrahepatic biliary tree, that is the part extending from the ducts of Hering to the septal bile ducts. The duct of Hering is the transitional segment located at the level of the limiting plate, connecting the network of the biliary canaliculi with the ductules. At this level, hepatocytes and cholangiocytes share a common lumen and common junctional complexes. *In situ*, the volume density of the biliary epithelium accounts for only about 0.14% of the total parenchymal area[10–13], representing about 3% of the nuclear population[10] when estimated on routine sections examined under the light microscope. This figure is probably underestimated, since ducts smaller than 10 μm escape observation under these conditions[13]. That the population of biliary cells is relatively small, when examined *in situ*, explains the small number of studies on biliary cells, for so long, as opposed to studies of hepatocytes. Preparations of isolated bile ducts allow recovery of the smallest ducts, up to 5 μm in diameter, lined by two cholangiocytes, but not the transitional area (duct of Hering) lined by both cholangiocytes and hepatocytes, which can be seen only *in situ*. In this area the passage is abrupt between hepatocytes and cholangiocytes, without evidence of transitional features in the normal liver. The morphological appearance of hepatocytes and cholangiocytes is distinct, whether for the size of the cells, the nucleocytoplasmic ratio, the organelle content and distribution, or the relationship with a basement membrane (Figure 1). The ducts of Hering are not easily seen in routine sections examined under the light microscope. They can be more readily detected by immunohistochemistry, allowing demonstration of specific cytokeratins even in cells apparently isolated in the parenchyma[14]. At the margin of the portal spaces, the bile ductules, less than 20 μm in cross-section, present a lumen surrounded by a homogeneous population of cholangiocytes resting on a continuous basement membrane. The lining cells are short, and with a high nucleocytoplasmic ratio. Well-developed tight junctions prevent communication between the ductular lumen and the surrounding tessutal spaces (Figure 2). Next to the tight junctions the membranes of adjacent cells are usually straight and closely apposed, while towards the base of the cells they show complex plications, suggesting that variations of cell volume may occur in response to various stimuli[5], as shown, for instance, with the 'emptying' of the cytoplasm after exposure to secretin[15]. Interlobular bile ducts are larger, 20–100 μm in cross-section, and are located at a distance from the edge of portal spaces. The lining cells are taller than in bile ductules, the nucleocytoplasmic ratio is lower and the cellular organelles are distributed in a somewhat similar fashion. However, the nucleus tends to migrate towards the basal pole of the cells, accompanied by the components of the Golgi apparatus[13]. In septal bile ducts, 100 μm and more in cross-section, the lining epithelium tends to assume a columnar pattern, with elongated cells exhibiting a nucleus located close to the basal area and a low nucleocytoplasmic ratio. It is remarkable that, despite the variable size and morphology of the cholangiocytes along the intrahepatic biliary tree, there is no significant difference concerning the volume density of the subcellular organelles, as shown by morphometric studies, with a paucity of rough endoplasmic reticulum, rare lysosomes and few, small mitochondria. The main variables are the gradual increase in cell size – which correlates with the diameter of the duct – together with a gradual decrease of the nucleocytoplasmic ratio from the smallest to the largest ducts (Figure 3), accompanied by a displacement of the nucleus towards the base of the cells[13].

In situ, as well as in isolated intrahepatic ductules, evidence of active endocytosis along the basolateral membrane is suggested by the presence of numerous pinocytic vesicles. This evidence is supported by the uptake of fluid-phase markers such as horseradish peroxidase, and the arrest of intracellular trafficking

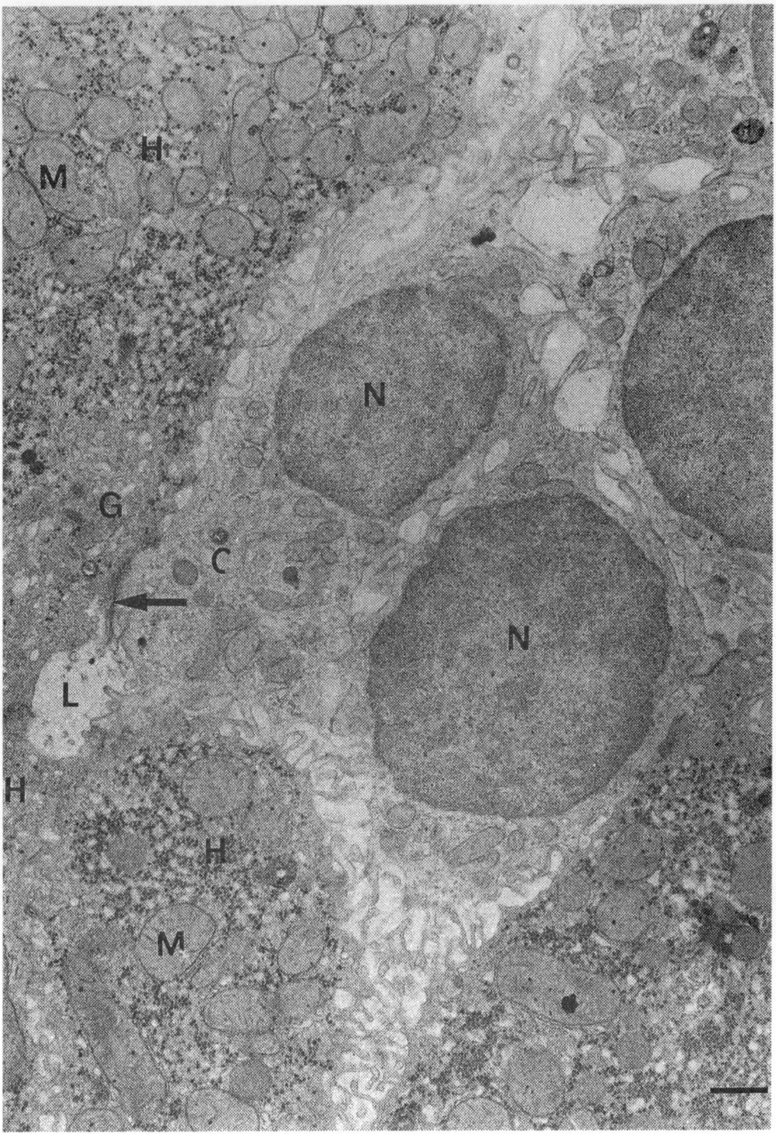

Figure 1 Part of human liver parenchyma showing a zone of transition in the biliary pathway. In this micrograph the lumen of the canalicular–ductular junction (L) is lined by three hepatocytes (H) and one cholangiocyte (C). On the right a small lumen is lined by one hepatocyte and one cholangiocyte. The subcellular organization is strikingly different in cholangiocytes and hepatocytes, with abundant glycogen, numerous mitochondria (M) and well-developed Golgi areas (G) in hepatocytes, smaller size, scarce endoplasmic reticulum and high nucleocytoplasmic ratio in cholangiocytes. Hepatocytes and cholangiocytes contribute to the formation of common tight junctions (arrow) around a common lumen. A basement membrane is already evident at this level along the cholangiocytes, running parallel to the basolateral aspect of the cells. N: nucleus, M: mitochondria. Bar = 1 μm

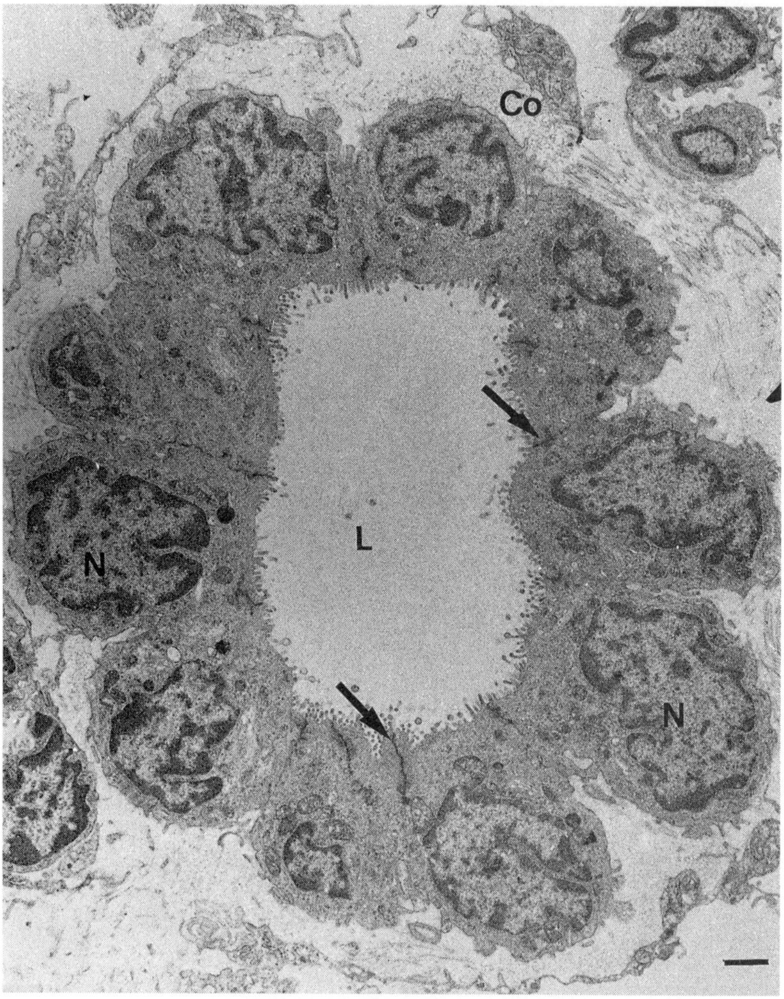

Figure 2 This micrograph illustrates the aspect of an isolated intrahepatic rat bile duct, about 20 μm in diameter. The duct is lined by cholangiocytes, remarkably homogeneous in size, with well-preserved tight junctions (arrows) and apical microvilli. There is also a good preservation of the basolateral aspect of the cells which is associated with some components of the extracellular matrix. L: lumen, N: nuclei, Co: collagen fibres. Bar = 1 μm

after exposure of cells to Brefeldin A[8,16]. The presence of specific receptors along the basolateral membrane has been detected by immunofluorescence and confirmed by immunoelectron microscopy, showing, for instance, the binding sites of antibodies to M35 muscarinic acetylcholine receptors. The special labelling of membrane invaginations exhibiting the structure of coated pits strongly suggests receptor-mediated endocytosis (unpublished). Although secondary lysosomes are scarce in the normal tissue, overload of these organelles may occur in some lysosomal storage diseases such as MPS type II[17] (Figure 4),

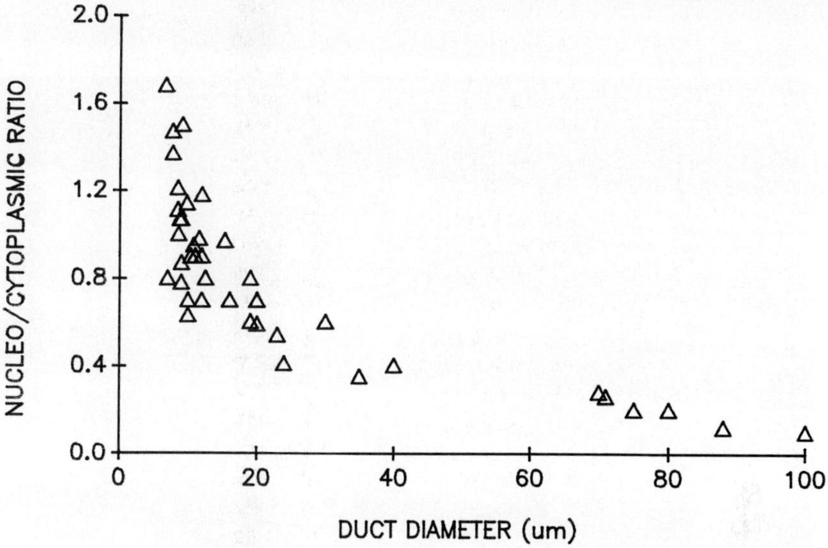

(a)

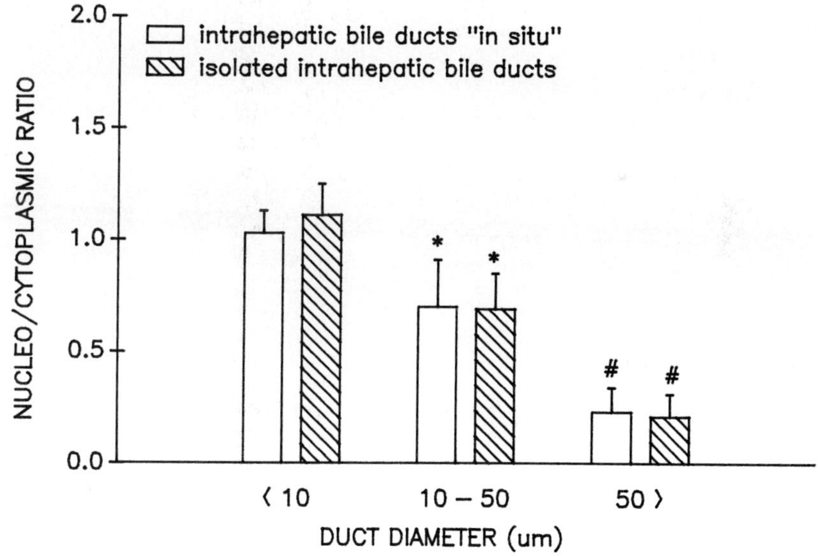

(b)

Figure 3 **(a)** Diagram illustrating the inverse relationship between the nucleocytoplasmic ratio in cholangiocytes and the diameter of the ducts ($p < 0.001$). **(b)** The inverse relationship is evident whether the observations are conducted on histological sections (white bars) or on ultrathin sections of isolated intrahepatic bile ducts (hatched bars) *$p < 0.002$ vs #. (Reproduced from ref. 13, with permission of the publisher)

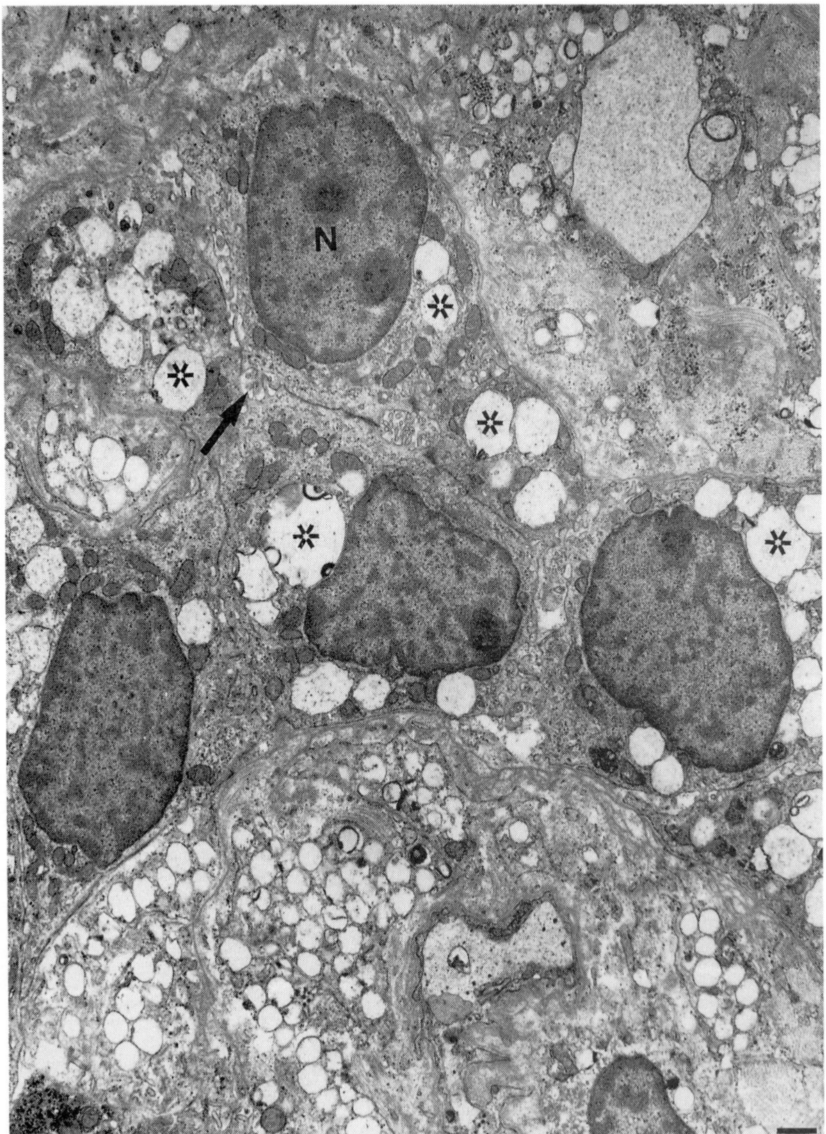

Figure 4 Structural changes of the biliary epithelium in a child with mucopolysaccharidosis type II (Hunter's disease). The micrograph illustrates the foamy appearance of the hepatocytes containing secondary lysosomes of variable size filled with electronlucent material (mucopolysaccharides). The cholangiocytes lining a small duct also show evidence of lysosomal overload similar to that seen in hepatocytes (asterisks). The arrow points to the lumen of the small ductule. N: nucleus. Bar = 1 μm

or in haemochromatosis. The presence of prominent residual bodies is also a constant feature of prolonged cholestasis (see below). Cisternae of the rough endoplasmic reticulum may be the site of storage of secretory products such as α_1-antitrypsin in α_1-antitrypsin deficiency[18]. The paucity of smooth endoplasmic reticulum is in agreement with the scarce involvement of biliary cells in drug biotransformation, and with the lack of microsomal phase I biotransformation enzymes[19,20]. In addition, it has been demonstrated that in patients undergoing long-term anticonvulsant therapy with microsomal enzymes inducers, there is a prominent proliferation of the endoplasmic reticulum in hepatocytes, but not in the cholangiocytes[21].

MODALITIES OF INJURY AND DEATH

There is little evidence of proliferation of cholangiocytes in human or animal liver in normal steady-state conditions whether demonstrated by [^{3}H]thymidine or bromodeoxyuridine incorporation[11,14], but an early proliferation of cholangiocytes occurs after bile duct ligation, preceding a small wave of replicative activity in hepatocytes[14]. This occurs along the whole intrahepatic ductal system[11] including the junctional areas (ducts of Hering)[14]. Cholangiocytes, however, keep their distinct subcellular configuration and cytokeratin pattern, without evidence of transitional features. The pattern appears different in the early stages of experimental hepatocarcinogenesis, where transitional or 'oval' cells have been described, These cells contain the cytoskeleton proteins of biliary epithelial cells, and show some ultrastructural features of hepatocytes and positivity for albumin[20]. In humans, similar cells have not been described, except for the presence of 'small cells' which may correspond to progenitor bipotential cells in chronic ductular reaction[22].

Injury to bile ducts may involve the epithelial lining, intercellular relationships, basement membrane or relationships between epithelium and the surrounding matrix. In all cholestatic conditions, especially long-lasting, a wide variety of structural changes may be observed. The earliest and more common alteration occurs at the level of microvilli which become shorter and swollen (Figure 5). In advanced stages there is evidence of accumulation of biliary pigment in residual bodies of cholangiocytes, probably due to reabsorption of bile. This may ultimately lead to destruction of the epithelial lining with lysis of the cell membrane, loss of tight junction integrity and leakage of necrotic material, both in the lumen and in the peribiliary tissue. Such a pattern is seen in advanced stages of primary biliary cirrhosis (Figure 6). In these cases the basement membrane surrounding the bile ductules often presents a complex branching pattern, entrapping biliary debris. By electron microscopy the changes observed in primary biliary cirrhosis are similar to those observed in graft-versus host disease[23]. In experimental models such as ligation of the common bile duct in the rat, the ductular proliferation is associated with structural damage, with altered microvilli at the apical membrane of cholangiocytes, but there is no reduplication of the basement membrane. Moreover, the ductular proliferation is reversible for some time, since removal of the obstruction is followed by the disappearance of newly formed ductules through apoptosis[24]. Prolonged exposure of the epithelium to bile acids probably accounts for the

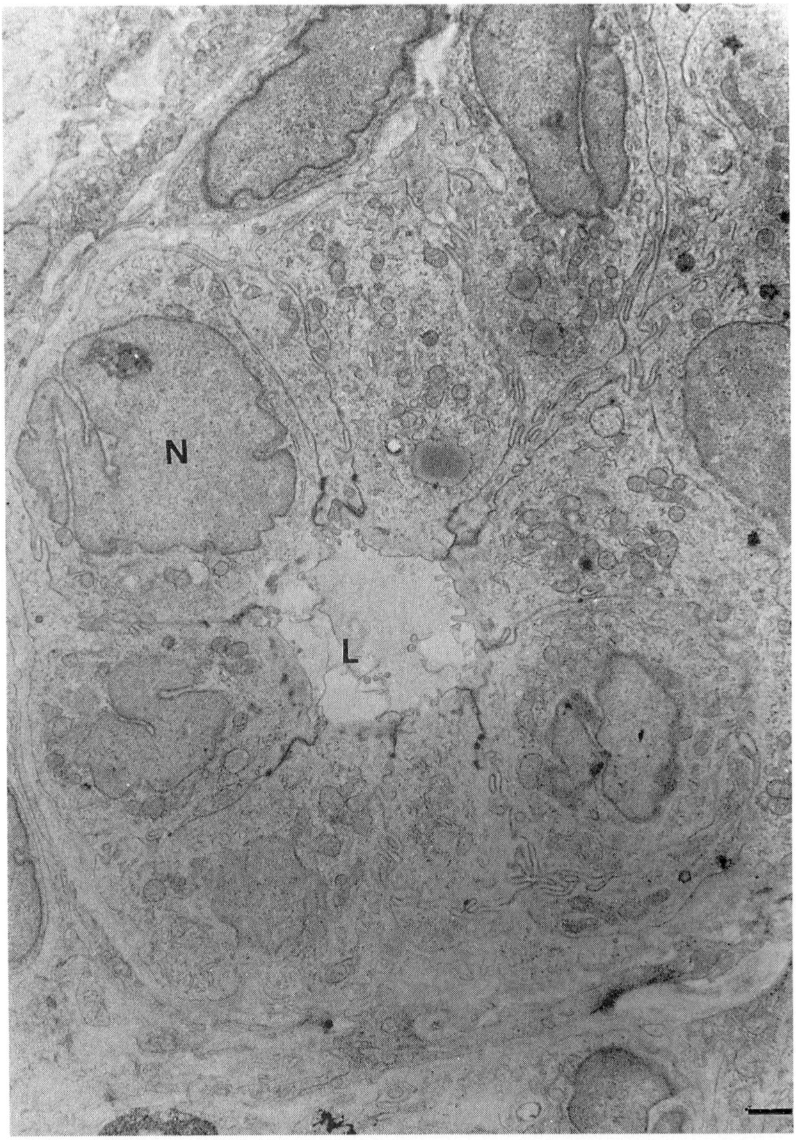

Figure 5 Intrahepatic bile duct, about 20 μm, in rat liver, seen *in situ* at 3 weeks after common bile duct ligation. The general architecture, the homogeneity and the subcellular organization of the lining cells, the integrity of the tight junctions and the relationship with the extracellular matrix are well preserved. However, damage to the cell membrane is evident at the apical pole of the cholangiocytes, with swelling of microvilli and formation of large blebs protruding into the lumen (L). N: nuclei. Bar = 1 μm

structural alterations associated with cholestasis. It has been shown that subcellular damage occurs in isolated bile ducts exposed *in vitro* to the more hydrophobic bile acids, and affects the mitochondria, which show prominent

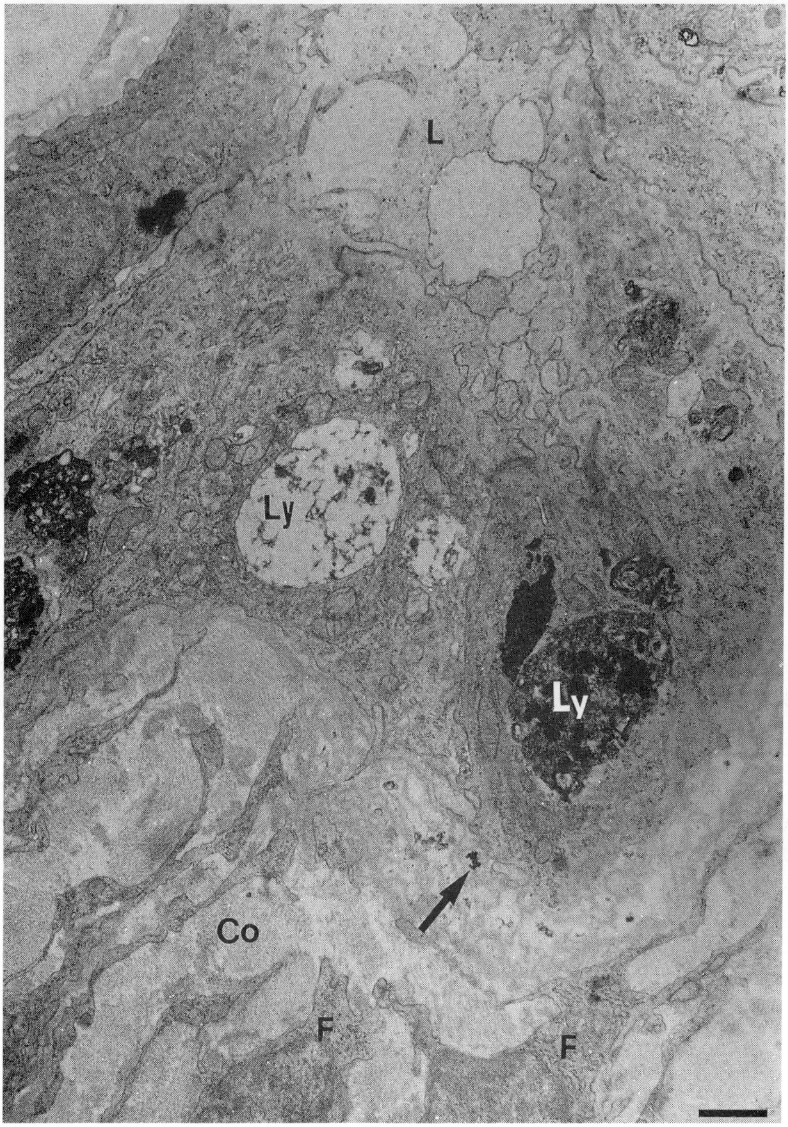

Figure 6 Part of a bile duct, about 30 μm in diameter, as seen in primary biliary cirrhosis, stage III. There are profound alterations of the duct architecture, the subcellular configuration of the lining cells and the relationships of the cells with the surrounding matrix. Damage to the apical pole of the cholangiocytes is shown, with absence of normal microvilli and formation of large blebs protruding into the lumen (L). The cytoplasm contains numerous heterogeneous residual bodies (Ly). There is also a complex, multilayered rearrangement of the basement membrane, entrapping electron-dense fragments of variable size, probably originating from lysis of cholangiocytes (arrow). The peribiliary tissue contains numerous fibroblasts (F) and large amounts of collagen (Co), Bar = 1 μm

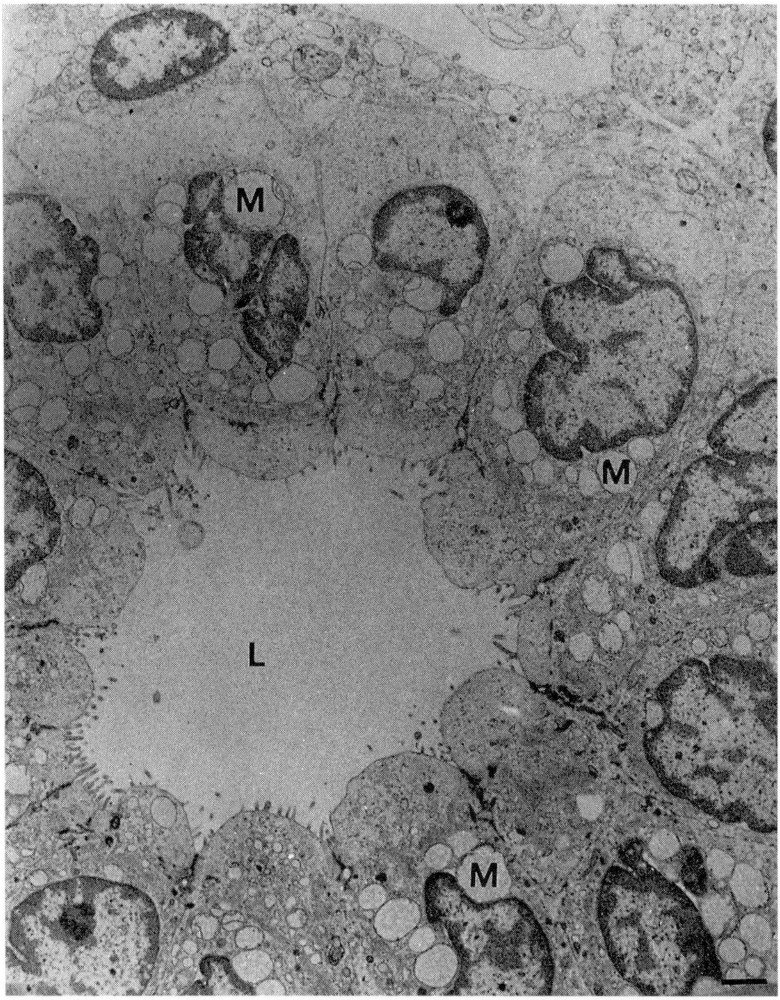

Figure 7 Part of an isolated rat bile duct, about 30 μm in diameter, after exposure to deoxycholic acid. The general architecture of the duct is preserved but there is a striking and diffuse alteration of the morphology of mitochondria (M) which assume a globular shape while short cristae are pushed against the outer membrane. A morphometric evaluation showed that, in ducts exposed to the more hydrophobic bile acids, the volume density of mitochondria increased two-fold compared to ducts exposed either to their tauroconjugates, to hydrophilic bile acids or to untreated controls

swelling and loss of cristae (Figure 7). These changes are reminiscent of the mitochondrial alterations commonly observed in hepatocytes during cholestasis, and have been related to the toxic effect of endogenous bile acids, especially hydrophobic bile acids retained in the hepatocytes[25]. However, such alterations could not be reproduced after perfusion with bile salts in isolated perfused liver, suggesting the existence of protective mechanisms *in vivo* in normal liver (Alvaro *et al.*, in press). In acute vanishing bile duct syndrome, with irreversible rejection after orthotopic liver transplantation, there is an invasion of the epithelium by inflammatory cells and ductal necrosis, but there is a minimal thickening of the basement membrane of the ductules[26]. In a number of other situations cholestasis is associated with damage to the intrahepatic biliary tree, such as in the cholestasis following therapy with various antibiotics[27]. In injury complicating benoxaprofen therapy the presence of ductal concretions is associated with degeneration of the epithelium[28] and also in cystic fibrosis-associated biliary cirrhosis, intraluminal aggregates of dense filamentous material are associated with loss of microvilli and flattening of biliary cells[18].

In summary, progress has been made in recent years with the definition of the subcellular arrangement of even the smallest branches of the intrahepatic biliary tree. The newly devised methods of isolation and *in-vitro* studies have also enriched our knowledge of the functional properties of the biliary epithelium. This information may be of help in understanding diseases in which the cholangiocytes appear as a specific target for injury.

References

1. Malpighi M. De viscerum structura exercitatio anatomica. London;1666.
2. Mascagni R. Prodromo della grande Anatomia. Firenze;1819.
3. Kiernan F. The anatomy and physiology of the liver. Phil Trans R Soc Lond. 1833;123:711.
4. Lereboullet A. Mémoire sur la structure intime du foie et sur la nature de l'altération connue sous le nom de foie gras. Paris: Baillière;1853.
5. Steiner JW, Carruthers JS. Studies on the fine structure of the terminal branches of the biliary tree. I. The morphology of normal bile canaliculi, bile pre-ductules (ducts of Hering) and bile ductules. Am J Pathol. 1961;38:639–61.
6. Ishii M, Vroman B, LaRusso NF. Isolation and morphologic characterization of bile duct epithelial cells from normal rat liver. Gastroenterology. 1989;97:1236–47.
7. Alpini G, Lenzi R, Zhai WR *et al.* Isolation of a nonparenchymal liver cell fraction enriched in cells with biliary phenotypes. Gastroenterology. 1989;97:1248–60.
8. Benedetti A, Marucci L, Bassotti C *et al.* Tubulovesicular transcytotic pathway in rat biliary epithelium: a study in perfused liver and in isolated intrahepatic bile duct. Hepatology. 1993;18:422–32.
9. Van Eyken P, Sciot R, Van Damme B, de Wolf-Peters, C, Desmet VS. Keratin immunohistochemistry in normal human liver. Cytokeratin pattern of hepatocytes bile ducts and acinar gradient. Virchows Archiv A. 1987;412:63–72.
10. Tavoloni N. The intrahepatic biliary epithelium: an area of growing interest in hepatology. Sem Liver Dis. 1987;7:280–92.
11. Slott PA, Liu MH, Tavoloni N. Origin, pattern and mechanism of bile duct proliferation following biliary obstruction in the rat. Gastroenterology. 1990;99:466–77.
12. Gall JAM, Bhathal PS. A quantitative analysis of the liver following ligation of the common bile duct. Liver. 1990;10:116–25.
13. Benedetti A, Bassotti C, Rapino K, Marucci L, Jezequel AM. A morphometric study of the epithelium lining the rat intrahepatic biliary tree. J Hepatol. 1996;24:335–42.
14. Marucci L, Svegliati Baroni G, Mancini R, Benedetti A, Jezequel AM, Orlandi F. Cell proliferation following extrahepatic obstruction. Evaluation by immunohistochemical methods. J Hepatol. 1993;17:163–9.
15. Buanes T, Grotmol T, Landsverk T, Reader MG. Secretin empties bile duct cell cytoplasm of vescicles when it initiates ductular HCO_3 secretion in the pig. Gastroenterology. 1992;102:963–8.
16. Benedetti A, Marucci L, Bassotti C, Guidarelli C, Jezequel AM. Brefeldin A inhibits the transcytotic vesicular transport of horseradish peroxidase in intrahepatic bile ductules isolated from rat liver. Hepatology. 1995;22:194–201.

17. Coppa GV, Gabrielli O, Zampini L *et al.* Bone marrow transplantation in Hunter syndrome (mucopolysaccharidosis type II). Two year follow-up of the first italian patient and review of the litterature. Ped Med Chir. 1995;17:227–35.
18. Phillips MJ, Poucell S, Patterson J, Valencia P. Cholestasis. In: Phillips MJ, Poucell S, Patterson J, Valencia P, editors. The liver: an atlas and text of ultrastructural pathology. New York: Raven Press;1987:101–8.
19. Parola M, Cheeseman KH, Biocca ME, Dianzani MU, Slater TF. Isolation and characterization of biliary epithelial cells from rat liver. J Hepatol. 1998;6:175–86.
20. Sirica AE, Mathis GA, Sano N, Elmore LW. Isolation, culture and transplantation of intrahepatic biliary epithelial cells and oval cells. Pathobiology. 1990;58:44–64.
21. Jezequel AM, Librari ML, Mosca P, Novelli G, Lorenzini I, Orlandi F. Changes induced in human liver by long-term anticonvulsant therapy. Functional and ultrastructural data. Liver. 1984;4:307–17.
22. De Vos R, Desmet V. Ultrastructural characteristics of novel epithelial cell types identified in human pathologic liver specimens with chronic ductular reaction. Am J Pathol. 1992;140:1441–50.
23. Berman D, Feldmann G, Degott C, Gisselbrecht C. Ultrastructural lesions of bile ducts in primary biliary cirrhosis. A comparison with the lesions observed in graft versus host disease. Hum Pathol. 1981;12:782–93.
24. Gall JAM, Bhathal PS. Origin and involution of hyperplastic bile ductules following total biliary obstruction. Liver. 1990;10:106–15.
25. Guan Lim A, Ahmed AA, Jazrawi RP, Levy JH, Northfield TC. Effect of bile acids on human hepatic mitochondria. Eur J Gastroenterol Hepatol. 1994;6:1157–63.
26. Ludwig J, Wiesner RH, Batts KP, Perkins JD, Kromm RAF. The acute vanishing bile duct syndrome (acute irreversible rejection) after orthotopic liver transplantation. Hepatology. 1987;7:476–83.
27. Degott C, Feldmann G, Larrey D *et al.* Drug-induced prolonged cholestasis in adults: a histological semiquantitative study demonstrating progressive ductopenia. Hepatology. 1992;15:244–51.
28. Portmann B, MacSween RNM. Diseases of the intrahepatic bile ducts In: McSween RNM, *et al.* editors. Pathology of the liver, 2nd edn. Edinburgh: Churchill Livingstone;1987:424–53.

4
Experimental models to study the physiology of biliary epithelium

S. A. LEVINE and N. F. LaRUSSO

INTRODUCTION

Bile duct epithelial cell physiology is a difficult field to study because cholangiocytes (i.e. the epithelial cells that line the bile ducts inside the liver) comprise only 3–5% of liver cells, they are in intimate contact with hepatocytes and are not easily separated, and they represent a heterogeneous cell population. In addition, these cells are involved in a variety of complex functions both in the normal and diseased state; these include modification of bile composition, secretion and absorption of ions, transport of water, bile acids, proteins, and carbohydrates, as well as proliferation during growth, development and liver regeneration. Cholangiocytes also display a proliferative response to certain chemicals or dietary manipulations under experimental conditions and in virtually all forms of human cholestatic liver diseases, such as extrahepatic biliary obstruction, primary biliary cirrhosis (PBC), primary sclerosing cholangitis (PSC), and alcoholic liver disease. They also undergo malignant transformation to form cholangiocarcinomas, tumours which are commonly fatal. Additionally, cholangiocytes express proteins of the major histocompatibility complex, can function in antigen presentation, and are the targets of immune-mediated diseases. Fortunately, the study of biliary physiology and pathophysiology has been enhanced by the recent development of a variety of novel *in vivo* and *in vitro* experimental models. This chapter will describe and review several of these models, with particular emphasis on the techniques with which we have experience or have developed in our laboratory.

IN VIVO MODELS

Cholangiocyte hyperplasia can be induced in the rat through dietary manipulation (e.g. α_1-naphthyl isothiocyanate (ANIT) feeding)[1,2], or through common bile duct ligation (BDL)[3,4], and provides a useful *in vivo* model with which to study physiological parameters of ductular bile secretion. When the common bile duct of a rat is ligated, type 1 or 'typical' ductular proliferation is observed[5]. This hyperplastic reaction is produced by an unknown mechanism that results in selective proliferation of cholangiocytes in bile ducts confined to portal areas. A similar proliferative response occurs after several weeks of ANIT feeding. In addition to providing an opportunity to study ductular bile secretion *in vivo*, these models can potentially contribute to our understanding of embryonic development of the biliary tract, allow investigation of the molecular mechanisms that regulate cholangiocyte proliferation, and facilitate study of the underlying processes in cholestatic liver diseases and biliary tract carcinogenesis. Importantly, these techniques to induce selective proliferation of cholangiocytes also increase the yield of cholangiocytes that can be harvested from liver[6]; the cells obtained are essentially a pure population of cholangiocytes which are useful for short-term primary culture, cell fractionation or plasma membrane vesicle studies.

Another *in vivo* experimental model studied in our laboratory is that of immune-mediated cholangitis, obtained by immunization of rats with cholangiocytes isolated from donor rats after BDL[7]. After immunization, recipient animals developed non-suppurative cholangitis without inflammation in other organs. Transfer of splenic lymphocytes from these cholangiocyte-immunized rats into recipients also caused cholangitis, and these lymphocytes were cytotoxic *in vitro* for cultured rat cholangiocytes. This unique rodent model of immune cholangitis will be invaluable in exploring the mechanisms by which the immune system targets and damages cholangiocytes.

IN VITRO MODELS

Perhaps the area in which the most important technological advances in the study of cholangiocyte biology have been made is the development of *in vitro* models, including: isolated bile duct units, freshly isolated cells for short-term culture or cell fractionation, and establishment of long-term non-malignant and malignant cell lines from both rats and humans. We and others recently reported a technique to harvest intact intrahepatic bile duct units from freshly isolated normal rat liver[8,9]. The cells within the bile duct units retain the morphological and cytochemical characteristics of cholangiocytes *in situ*, and provide an important experimental tool with which to study ductal ion secretion. These bile duct units form closed compartments after 36 hours in culture, and can be microinjected with fluorescent probes to measure lumenal pH and ion concentrations. Our studies with this model have demonstrated cAMP-dependent active lumenal bicarbonate secretion, and the data support the involvement of an apical Cl^-/HCO_3^- exchanger in this process.

In addition to the intact bile duct units, cholangiocytes can be isolated as individual cells from freshly perfused rat liver using a series of enzyme digestions and mechanical disruptions of the portal tract[10,11]. Subpopulations of cells are isolated by serial counterflow elutriation, isopycnic centrifugation or immunoaffinity separation. When cells are prepared by these techniques the purity of preparation can be greater than 95% cholangiocytes. In this preparation the cells are positive by cytochemistry for the cholangiocyte specific proteins,

γ-glutamyltranspeptidase and cytokeratin 19, and negative for the mesenchymal marker, vimentin. Although the purity is high, the yield is low, with less than 20% of the total bile duct cells harvested. These cells are useful for short-term studies, as polarity is maintained for at least 60 minutes following isolation, although it is lost overnight. The technique for isolation of cholangiocytes can also be modified such that subpopulations of cholangiocytes which differ in size, and which are derived from different portions of the biliary tree, can be harvested. These subpopulations are functionally distinct, and are currently being used to map the geographic distribution and the proposed proximal-to-distal gradient of functional activities of the biliary tree[12].

Freshly isolated cholangiocytes have also been used to study both receptor-mediated and fluid-phase endocytosis[13,14]. The cells internalize epidermal growth factor by endocytosis via coated pits containing receptors in the basal domain. In addition, horseradish peroxidase, a marker of fluid-phase endocytosis, is taken up exclusively at the apical domain and either routed to secondary lysosomes or carried in phosphatase-negative vesicles to the basal domain and discharged.

In addition, freshly isolated cholangiocytes have been used to demonstrate that there is reversible, specific binding of the peptide hormone, secretin, to biliary epithelial cells, and that this binding is enhanced in cells isolated from BDL rats compared with non-ligated control animals[15]. In these cells, secretin caused a dose-dependent increase in cAMP levels, which paralleled an increase in exocytic activity, as indicated by a fluorescence unquenching assay using acridine orange. In conjunction with the functional response to secretin in BDL rat cholangiocytes, an increase in secretin receptor mRNA levels suggests that up-regulation after bile duct ligation may contribute to secretin-induced hypercholeresis. The secretin-induced exocytosis could be inhibited by somatostatin, as could the secretin-induced increase in cAMP. The results of these studies suggest that somatostatin interacts directly with receptors located in liver exclusively on cholangiocytes and, in concert with secretin, regulates ductal bile secretion by alterations in cAMP-dependent exocytosis. In addition to the functional significance of the somatostatin receptors on normal cholangiocytes to bile secretion, the presence of these receptors on cholangiocarcinoma cells may provide a tool for diagnostic localization and treatment of biliary tract malignancies[16].

Isolated rat cholangiocytes have also been used to study water movement across the biliary epithelium[17]. These cells increased in volume in hypotonic extracellular buffers; this increase was inversely proportional to buffer osmolarity, was temperature-independent, and was reversibly blocked by $HgCl_2$, all features of channel-mediated water transport. RNAse protection assays, immunoblots, and immunocytochemistry confirmed the presence of the water-selective channel, aquaporin-CHIP. This channel is thought to play a pivotal role in the transcellular movement of water across cholangiocytes, and to provide a mechanism for ductal water secretion. Currently, studies are under way to further characterize the channel activity and possible hormonal regulation of the water transport process.

Although freshly isolated cells have proved useful for a variety of studies, they are difficult to harvest in substantial numbers, and they have a short lifespan. Thus, efforts have been made to establish biliary epithelial cell lines in culture. We and others[18,19] have developed techniques to culture gallbladder epithelial cells. We have recently described the isolation and culture of human gallbladder epithelial cells which were harvested from normal tissue by mechanical and enzymatic dissociation[20]. These cells, when plated on an appropriate extracellular matrix, grow to confluence and retain the polarity and ultrastructural features of these cells *in vivo*. Although these cells have a limited lifespan (five or six population doublings), large numbers of cells can be generated and are useful for experimental study.

Advances have also been made in techniques to establish cholangiocyte cells in culture[21–27]. A rat cholangiocyte cell line that has been passaged and maintained in culture for over 2 years was developed from intrahepatic bile duct epithelial cells isolated from normal rats using enzyme digestion of a portal tract[28]. These cells grow on a thick rat-tail collagen gel, and require hormonally supplemented media with forskolin and dexamethasone. They are epithelial in appearance, with dense apical membrane microvilli with occasional tufts of cilia, and they express cholangiocyte-specific markers. These cells are useful for transport studies, as they form polarized monolayers on permeable supports, with transepithelial electrical resistance ~625 $\Omega \cdot cm^2$ within a week following confluence. Recent studies have shown that these cells absorb glucose from the apical surface; uptake of a non-metabolizable form of glucose is inhibited by removal of sodium and by phlorizin, a competitive inhibitor of Na^+/glucose co-transport[29]. In addition, the cells respond to forskolin with an increase in intracellular cAMP, and this response is inhibited by basolateral, but not apical, somatostatin.

Several human cell lines have also proved useful for the study of biliary physiology. A human cholangiocyte cell line derived from normal liver and immortalized with the SV40 large T antigen[30] is being used to establish a model of microbial cholangitis, and several human cholangiocarcinoma cell lines are currently used in our laboratory for a variety of studies. These cell lines provide invaluable tools to study and compare the physiology of normal and cancerous cells[31]. A current project in our laboratory involves the development and characterization of experimentally induced models of apoptosis in the normal human and rat cholangiocyte cell lines in parallel with studies of this process in cholangiocarcinoma cell lines[32]. This work will elucidate the stimuli and pathways involved in 'programmed cell death' in normal cholangiocytes, and may yield useful information regarding failure of this normal process that is thought to be a key step in development of malignancy and growth of tumours.

The new techniques and tools available now allow study of biliary epithelial cell physiology at the subcellular as well as cellular and organ level, and the ability to isolate plasma membrane from apical and basolateral domains has allowed study of receptors, transporters, and channels in each domain. The technique, developed in our laboratory, has been used successfully in both freshly isolated and cultured cholangiocytes[33,34]. When freshly isolated cells are used they are taken from rats in which the common bile duct has been ligated 3 weeks prior to cell isolation, in order to induce selective cholangiocyte proliferation and increase the number of cells harvested. A cholangiocyte-enriched cell population is obtained following a series of enzymatic digestions and mechanical disruptions. A plasma membrane fraction is prepared via a series of differential gradient centrifugation steps, with marker enzymes used to identify plasma membranes. Mixed cholangiocyte plasma membranes are separated into apical and basolateral plasma membranes via a three-step sucrose gradient. The preparation is confirmed by biochemical characterization, including alkaline phosphatase, leucine aminopetidase and γ-glutamyltranspeptidase for apical markers, and Na^+,K^+,ATPase for the basolateral domain. Transmission electron microscopy, membrane lipid analysis, one- and two-dimensional SDS PAGE, and Western blotting for CFTR have been used to further characterize the vesicles which form from apical and basolateral membrane domains. We have recently modified this technique so that vesicles enriched in apical and basolateral plasma membrane domains can be generated from cholangiocytes in culture, an approach which greatly facilitates their preparation[34]. These vesicles can then be used for transport studies, and will provide insight into the regulation and kinetics of ion channels, transporters and exchangers.

SUMMARY

Recently there have been advances in the development of a variety of experimental models which should lead to a more complete understanding of cholangiocyte physiology, and improvements in the diagnosis and treatment of a large number of clinically significant biliary tract diseases. Further progress in the field of cholangiocyte physiology will be dependent on the development of new *in vivo* and *in vitro* experimental models. These may include three-dimensional reconstruction and imaging of the biliary tract, development of transgenic animals, creation of cDNA libraries from pure cholangiocyte populations, and production of monoclonal antibodies to cholangiocyte-specific proteins.

Acknowledgements

This work was supported by Grant DK24031 from the National Institutes of Health and by the Mayo Foundation.

References

1. Lopez M, Mazzanti L. Experimental investigation on alpha-naphthylisothiocyanate as a hyperplastic agent of the biliary ducts of the rat. J Pathol Bacteriol. 1955;69:243–50.
2. Goldfarb S, Singer EJ, Popper H. Experimental cholangitis due to α-naphthylisothiocyanate (ANIT). Am J Pathol. 1962;40:685–98.
3. Accatino L, Contreras A, Fernandez S, Quintana C. The effect of complete biliary obstruction on bile flow and bile acid excretion: postcholestatic choleresis in the rat. J Lab Clin Med. 1979;93:706–17.
4. Steiner JW, Carruthers JS, Kalefat SR. The ductular cell reaction of rat liver in extrahepatic cholestasis. I. Proliferated biliary epithelial cells. Exp Mol Pathol. 1962;1:162–85.
5. Slott PA, Liu MH, Tavoloni N. Origin, pattern and mechanism of bile duct proliferation following biliary obstruction in the rat. Gastroenterology. 1990;99:466–77.
6. Alpini G, Phillips JO, Vroman B, LaRusso NF. Recent advances in the isolation of liver cells. Hepatology. 1994;20:494–514.

7. Ueno Y, Phillips JO, Ludwig J, Lichtman SN, LaRusso NF. Development and characterization of a rodent model of immune-mediated cholangitis. Proc Natl Acad Sci USA. 1996;92:216–20.
8. Roberts SK, Kuntz SM, Gores GJ, LaRusso NF. Regulation of bicarbonate-dependent ductular bile secretion assessed by lumenal micropuncture of isolated rodent intrahepatic bile ducts. Proc Natl Acad Sci USA. 1993;90:9080–4.
9. Mennone A, Alvaro D, Cho W, Boyer JL. Isolation of small polarized bile duct units. Proc Natl Acad Sci USA. 1995;92:6527–31.
10. Ishii M, Vroman B, LaRusso NF. Isolation and morphologic characterization of bile duct epithelial cells from normal rat liver. Gastroenterology. 1989;97:1236–47.
11. Gall JA, Bhathal PS. The isolation of intrahepatic biliary epithelial cells from normal rat livers. Cell Biol Int Rep. 1985;9:315–22.
12. Alpini G, Phillips JO, LaRusso NF. The biology of biliary epithelia. In: Arias IM, Boyer JL, Fausto N, Jakoby WB, Schachter DA, Shafritz DA, editors. The liver: biology and pathobiology, 3rd edn. New York: Raven Press;1994:623–53.
13. Ishii M, Vroman B, LaRusso NF. Morphologic demonstration of receptor-mediated endocytosis of epidermal growth factor by isolated bile duct epithelial cells. Gastroenterology. 1990;98:1284–91.
14. Ishii M, Vroman B, LaRusso NF. Fluid-phase endocytosis by intrahepatic bile duct epithelial cells isolated from normal rat liver. J Histochem Cytochem. 1990;38:515–24.
15. Kato A, Gores GJ, LaRusso NF. Secretin stimulates exocytosis in isolated bile duct epithelial cells by a cyclic AMP-mediated mechanism. J Biol Chem. 1992;267:15523–9.
16. Tan CK, Podila PV, Taylor JE *et al.* Human cholangiocarcinomas express somatostatin receptors and respond to somatostatin with growth inhibition. Gastroenterology. 1995;108:1908–16.
17. Roberts SK, Yano M, Ueno Y *et al.* Cholangiocytes express aquaporin-CHIP and transport water via a channel-mediated mechanism. Proc Natl Acad Sci USA. 1994;91:13009–13.
18. Purdum RP, Alessandra U, Hylemon PB, Shiffman ML, Moore EW. Cultured human gallbladder epithelium. Lab Invest. 1993;68:345–53.
19. Oda D, Lee SP, Hayashi A. Long-term culture and partial characterization of dog gallbladder epithelial cells. Lab Invest. 1991;682–92.
20. Hoerl BJ, Vroman BJ, Kasperbauer JL, LaRusso NF, Scott RE. Biological characteristics of primary cultures of human gallbladder epithelial cells. Lab Invest. 1992;66:243–50.
21. Kumar U, Jordan TW. Isolation and culture of biliary epithelial cells from the biliary tract fraction of normal rats. Liver. 1986;6:369–78.
22. Joplin R, Hishida T, Tsubouchi H *et al.* Human intrahepatic biliary epithelial cells proliferate *in vitro* in response to human hepatocyte growth factor. J Clin Invest. 1992;90:1284–9.
23. Strain AJ, Wallace L, Joplin R *et al.* Characterization of biliary epithelial cells isolated from needle biopsies of human liver in the presence of hepatocyte growth factor. Am J Pathol. 1995;146:537–45.
24. Sirica AE, Sattler CA, Cihala HC. Characterization of a primary bile ductular cell culture from the livers of rats during extrahepatic cholestasis. Am J Pathol. 1985;120:67–78.
25. Yang LI, Faris RA, Hixson DC. Long-term culture and characteristics of normal rat liver bile duct epithelial cells. Gastroenterology. 1993;104:840–52.
26. Okamoto H, Ishii M, Mano Y *et al.* Confluent monolayers of bile duct epithelial cells with tight junctions. Hepatology. 1995;22:153–9.
27. Li Y, Faris RA, Hixson DC. Long-term culture and characteristics of normal rat liver bile duct epithelial cells. Gastroenterology 193;104:840–50.
28. Vroman B, LaRusso NF. Development and characterization of polarized primary cultures of rat intrahepatic bile duct epithelial cells. Lab Invest. 1996;74:303–13.
29. Lazaridis K, Vroman B, Pham L, LaRusso NF. Molecular characterization of a sodium-dependent, glucose co-transporter in normal rat cholangiocytes. Gastroenterology. 1996;110:A1247.
30. Grubman SA, Perrone RD, Lee DW *et al.* Regulation of intracellular pH by immortalized human intrahepatic biliary epithelial cell lines. Am J Physiol. 1994;266:G1060–70.
31. Knuth A, Gabbert H, Dippold W *et al.* Biliary adenocarcinoma: characterization of three new human tumor cell lines. J Hepatol. 1985;1:579–96.

32. Harnois D, Que F, Gores GJG, Pham LD, Kuntz SM, LaRusso NF. BCL-2 is overexpressed and alters the threshold for apoptosis in a cholangiocarcinoma cell line. Gastroenterology. 1996;110:A1205.
33. Tietz PS, Holman RT, Miller LJ, LaRusso NF. Isolation and characterization of rat cholangiocyte vesicles enriched in apical or basolateral plasma membrane domains. Biochemistry. 1995;34:15436–43.
34. Tietz P, Vroman B, Levine S, LaRusso NF. Characterization of plasmal membrane vesicles enriched in apical or basolateral domains derived from rat cholangiocytes in primary culture. Gastroenterology. 1996;110:A1346.

5
Morphological and functional heterogeneity of the rat intrahepatic biliary tree

G. ALPINI, S. GLASER, R. E. D. RODGERS, W. ROBERTSON, J. L. PHINIZY, O. COLEGIO, S. ROBERTS, L. PHAM, G. LeSAGE and N. F. LaRUSSO

INTRODUCTION

The intrahepatic biliary tree is composed of a three-dimensional complex network of interconnecting conduits of different diameters lined by simple epithelia, intrahepatic bile duct epithelial cells or cholangiocytes[1,2]. Cholangiocytes modify bile of canalicular origin by a series of reabsorptive and secretory processes under basal and hormone-regulated conditions[3–31]. For example, the gastrointestinal hormone, secretin, stimulates ductal bile secretion of water and electrolytes by interacting with specific receptors on cholangiocytes through an increase in adenosine 3′,5′-cyclic monophosphate (cAMP) synthesis[8,9,19,20,21,23,31]. Similarly, vasoactive intestinal peptide and bombesin, two gastrointestinal hormones, stimulate ductal bile secretion both *in vivo* and in isolated cholangiocytes[13,14]. On the other hand, somatostatin inhibits: (a) both basal and secretin-induced choleresis *in vivo*; and (b) both secretin-stimulated cAMP levels and exocytosis *in vitro*[31]. Moreover, Glaser *et al.*[19] have shown that the gastrointestinal hormone, gastrin, inhibits in bile duct ligated (BDL) rat liver: (a) secretin-induced choleresis and bicarbonate output *in vivo*; and (a) secretin receptor (SR) gene expression and secretin-stimulated cAMP levels *in vitro* through interaction with specific receptors on cholangiocytes.

Cholangiocytes markedly and selectively proliferate in a number of experimental models of cholestasis such as BDL, α-naphthylisothiocyanate feeding, carcinogenic dietary regimens (i.e. choline-deficient diet containing 0.5% ethionine), 70% partial hepatectomy or combined BDL/furan treatment[3–8,19,20,23,24,28,31–36]. In these cholestatic liver models, cholangiocyte proliferation is closely associated with an increase in ductal secretory activity[3–8,19,20,22–24,28,31].

Regional specialization of secretory functions, similar to that occurring in the intestine[37] or kidney[38,39], has also been proposed in the liver[40]. For example, enzymes involved in oxidative events – such as glycogenolysis fatty acid oxidation and ureagenesis from amino acids – are detected in greater amounts in periportal hepatocytes where oxygen tension is greater[40]. On the other hand, enzymes associated with a lower oxygen tension – including those involved in glucose uptake, lipogenesis and ureagenesis – are localized in pericentral hepatocytes[40]. There is an increasing amount of information supporting the concept that cholangiocytes lining the intrahepatic biliary tree are functionally heterogeneous[9,25,41–47]. For example, human cholangiocytes differentially express blood-group-related antigens with sialylated Le^a antigens expressed principally in large, septal bile ducts[46,47]. In human liver, small and medium cholangiocytes (lining small and medium ducts) principally express the protein for Cl^-/HCO_3^- exchanger[25]. Moreover, hyperplastic rodent cholangiocytes differentially express enzymes including alkaline phosphatase and leucine amino peptidase[43–45]. Moreover, Benedetti *et al.*[48] have shown morphological heterogeneity of cholangiocytes along the rat intrahepatic biliary tree, with higher nucleocytoplasmic ratio being present in small cholangiocytes lining small ducts. The latter morphological parameter may indeed represent an important tool for identifying small cholangiocytes along the intrahepatic biliary tree.

Thus, to extend the concept of functional heterogeneity of cholangiocytes along the normal intrahepatic biliary tree we first assessed whether cholangiocytes are morphologically heterogeneous *in situ*. We then isolated pure subpopulations of small, medium and large cholangiocytes from different portions of the normal intrahepatic biliary tree and assessed: (a) steady-state levels of the messages for SR, chloride bicarbonate (Cl^-/HCO_3^-) exchanger and cystic fibrosis transmembrane regulator (CFTR); and (b) secretin-altered changes in cAMP formation. To further extend these studies we also isolated small, medium and large cholangiocytes from BDL rat liver and assessed: (a) the genetic and functional expression of SR, Cl^-/HCO_3^- exchanger activity and CFTR; and (b) proliferative capacity of cholangiocytes. The rationale for using the BDL rat is based on the following observations: (a) the BDL rat model is a physiologically important model of cholestasis[3–8,31]; (b) cholangiocyte proliferation, in response to BDL, is associated with an increase in both basal and secretin-induced ductal bile secretion[4–6,31]; (c) *in-vivo* secretory response to a number of gastrointestinal hormones (e.g. secretin, somatostatin, gastrin etc.) occurs only in pathophysiological conditions associated with cholangiocyte proliferation[4–6,19,20,31]; and (d) proliferating cholangiocytes display phenotypes of normal cholangiocytes[32]. Taken together, all these observations support the importance and use of the BDL rat model for studying the functional heterogeneity of cholangiocytes. In the current studies our general hypothesis is that along the intrahepatic biliary tree agonist-stimulated transport of water and electrolytes is solely limited to specific duct-sized ducts (i.e. medium and large). We also propose that following BDL cholangiocytes are also heterogeneous with regard to proliferative capacity with proliferative processes present in medium and large but not small cholangiocytes.

MATERIALS AND METHODS

Animals and materials

Male Fisher 344 rats (225–250 g) were obtained from Harlan Sprague Dawley, Inc. (Indianapolis, IN), maintained in a temperature-controlled enviornment (22°C) with a 12 hour light–dark cycle and fed standard rat chow. Before each experiment the animals were anaesthetized with sodium pentobarbital (50 mg/kg i.p.). Our experiments were performed in normal rats and rats with BDL for 28 days performed as previously described by us[5,6,31] and others[4,22]. Reagents were purchased from Sigma Chemical Co. (St Louis, MO) unless otherwise indicated. The mouse anti-CK-19 antibody was obtained from Dako, Clostrup, Denmark. The secondary antibody (peroxidase-labelled goat anti-mouse IgG) was obtained from Tago Inc., Burlingame, CA. Guanidinium thiocyanate was obtained from Fluka Chem. Corp., New York.

In situ immunohistochemistry in normal and BDL rat livers

The extent of cholangiocyte hyperplasia was assessed by immunohistochemistry for cytokeratin-19 (CK-19), a cholangiocyte specific marker in rat liver[7,24,32,41,49]. Tissue liver blocks (1–2 cm) from both normal and BDL rats were embedded in Tissue Tek OCT compound (Miles Inc. Diagn. Division, Elkhart, IN), forzen in isopentane, cut into 4–6 μm thick sections and stained for CK-19 as previously described[49]. Briefly, following the blocking of non-specific binding sites by incubation with 1.5% normal horse serum, frozen liver sections (4–6 μm thick) were incubated in a humidified chamber for 2 h at room temperature with a 1 : 10 dilution of mouse anti-CK-19 antibody. Following several washes with Dulbecco's PBS, the liver sections were incubated in a humidified chamber for 30 min at room temperature with a 1 : 200 dilution of a secondary antibody, a biotin-labelled horse anti-mouse IgG rat adsorbed. The final peroxidase product was developed using the substrate 3-amino-9-ethylcarbazole. Following light counterstaining with haematoxylin, sections were examined in a coded fashion with a Zeiss microscope.

In situ morphometric analysis of the intrahepatic biliary tree

In situ morphometry of the intrahepatic biliary tree was performed as previously described by us[9]. After 10-min perfusion with solution A [140 mmol/L NaCl, 5.4 mmol/L KCl, 0.8 mmol/L Na_2HPO_4, 25 mmol/L N-(2-hydroxyethyl) piperazine-N′-2-ethanesulphonic acid (HEPES), 0.8 mmol/L $MgSO_4$, pH 7.4], normal rat livers were fixed at 4°C with 2% paraformaldehyde, 2.5% glutaraldehyde in Dulbecco's PBS, pH 7.4. After fixation, blue agar was injected into the portal vein to allow light microscopic identification of portal areas in the liver. The entire liver from two normal rats was cut into 3-mm thick slices that were subsequently dissected into 300 blocks of 2–4 mm^2. Following fixation for 2 h at 4°C, liver blocks were immersed for 1 h at 4°C in 2% tannic acid solution, post-fixed with 2% OsO_4 in 1% Dulbecco's PBS and embedded in Spurr's resin. Portal areas within these blocks were identified by light microscopy and sectioned in 90 nm thick slices. Following staining with 2% uranyl acetate, samples were randomly analysed by transmission electron microscopy. After staining with toluidine blue, 1-μm sections of larger ducts (150–200 μm) were analysed by light microscopy. Both external bile duct diameter and individual cholangiocyte areas were assessed by point-counting analysis on transmission electron microscopy photographs using a grid of 250 points, an approach analogous to that used in the rat inner medullary collecting ducts[39]. The magnification of the transmission electron microscopy photographs (7500–30 000×) was inversely related to the diameter of the cell and duct under analysis.

Isolation and phenotypic characterization of cholangiocyte subpopulations from normal and BDL rat liver

A mixed non-parenchymal cell fraction [40–55% pure by γ-glutamyl-transpeptidase (γ-GT) staining][5,8,9,21,49,50] was obtained from portal tracts isolated from both normal and BDL rat livers and fractionated in three subpopulations of small, medium and large cholangiocytes by counterflow elutriation (CFE) using a Beckman J6-MI centrifuge equipped with a JE-5.0 rotor (Beckman Instruments Inc., Fullerton, CA)[9,24,32,49,50]. The three subpopulations were obtained at the flow rates of 25, 36 and 55 ml/min, respectively, and subsequently purified by immunoaffinity separation[8,9,31,50]. Cell number and viability was assessed by trypan blue exclusion. The purity of the three subpopulations was determined by positive reaction for both γ-GT and CK-19 as previously described[24,32,49,50].

Mean diameters of the three subpopulations obtained from both normal and hyperplastic rat livers were assessed by both light microscopy and computerized image analysis as previously described by us[9]. For each subpopulation at least 300 cells were examined.

Cholangiocyte gene expression

Total cellular RNA was extracted from tissues ($\approx$ 1.0 g) and cholangiocyte subpopulations ($\approx 5.0 \times 10^6$) by the single-step extraction method of Chomczynsky and Sacchi[51]. Yield of the total RNA assayed was determined by both UV detection of ethidium bromide stained blots and absorption at 260 nm. The quality of the RNA samples was assessed by $A_{260} : A_{280}$ ratio.

Steady-state levels of selected messages were measured in total RNA (10 μg) by the RPA II™ RNase protection assay kit (Ambion Inc., Austin, TX), a technique previously used by us for determining the expression of selected genes[8,9]. The comparability of the total cellular RNA assayed was determined by hybridization with glyceraldehyde-3-phosphate dehydrogenase (GAPDH), a housekeeping gene[8,9]. Antisense riboprobes were transcribed from linearized DNA templates with either T_7 or SP_6 RNA polymerase using [α-^{32}P UTP] (800 Ci/mmol, Amersham, Arlington Heights, IL).

We used the following [^{32}P]-labelled antisense riboprobes: pGEM4ZgGT139, encoding sequence from MP 170–1799 of the rat γ-GT gene (a gift from M. N. Chobert, Crétel, France): a 157 bp single-stranded riboprobe (MP 1638–1799) was transcribed by T_7 RNA polymerase from the linearized plasmid, **Ava I** cleaved; a 350 bp antisense riboprobe, encoding the message for rat CK-19, was generated by T_7 RNA polymerase from pBlueScriptSKCK19, **EcoR I** linearized (a gift from A. Quaroni, Ithaca, NY); a probe 139 bases long, encoding for rat GAPDH mRNA, was obtained from the United States Biochemical Corporation, Cleveland, OH; our rat SR cDNA clone[8] containing a 318 bp fragment, MP 380–698: the antisense riboprobe was transcribed by T_7 RNA polymerase from pGEM4ZSR **EcoR I** cleaved; pGEM3Z containing a 695 bp cDNA fragment (MP 341–1036) of the rat CFTR gene was generated by RT-PCR: a 217 bp antisense riboprobe (MP 819–1036) was generated with SP_6 RNA polymerase and **Apa I** which cleaves the CFTR gene at position 819; a rat pCR ^{TM}IICl^-/HCO_3^- (chloride bicarbonate) exchanger containing a 349 bp cDNA fragment (MP 111–459) was generated by RT-PCR: an antisense riboprobe of 349 bp was generated from the pCR ^{TM}IICl^-/HCO_3^-, **Xho I** cleaved, using SP_6 RNA polymerase; a rat riboprobe encoding for H_3 histone (an index of DNA synthesis) was a gift from Sunjev Gupta (Albert Einstein Hospital, Bronx, NY).

Functional cholangiocyte heterogeneity

Determination of intracellular cAMP levels in cholangiocytes from normal and proliferating cholangiocytes

In cholangiocytes from both normal and BDL rat livers we determined basal and agonist-induced cAMP levels by radioimmunoassay according to the instructions from the vendor[9,21,23,31]. After immunopurification each subpopulation (1×10^5) was incubated for 2 h at 37°C to regenerate surface proteins (damaged by digestion with proteolytic enzymes[21] and subsequently stimulated with either secretin (10^{-7} mol/L) or forskolin (10^{-4} mol/L, positive control) for 5 min at 22°C. In each experiment 0.5 mmol/L 3-isobutylmethylxanthine, an effective inhibitor of phosphodiesterase, was added.

Measurement of membrane Cl^- efflux in cholangiocyte subpopulations from BDL rat liver

In subpopulations of small, medium and large cholangiocytes purified from BDL rat liver, we measured basal and agonist-induced Cl^- efflux according to the methodology of Fitz *et al.*[18]. Prior to exposure to secretin (10^{-6} mol/L), each subpopulation (attached to the beads used for the isolation) was incubated at 37°C for 2 h to regenerate the secretin receptor damaged by digestion with trypsin[21]. Each cholangiocyte aliquot ($\approx 3 \times 10^6$) was incubated for 1 h at room temperature in Cl^--rich buffer (140 mmol/L NaCl, 4 mmol/L KCl, 2 mmol/L $MgCl_2$, 1 mmol/L $CaCl_2$, 1 mmol/L KH_2PO_4, 10 mmol/L glucose, 10 mmol/L HEPES pH 7.4) with 5 mCi/ml of $^{36}Cl^-$ isotope (Amersham). After loading, cholangiocyte subpopulations were washed with 2 ml isotope-free buffer four times over 4 min using a magnetic bead-holder. The studies were initiated by adding 1 ml isotope-free buffer; after 60 s the buffer was removed and changed every 60 s. After 180 s the effect of agonists on Cl^- efflux among these cholangiocyte subpopulations was assessed by adding either secretin (10^{-6} mol/L containing 0.02% bovine serum albumin) or forskolin (10 mmol/L) containing [8-(4-chloro-phenylthio)-cAMP (cpt-cAMP) at 500 mmol/L], a membrane permeant analogue of cAMP. At the end of the studies, cells were lysed with NaOH 0.1 mol/L and the remaining radioactivity was counted. The rate of isotope efflux was also assessed in the presence of the Cl^- channel blocker 5-nitro-2-(3-phenylpropylamino)-benzoic acid (NPPB) at 50 mmol/L. Each experiment was performed in triplicate. The efflux of $^{36}Cl^-$ at each time-point was expressed as a ratio of counts at that time-point over the remaining counts. The rate of agonist-induced Cl^- efflux was compared to their basal values at the same time-point.

Measurement of cholangiocyte proliferation

DNA synthesis, assessed by measurement of both [^{3}H]thymidine incorporation and H_3 histone gene expression, was determined as previously described by us[41] and others[52]. Ninety minutes after an intraperitoneal injection of 1 μCi/g body weight of [methyl-[^{3}H]thymidine] (6.70 Ci/mmol, DuPont NEN Products, Boston, MA), we isolated subpopulations of small, medium and large cholangiocytes from normal rats and rats with BDL at 28 days. After isolation, each subpopulation ($\approx 2.0 \times 10^6$, $\geqslant$ 97% pure) was first treated with 3 mol/L KOH at 37°C for 30 min, then with a solution containing 15% trichloroacetic acid and 6 N HCl at 4°C for 12 h. After centrifugation at 10 000***g*** for 20 min at 4°C, DNA was extracted from the cell pellet with $HClO_4$ at 80°C for 15 min. After spinning, the supernatant was transferred into a clean tube and the radioactivity incorporated into DNA was measured in triplicate. The results were expressed as cpm per million cholangiocytes.

RESULTS

In situ immunohistochemistry

In normal rat liver, only two or three bile ducts staining for CK-19, the cholangiocyte-specific marker[7,24,32,49], were present in a section of normal rat liver (Figure 1a). Following BDL for 28 days, there was a marked and selective proliferation of intrahepatic bile ducts and at least 20 bile ducts, stained for CK-19, were present per portal area (Figure 1b). Neither portal inflammation nor peribiliary fibrosis was observed in BDL rat livers.

In situ morphometry

In situ morphometry of 142 intrahepatic ducts from normal rat liver showed that intrahepatic bile ducts are heterogeneous in external diameter ranging from 5 to 200 μm (Figure 2a); approximately 85% of these ducts range from 5 to 40 μm in diameter. *In situ* frequency distribution of 645 individual cholangiocytes from two normal rat livers demonstrated that cholangiocytes in normal rat liver range in area from 3 to 80 μm^2 (Figure 2b), thus demonstrating that cholangiocytes in

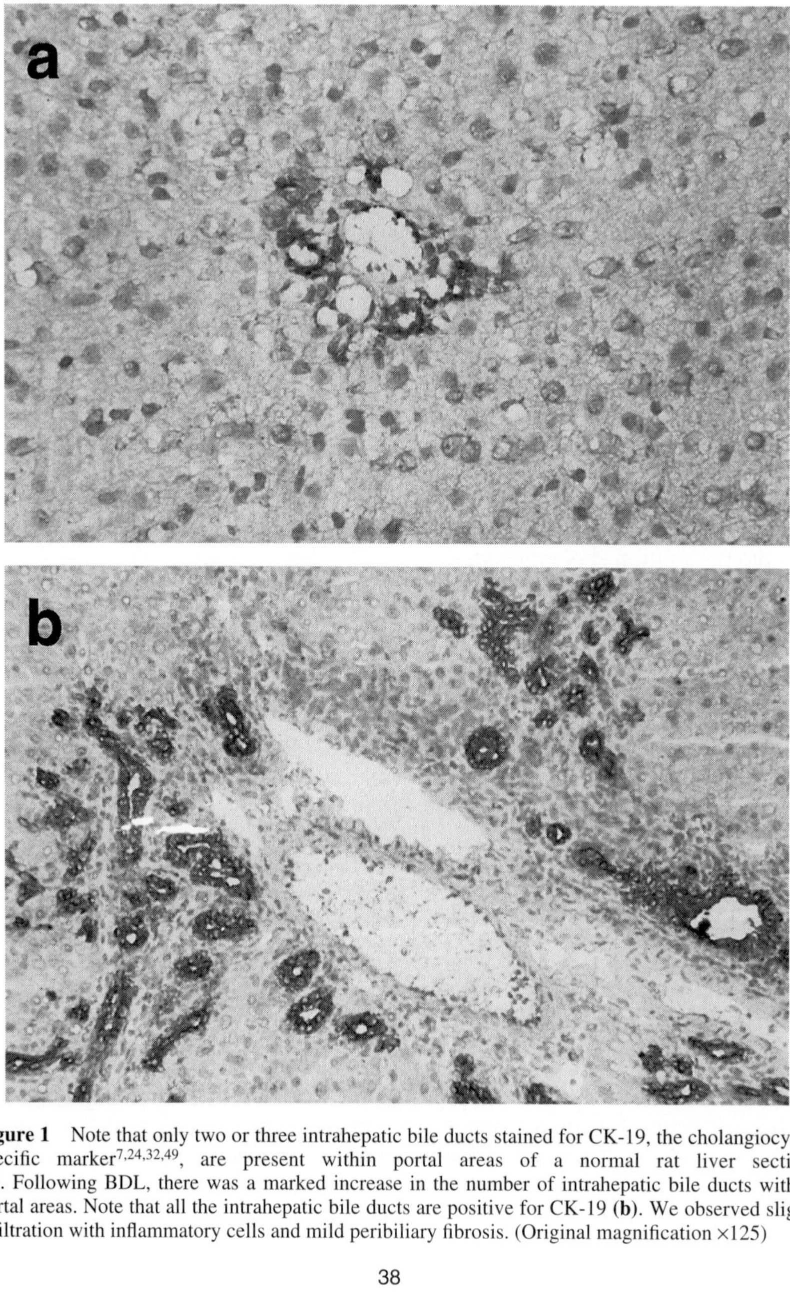

Figure 1 Note that only two or three intrahepatic bile ducts stained for CK-19, the cholangiocyte-specific marker[7,24,32,49], are present within portal areas of a normal rat liver section (**a**). Following BDL, there was a marked increase in the number of intrahepatic bile ducts within portal areas. Note that all the intrahepatic bile ducts are positive for CK-19 (**b**). We observed slight infiltration with inflammatory cells and mild peribiliary fibrosis. (Original magnification ×125)

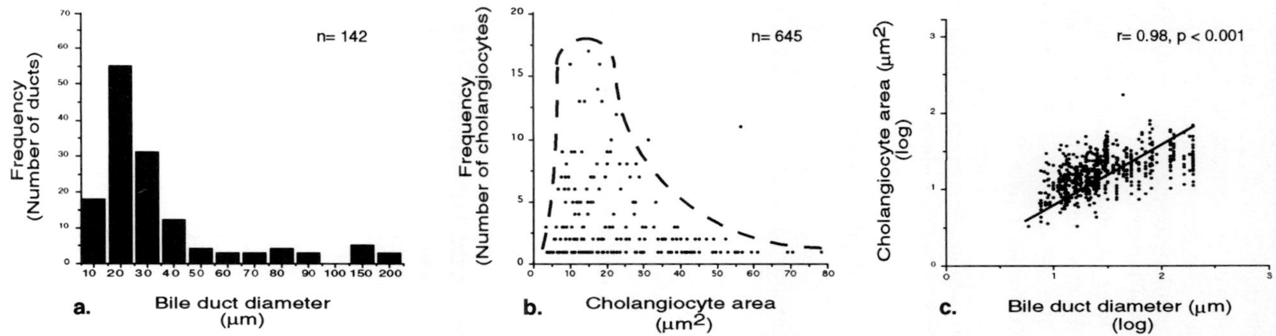

Figure 2 *In situ* morphometry of the normal intrahepatic biliary tree. Intrahepatic bile ducts are randomly selected from two rat livers and analysed as described in Materials and Methods. Both external bile duct diameter and individual cholangiocyte areas were assessed by point-counting analysis on transmission electron microscopy photographs. **(a)** *In situ* diameter distribution of 142 intrahepatic bile ducts from two rat livers. Intrahepatic bile ducts in normal rat liver range in diameter from 5 to 200 μm. **(b)** *In situ* frequency distribution of 645 individual cholangiocyte areas in normal rat liver. Cholangiocytes in normal rat liver range in area from 3 to 80 μm^2. **(c)** Regression analysis between individual cholangiocyte areas and bile duct diameter in normal rat liver. A highly significant relationship ($r = 0.98$, $p < 0.001$) exists between cholangiocyte area and bile duct diameter. (Reproduced with permission from ref. 9)

normal rat liver are also heterogeneous in cell area. To address the question whether small bile ducts are lined by small cholangiocytes and large ducts by large cholangiocytes we studied the relationship between the areas of individual cholangiocytes and external bile duct diameter. The data (Figure 2c) showed that a highly significant relationship exists between the log of cholangiocyte area and the log of bile duct diameter. The data represent the first evidence that, in normal rat liver, small rodent cholangiocytes line small bile ducts, whereas larger cholangiocytes line ducts of larger diameter. Furthermore, *in situ* morphometric analysis of BDL rat liver (Alpini and LeSage, unpublished observations, 1996) indicates that: (a) the diameter of intrahepatic bile ducts ranges in size between 10 and 75 μm; and (b) there is a direct relationship between cholangiocyte size and bile duct diameter ($R = 0.92$) (results not shown). In a fashion analogous to that seen in normal rat liver, the data indicate that small bile ducts are lined by small cholangiocytes whereas larger ducts are lined by larger hyperplastic cholangiocytes (results not shown).

Isolation and characterization of cholangiocyte subpopulations from normal and BDL rat livers

By CFE followed by immunoaffinity separation we isolated from normal rat liver three subpopulations of small (average number 0.5×10^6 per liver), medium (average number 0.9×10^6 per liver) and large (average number 1.7×10^6 per liver) cholangiocytes. Following BDL, the number of isolated cholangiocytes markedly increased as a consequence of cholangiocyte proliferation. The mean number of the three subpopulations of small, medium and large cholangiocytes were 4.5, 6.6 and 4.8 million per liver, respectively. The viability of each subpopulation was $\geqslant 97\%$. The purity of the three subpopulations from both normal and hyperplastic rat livers was $\geqslant 97\%$ by positive reaction for γ-GT and CK-19 (results not shown).

Both light microscopic and computerized image analyses were performed to accurately determine the diameters of the three subpopulations of small, medium and large cholangiocytes obtained from normal (Figure 3a–f) and BDL rat liver (results not shown). The cells clearly differ in size among the three subpopulations of small, medium and large cholangiocytes from both normal (Figure 3a–f) and BDL (results not shown) rat livers. In normal rat liver the diameters of the three subpopulations of small, medium and large cholangiocytes were 8.49 ± 0.05, 11.86 ± 0.05 and 14.53 ± 0.05 μm (mean ± SE, $p < 0.05$ by unpaired *t*-test when compared to each other). However, there was a small degree of overlap in diameter between medium and large (9.2%, Figure 3a–f) and between small and medium cholangiocytes (3.7%, Figure 3a–f). The data suggest that small cholangiocytes were isolated from small intrahepatic bile ducts ($\leqslant 15$ μm), medium cholangiocytes from medium-sized ducts (15–100 μm in diameter) and large cholangiocytes from large bile ducts (100–200 μm in diameter). No increase in diameter was seen in cholangiocytes from BDL rat liver as compared to normal cholangiocytes (results not shown). This correlates with our previous studies[5,32,49] showing that the diameter of hyperplastic cholangiocytes is similar to that of normal cholangiocytes. Diameters of the three subpopulations of hyperplastic cholangiocytes were 8.75 ± 0.01, 12.12 ± 0.01 and

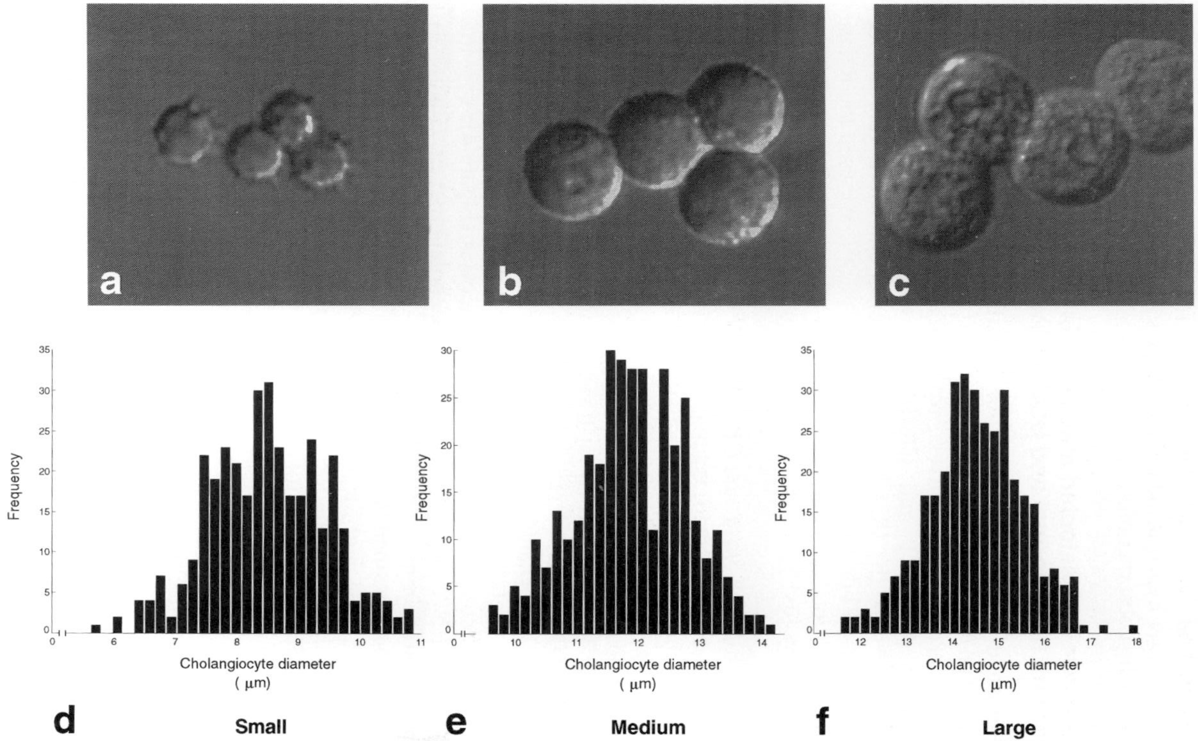

Figure 3 Frequency diameter distribution of subpopulations of small, medium and large cholangiocytes isolated from normal rat liver by CFE followed by immunoaffinity separation[8,9,54]. By this approach we were able to isolate three distinct subpopulations of cholangiocytes from normal rat liver. Mean diameter of each cholangiocyte subpopulation was determined by computerized image analysis as previously described by us[9]. (Original magnification ×625; reproduced with permission from ref. 9)

14.83 ± 0.01 μm (mean ± SE, $p < 0.05$ by unpaired t-test when compared with each subpopulation). There was a small degree of overlap in diameter between medium and large cholangiocytes (10.2%, results not shown) and between small and medium cholangiocytes (1.7%, results not shown). Similar to what we observed in normal rat liver, small cholangiocytes from BDL rat liver line small bile ducts while larger hyperplastic cholangiocytes line larger ducts (Alpini and LeSage, unpublished observation, 1996).

Steady-state levels of selected messages in cholangiocyte subpopulations from normal and BDL rat livers

Having established a novel technique for isolating pure subpopulations of small, medium and large cholangiocytes from different portions of the biliary tree of both normal and BDL rat livers, we studied the expression of selected genes including: (a) γ-GT and CK-19, the two cholangiocyte-specific genes[5,7,9,24,28,32,49,50]; and (b) SR, Cl^-/HCO_3^- exchanger and CFTR genes which are important to ductal bile secretion[3,5–12,15–18,21,23–32,41,42]. We used the RNase protection assay on total cellular RNA (10 μg), a very sensitive technique previously used by us[8,9] for determining state-steady levels of selected messages.

The transcripts for both γ-GT and CK-19 genes were similarly expressed by the three subpopulations of small, medium and large cholangiocytes from both normal (Figure 4) and BDL rat liver. Similarly, GAPDH, the housekeeping gene used to measure the comparability of the RNA assayed, was equally expressed in the three subpopulations from both normal (Figure 4) and proliferating rat liver. On the other hand, in normal rat liver, SR was principally expressed in both medium (≈ 3.0-fold) and large (≈ 1.5-fold) but not small cholangiocytes (Figure 4). Parallel with changes in SR gene expression, steady-state levels of CFTR mRNA were higher in both medium (≈ 1.5-fold) and large cholangiocytes (≈ 1.1-fold) as compared with small cholangiocytes (Figure 4); very low levels of CFTR mRNA were detected in small cholangiocytes (Figure 4). Furthermore, the transcript for Cl^-/HCO_3^- exchanger was detected in both medium and large but not small cholangiocytes (Figure 4). Following BDL there was an increased expression of SR, CFTR and Cl^-/HCO_3^- exchanger mRNA in both medium and large cholangiocytes (results not shown). Similar to the normal rat liver, the transcripts for these genes were not detected in small cholangiocytes from BDL rats (results not shown).

Functional cholangiocyte heterogeneity

Agonist-induced cAMP levels

To extend these studies to the level of protein expression for the secretin receptor, we measured secretin-induced cAMP levels among the three subpopulations of small, medium and large cholangiocytes isolated from both normal and BDL rat livers. In normal rat liver, while the basal cAMP levels were similar among the three subpopulations of small, medium and large cholangiocytes [6.27 ± 2.4, 5.8 ± 1.1 and 8.8 ± 3.2 (mean ± SE) fmol/100 000

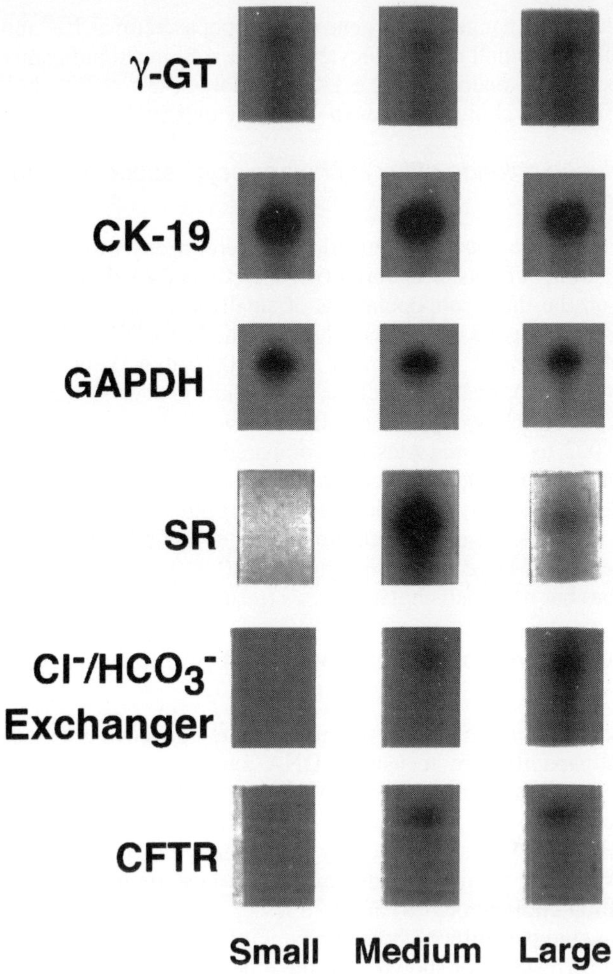

Figure 4 Steady-state levels of selected messages among subpopulations of small, medium and large cholangiocytes purified from normal rat liver by CFE followed by immunoaffinity separation[8,9,49,50]. Molecular analysis was performed by RNase protection assay on total cellular RNA (10 μg) extracted from cholangiocytes by the single-step extraction method of Chomczynsky and Sacchi[51]. Total RNA was hybridized to ^{32}P-labelled antisense riboprobes transcribed from selected cDNA templates as described in Materials and Methods. Gels were exposed for 2–4 h and autoradiograms were quantified by laser densitometry. (Reproduced with permission from ref. 9)

cells, respectively], secretin (10^{-7} mol/L) stimulated cAMP levels to different degrees with levels being much higher in medium (45.2 ± 24.0) and large (46.2 ± 13.0) cholangiocytes than in small cholangiocytes (15.2 ± 6.5). Following BDL there was an increase (2–3-fold) in basal cAMP levels among small, medium and large cholangiocytes (14.13 ± 3.2, 16.106 ± 3.4 and 21.4 ± 8.0, respectively) as compared to normal cholangiocytes ($p < 0.05$ by unpaired *t*-test). Parallel with changes in SR gene expression, secretin at 10^{-7} mol/L had no significant effect in small cholangiocytes (24.8 ± 4.5) but significantly increased cAMP levels in both medium (81.1 ± 17.8) and large (43.6 ± 7.2) cholangiocytes compared with small cholangiocytes ($p < 0.02$ by unpaired *t*-test).

Agonist-induced chloride efflux in cholangiocyte subpopulations from BDL rat liver

To further extend the concept of functional heterogeneity of cholangiocytes we measured the direct effects of agonists (i.e. secretin and forskolin) on the rates of $^{36}Cl^-$ efflux on the three subpopulations of small, medium and large cholangiocytes from BDL rat livers (results not shown). The basal $^{36}Cl^-$ efflux rates among the three subpopulations were similar (i.e. $\leqslant$ 0.10 min^{-1}). In the presence of secretin (10^{-6} mol/L), peak $^{36}Cl^-$ efflux rates were greater in medium (0.252 ± 0.005 min^{-1}, $p < 0.002$ by unpaired *t*-test) and large cholangiocytes (0.210 ± 0.005 min^{-1}, $p < 0.002$ by unpaired *t*-test) as compared with their corresponding basal values (results not shown); no effect was seen in small cholangiocytes (results not shown). When exposed to forskolin (10^{-4} mol/L) plus cpt-cAMP (500 μmol/L), $^{36}Cl^-$ efflux rates increased in medium (0.261 ± 0.0059 min^{-1}, $p < 0.002$ by unpaired *t*-test) and large cholangiocytes (0.280 ± 0.018 min^{-1}, $p < 0.002$ by unpaired *t*-test) but not small cholangiocytes (results not shown).

Proliferative activity of cholangiocyte subpopulations from BDL rat livers

To determine whether cholangiocytes are also heterogeneous with regard to their proliferative capacity, we measured DNA synthesis among the three subpopulations by measurement of both [^{3}H]thymidine incorporation and H_3 histone gene expression. As shown in Figure 5, DNA synthesis in cholangiocytes from BDL rat livers (assessed by measurement of [^{3}H]thymidine incorporation) was greater in medium cholangiocytes [186.05 ± 13.63 (mean ± SE) cpm per million cholangiocytes] and to a lesser degree by large cholangiocytes (42.51 ± 9.34 cpm per million cholangiocytes) (Figure 5) as compared to normal cholangiocytes (results not shown). On the other hand, DNA synthesis was virtually absent in small cholangiocytes (Figure 5) and comparable to that of normal cholangiocytes (results not shown). The genetic expression of H_3 histone gene expression (an index of DNA synthesis) parallels the findings obtained by measurement of [^{3}H]thymidine incorporation. Specifically, the transcript for the H_3 histone gene was detected in both medium and large, but not small, cholangiocytes isolated from BDL rat livers.

DISCUSSION

The major findings of the studies relate to the morphological, molecular and functional diversity of cholangiocytes lining the rat intrahepatic biliary tree. Using *in-situ* morphometry we have demonstrated in normal rat liver that: (a) intrahepatic bile ducts are heterogeneous in external bile duct diameter;

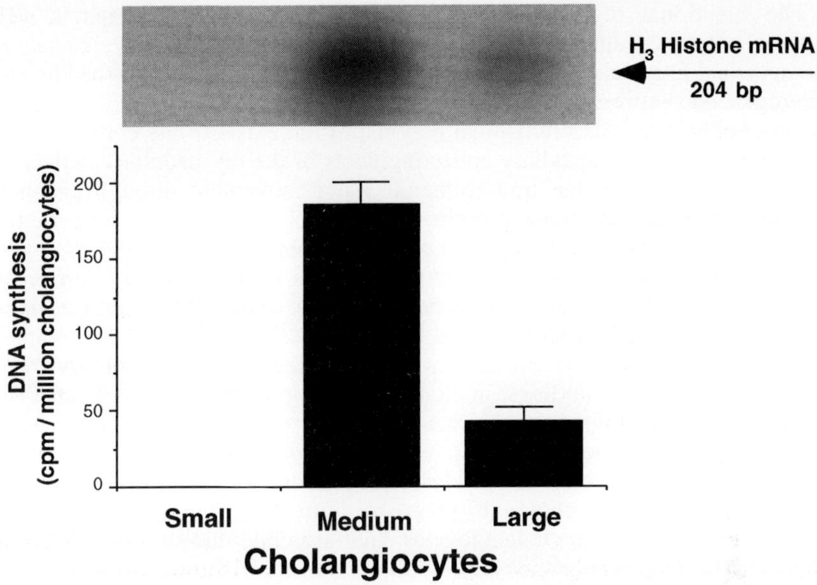

Figure 5 Proliferative activity of subpopulations of small, medium and large cholangiocytes isolated from BDL rat liver. Ninety minutes after an intraperitoneal injection of 1 μCi/g body weight of [methyl-[^{3}H]thymidine] the radioactivity incorporated into DNA was measured in purified liver cells (5.0×10^6, $\geq 97\%$ pure) as described in Materials and Methods. Steady-state levels of H_3 histone mRNA were determined by RNase protection assay using total cellular RNA (10 μg). The comparability of the total RNA used was assessed by hybridization for GAPDH, the housekeeping gene. Autoradiograms were quantified by densitometry

(b) cholangiocytes lining intrahepatic bile ducts are heterogeneous in area; and (c) a linear significant relationship exists between cholangiocyte area and external bile duct diameter along the intrahepatic biliary tree of normal rat liver. Furthermore, *in situ* morphometric studies in BDL rat liver (Alpini and LeSage, unpublished observations, 1996) also demonstrate a linear relationship between external bile duct diameter and cholangiocyte areas. Taken together, the data suggest that in both normal and BDL rat liver small bile ducts are lined by small cholangiocytes, whereas large intrahepatic bile ducts are lined by large cholangiocytes. To extend these *in situ* studies we isolated three subpopulations of small, medium and large cholangiocytes from both normal and BDL rat liver and have shown that: (a) the transcripts for SR, CFTR and Cl^-/HCO_3^- exchanger genes were present in both medium and large (but not small) cholangiocytes; (b) similarly, at the level of protein, secretin-induced cAMP response increased in medium and large, but not small, cholangiocytes; (c) both secretin- and forskolin-stimulated $^{36}Cl^-$ efflux rates were increased in both medium and large cholangiocytes from BDL rat liver; no increase in $^{36}Cl^-$ efflux rates was seen in small cholangiocytes; and (d) DNA synthesis was detected in both medium and large cholangiocytes; no active DNA synthesis was detected in small cholangiocytes.

The functional regionalization of epithelia lining other organs is well defined[37–39]. For example, Cohn *et al.*[37] have shown that *cis*-acting elements in the intestinal fatty acid-binding protein gene control its cell lineage-specific and heterogeneous expression along the duodenal–colonic and crypt–villus axes of the gut epithelium. Also functional regionalization exists in the cortical, outer medullary and inner medullary collecting ducts of the rat medullary collecting ducts[39]. Furthermore, the transepithelial water movement through channel-forming integral membrane protein 28 water channels occurs only in the proximal tubule and descending limb of Henle's loop[38].

In normal rat liver, morphometric analysis has been previously performed both *in situ*[48] and in isolated intrahepatic bile duct units[12,27,29]; however, these studies fail to specify a well-defined terminology for classifying the complex network of ducts of different sizes which form the intrahepatic biliary tree[2]. Parallel to previous findings in human liver[1], our morphometric analysis demonstrates that bile ducts are heterogeneous in external diameter. Also, cholangiocytes are heterogeneous in cell areas (Figure 6). On the basis of these observations, we conclude that *in situ* small bile ducts ($\leqslant$ 15 μm in diameter) are lined by small cholangiocytes, medium bile ducts (15–100 μm in diameter) by medium cholangiocytes, and large bile ducts (100–200 μm in diameter) by large cholangiocytes. Similarly, we have shown in isolated bile duct fragments from BDL rat liver (Alpini and LeSage, unpublished observations, 1996) that: (a) the diameter of intrahepatic bile ducts ranges in size between 10 and 75 μm; and (b) there is a direct relationship between cholangiocyte size and bile duct diameter (R = 0.92) (results not shown). In a fashion analogous to that seen in normal rat liver, the data indicate that small bile ducts are lined by small cholangiocytes, whereas larger ducts are lined by larger hyperplastic cholangiocytes (results not shown).

CFE has been used to isolate cholangiocytes of different sizes from both normal and proliferating rat liver[3,23,24,32,49], but the purity achieved in these studies was modest (40–75%). In the present studies we further refined the applicability of CFE which, in combination with immunoaffinity purification (an approach developed by us to purify normal rat cholangiocytes[50], yielded three distinct subpopulations of small, medium and large cholangiocytes (see Figure 3). In agreement with previous reports[5,7,32,35,43–45,49,50,53], we assessed purity and phenotypes of the three subpopulations by positive detection, at both genetic and protein levels, of γ-GT and CK-19.

To begin to test the hypothesis of the possible functional heterogeneity of cholangiocytes along the intrahepatic biliary tree we studied the molecular and functional expression of CFTR and Cl^-/HCO_3^- exchanger which, in concert with secretin, regulate ductal bile secretion[5–8,10,11,15,18,21–25,27–31]. For example, Alvaro *et al.*[10] have shown that secretin stimulates biliary HCO_3^- secretion in cholangiocytes by activating an apical localized Cl^-/HCO_3^- exchanger as a secondary consequence of cAMP-dependent protein kinase A Cl^- channel activation (presumably CFTR), a mechanism also demonstrated in other epithelia[54]. Cl^-/HCO_3^- exchanger activity has also been localized immunohistochemically in the apical domain of human epithelial cells where it regulates intracellular pH and transport of bicarbonate into the bile[25].

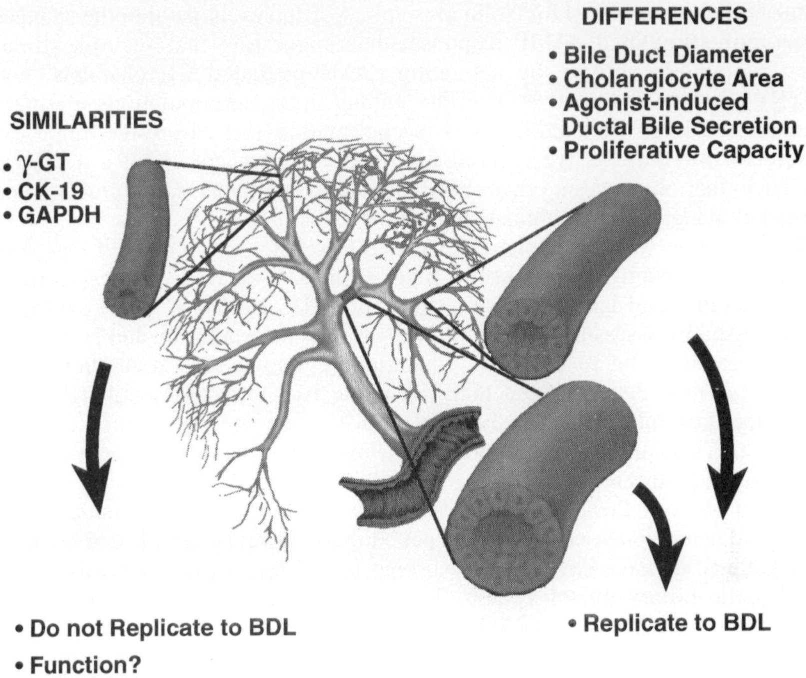

Figure 6 Working model for the heterogeneity of the intrahepatic biliary ductal system. The model proposes that cholangiocytes along the normal intrahepatic biliary ductal system are similar with regard to their expression of γ-GT, CK-19 and GAPDH genes, but are different with regard to cell area, secretin receptor gene expression and agonist-stimulated cAMP levels. The model implies that the major sites of secretin-induced water and electrolyte transport involve cholangiocytes in medium and large bile ducts, which contain secretin receptors and participate in secretin-induced choleresis. The model also implies that cholangiocytes in small ducts do not contain significant amounts of secretin receptors, and do not participate extensively in secretin-induced choleresis. The major function of these small cholangiocytes remains to be destermined

We next determined whether SR gene expression among the three subpopulations is closely related to changes in SR protein expression. To date, antibodies against the secretin receptor are not available, antibodies which will allow direct study of the expression of this protein among cholangiocyte subpopulations. Alternatively, to extend the aforementioned molecular studies to the level of protein expression for the secretin receptor, we determined the effect of secretin on cAMP synthesis, a functional assay for the secretin receptor[7,9,21,23]. These data further support the concept of functional heterogeneity of cholangiocytes, and indicate that heterogeneity of cholangiocytes along the intrahepatic biliary tree exists not only at the genetic but also at the translational level. To extend these studies to the level of functional expression of CFTR we studied the effect of agonists (i.e. secretin and forskolin plus cpt-cAMP) on Cl^- efflux among the three subpopulations of small, medium and large cholangiocytes from BDL rat liver. The increases in $^{36}Cl^-$ efflux rates in response to agonists (i.e. secretin and forskolin plus cpt-cAMP) closely parallel the changes in secretin-stimulated cAMP response, thus suggesting that secretin stimulates ductal bile activity by activating cAMP-mediated Cl^- channels (e.g. CFTR)[11,15,16,18]. The peak $^{36}Cl^-$ efflux among these subpopulations of small, medium and large cholangiocytes is reached within 180 s from the initial exposure to the agonists (i.e. secretin or forskolin plus cpt-cAMP), a kinetic similar to that observed in other cholangiocyte preparations (i.e. unfractionated normal cholangiocytes or human cholangiocyte cell lines)[11,18].

To determine whether cholangiocytes are also heterogeneous with regard to proliferative capacity in response to BDL we measured DNA synthesis among small, medium and large cholangiocytes from BDL rat livers. DNA synthesis was assessed by assessment of both [^{3}H]thymidine incorporation and H_3 histone gene expression. Our results closely parallel previous *in vivo* autoradiographic studies[34], which demonstrated that, following BDL, medium cholangiocytes lining medium bile ducts are the only cells to replicate, thus supporting the concept that cholangiocytes are heterogeneous in their capacity to respond to a proliferative perturbation.

On the basis of these observations we developed a model for mapping the functional heterogeneity of the intrahepatic biliary ductal system. Based on these observations we have developed a working model for the heterogeneity of the intrahepatic biliary ductal system. This model proposes that cholangiocytes along the normal intrahepatic biliary ductal system are similar with regard to their expression of γ-GT, CK-19 and GAPDH genes, but are different with regard to cell area, SR, CFTR and Cl^-/HCO_3^- exchanger gene expression, agonist-stimulated cAMP levels and Cl^- transport and proliferative capacity. The model implies that the major sites of secretin-induced water and electrolyte transport involve cholangiocytes in medium and large bile ducts, which contain secretin receptors and participate in secretin-induced choleresis. The model also implies that cholangiocytes in small ducts do not contain significant amounts of secretin receptors, and do not participate in secretin-induced choleresis. The major function of these small cholangiocytes remains to be determined.

Acknowledgements

This work was supported by a Grant Award to both Dr Alpini and Dr LeSage from Scott & White and Texas A&M University Health Science Center, and by a Grant Award to Dr LaRusso from the National Institutes of Health and by the Mayo Foundation.

References

1. Schaffner F, Popper H. Electron microscopic studies of normal and proliferated bile ductules. Am J Pathol. 1961;38:393–410.
2. Healey JE, Schroy PC. Anatomy of the biliary ducts within the human liver. Arch Surg. 1953;66:599–616.
3. Tavoloni N. The intrahepatic biliary epithelium: an area of growing interest in hepatology. Sem Liv Dis. 1987;7:280–92.

4. Accatino L, Contreras A, Fernandez S, Quintana C. The effect of complete biliary obstruction on bile flow and bile acid excretion: postcholestatic choleresis in the rat. J Lab Clin Med. 1979;93:706–17.
5. Alpini G, Lenzi R, Sarkozi L, Tavoloni N. Biliary physiology in rats with bile ductular cell hyperplasia. Evidence for a secretory function of proliferated bile ductules. J Clin Invest. 1988;81:569–78.
6. Alpini G, Lenzi R, Zhai W-R, Slott PA, Liu MH Tavoloni N. Bile secretory function of intrahepatic biliary epithelium in the rat. Am J Physiol. 1989;257:G124–33.
7. Alpini G, Phillips JO, LaRusso NF. The biology of the biliary epithelia. In: Arias I, Boyer J, Fausto N, Jakoby W, Schachter D, Shafritz DA, editors. The liver: biology and pathology, 3rd edn. New York: Raven Press;1994:623–53.
8. Alpini G, Ulrich II C, Phillips J, Pham L, Miller L, LaRusso N. Upregulation of secretin receptor gene expression in rat cholangiocytes after bile duct ligation. Am J Physiol. 1994;266:G922–8.
9. Alpini G, Roberts SK, Kuntz SM *et al.* Morphologic, molecular and functional heterogeneity of cholangiocytes from normal rat liver. Gastroenterology. 1996:110:1636–43.
10. Alvaro D, Cho WKC, Mennone A, Boyer JL. Effect of secretin on intracellular pH regulation in isolated rat bile duct epithelial cells. J Clin Invest. 1993;92:1314–25.
11. Basavappa S, Middleton J, Mangel AW, McGill JM, Cohn JA, Fitz JG. Cl^- and K^+ transport in human biliary cell lines. Gastroenterology. 1993;104:1796–1805.
12. Benedetti A, Marucci L, Bassotti C *et al.* Tubulovesicular transcytotic pathway in rat biliary epithelium: a study in perfused liver and in isolated intrahepatic bile ducts. Hepatology. 1993;18:422–32.
13. Cho WK, Mennone A, Boyer JL. Effect of bombesin on secretion in isolated polarized intrahepatic bile ductular units (IBDU). Gastroenterology. 1995;108:A1049.
14. Cho WK, Mennone A, Rydberg SA, Boyer JL. VIP is a potent stimulus of bicarbonate and fluid secretion in bile ducts. Hepatology. 1995;22:A752.
15. Cohn JA, Strong TV, Picciotto MR, Nairn AC, Collins FS, Fitz JG. Localization of the cystic fibrosis transmembrane conductance regulator in human bile duct epithelial cells. Gastroenterology. 1993;105:1857–64.
16. Cohn JA, Nairn AC, Marino CR, Melhus D, Kole J. Characterization of the cystic transmembrane conductance regulator in a colonocyte cell line. Proc Natl Acad Sci USA. 1992;89:2340–4.
17. Farouk M, Vigna SR, McVey DC, Meyers WC. Localization and characterization of secretin binding sites expressed by rat bile duct epithelium. Gastroenterology. 1992;102:963–8.
18. Fitz JG, Basavappa S, McGill J, Melhus O, Cohn JA. Regulation of membrane chloride currents in rat bile duct epithelial cells. J Clin Invest. 1993;91:319–28.
19. Glaser SS, Rodgers R, Phinizy JL *et al.* Gastrin inhibits secretin-induced hypercholeresis in the bile duct ligated rat liver through the cAMP system. Gastroenterology. 1996;110:A1197.
20. Gubba S, Glaser S, Robertson WE, Lasater J, LeSage G, Alpini G. Compensatory cholangiocyte proliferation in rats with 70% partial hepatectomy is associated with increased ductal secretion. Hepatology. 1995;22:A867.
21. Kato A, Gores GJ, LaRusso NF. Secretin stimulates exocytosis in isolated bile duct epithelial cells by a cyclic AMP-mediated mechanism. J Biol Chem. 1992;267:15523–9.
22. Kountouras J, McKavanagh S, Burmicky M, Billing BH. The effect of secretin on bile flow and bile acid and bilirubin excretion following relief of prolonged bile duct obstruction in the rat. J Hepatol. 1986;4:198–205.
23. Lenzen R, Alpini G, Tavoloni N. Secretin stimulates bile ductular secretory activity through the cAMP system. Am J Physiol. 1992;263:G527–32.
24. Lenzi R, Liu MH, Tarsetti F *et al.* Histogenesis of bile duct-like cells proliferating during ethionine hepatocarcinogenesis. Lab Invest. 1992;66:390–402.
25. Martinez-Anso' E, Castillo JE, Diez J, Medina JF, Prieto J. Immunohistochemical detection of chloride/bicarbonate anion exchanger in human liver. Hepatology. 1994;19:1400–6.
26. McGill JM, Basavappa S, Gettys TW, Fitz JG. Secretin activates Cl^- channels in bile duct epithelial cells through a cAMP-dependent mechanism. Am J Physiol. 1994;266:G731–6.
27. Mennone A, Alvaro D, Cho W, Boyer JL. Isolation of small polarized bile duct units. Proc Natl Acad Sci USA. 1995;92:6527–31.
28. Roberts SK, LaRusso NF. Pathobiology of biliary epithelia. Curr Opin Gastroenterol. 1994;10:526–33.

29. Roberts S, Kuntz S, Gores G, LaRusso N. Regulation of bicarbonate-dependent ductular secretion assessed by lumenal micropuncture of isolated rodent intrahepatic bile ducts. Proc Natl Acad Sci. 1993;90:9080–4.
30. Strazzabosco M, Mennone A, Boyer JL. Intracellular pH regulation in isolated rat bile duct epithelial cells. J Clin Invest. 1991;87:1503–12.
31. Tietz P, Alpini G, Pham LD, LaRusso NF. Somatostatin inhibits secretin-induced ductal choleresis *in vivo* and exocytosis by cholangiocytes. Am J Physiol. 1995;269:G110–18.
32. Alpini G, Aragona E, Dabeva M, Salvi R, Shafritz DA, Tavoloni N. Distribution of albumin and alpha-fetoprotein mRNAs in normal, hyperplastic, and preneoplastic rat liver. Am J Pathol. 1993;141:623–32.
33. Yaswen P, Hayner NT, Fausto N. Isolation of oval cells by centrifugal elutriation and comparison with other cell types from normal and preneoplastic rat liver. Cancer Res. 1984;44:324–31.
34. Slott PA, Liu MH, Tavoloni N. Origin, pattern, and mechanism of bile duct proliferation following biliary obstruction in the rat. Gastroenterology. 1990;99:466–77.
35. Sirica AE, Cihla HP. Isolation and partial characterizations of oval and hyperplastic bile ductular cell-enriched populations from the livers of carcinogen and noncarcinogen-treated rats. Cancer Res. 1984;44:3454–66.
36. Sirica AE, Gainay TW, Mumaw VR. Ductular hepatocytes. Evidence for a bile ductular cell origin in furan-treated rats. Am J Pathol. 1994;145:375–83.
37. Cohn S, Simon T, Roth K, Birkenmeier E, Gordon J. Use of transgenic mice to map *cis*-acting elements in the intestinal fatty acid binding protein gene (Fabpi) that control its cell lineage-specific and regional patterns of expression along the duodenal-colonic and crypt-villus axes of the gut epithelium. J Cell Biol. 1992;119:27–44.
38. Nielsen S, Smith BL, Christensen EI, Knepper MA, Agre P. CHIP28 water channels are localized in constitutively water-permeable segments of the nephron. J Cell Biol. 1993;120:371–83.
39. Clapp WL, Madsen KM, Verlander JW, Tisher CG. Morphological heterogeneity along the rat inner medullary collecting duct. Lab Invest. 1989;60:219–30.
40. Katz N, Jungermann K. Metabolic heterogeneity of the liver. In: Tavoloni N, Berk, PD, editors. Hepatic transport and bile secretion: physiology and pathophysiology. New York: Raven Press; 1993:55–70.
41. Alpini G, Roberts S, Phinizy J *et al.* Heterogeneity of the proliferative capacity of rat cholangiocytes. Gastroenterology. 1995;109:A1025.
42. Alpini G, Glaser SS, Robertson WE, Phinizy JL, Rodgers R, LeSage G. Large but not small intrahepatic bile duct units (IBDU) are involved in somatostatin-inhibition of secretin-stimulated ductal secretion. Gastroenterology. 1996;110:A1141.
43. Mathis GA, Walls SA, Sirica AE. Biochemical characteristics of hyperplastic rat bile ductular epithelial cells cultured 'on top' and 'inside' different extracellular matrix substitutes. Cancer Res. 1988;48:6145–53.
44. Mathis GA, Walls SA, D'Amico P, Gengo TF, Sirica AE. Enzyme profile of rat bile ductular epithelial cells in reference to the resistence phenotype in hepatocarcinogenesis. Hepatology. 1989;9:477–85.
45. Mathis GA, Wyss PA, Schuetz EG, Hughey RP, Sirica AE. Expression of multiple proteins structurally related to gamma-glutamyl transpeptidase in non-neoplastic adult rat hepatocytes *in vivo* and in culture. J Cell Physiol. 1991;146:234–41.
46. Sasaki M, Kono N, Nakanuma Y. Neoexpression of Lewis Y antigen is a sensitive change of the damage intrahepatic bile ducts. Hepatology. 1994;19:138–44.
47. Okada Y, Jinno K, Moriwaki S *et al.* Blood group antigens in the intrahepatic biliary tree. J Hepatol. 1988;6:63–70.
48. Benedetti A, Bassotti C, Rapino K, Marucci L, Jezequel AM. A morphometric study of the epithelium lining the rat intrahepatic biliary tree. J Hepatol. 1996;24:335–42.
49. Alpini G, Lenzi R, Zhai W-R *et al.* Isolation of a nonparenchymal liver cell fraction enriched in cells with biliary epithelial phenotypes. Gastroenterology. 1989;97:1248–60.
50. Ishii M, Vroman B, LaRusso NF. Isolation and morphological characterization of bile duct epithelial cells from normal rat liver. Gastroenterology. 1989;97:1236–47.
51. Chomczynski P, Sacchi N. Single-step method of RNA isolation by acid guanidium thiocyanate-phenol chloroform extraction. Anal Biochem. 1987;162:156–9.

52. Edwards AM, Lucas CM. Phenobarbital and some other liver tumor promoters stimulate DNA synthesis in cultured rat hepatocytes. Biochem Biophys Res Commun. 1985;131:103–8.
53. Alpini G, Vroman BS, Phillips JO, LaRusso NF. Recent advances in the isolation of liver cells. Hepatology. 1994;20:494–514.
54. Dunk CR, Brown CDA, Turnberg LA. Stimulation of Cl^-/HCO_3^- exchange in rat duodenal brush border membrane vesicles by cAMP. Pflügers Arch Eur J Physiol. 1989;414:701–5.

6
Hormonal regulation of electrolyte transport in biliary epithelial cells

D. ALVARO, A. GIGLIOZZI, T. LA ROSA, L. CARLI, S. FURFARO, F. FRAIOLI, C. FRANCIA, R. ROMEO and L. CAPOCACCIA

INTRODUCTION

Although representing only 3–5% of the total liver cell population, bile duct epithelial (BDE) cells produce from 10% to 40% of the daily bile output in different animal species[1–3]. In addition, BDE cells play a major role in the regulation of final bile composition through secretion or reabsorption of organic and inorganic bile components[1–3].

In the past few years enormous headway has been made in the physiology and biology of biliary epithelium, thanks to newly developed experimental models. First was the development of the bile duct ligated rat, an experimental model which, through the selective proliferation of BDE cells, allows us to highlight the role of biliary epithelium in the process of bile formation[4]. Therafter techniques were developed which, by combining isopycnic centrifugation, counterflow elutriation, free-flow electrophoresis and immunoaffinity separation, permit the isolation and short-term culture of BDE cells, with sufficient yield and purity for functional studies[5–10]. Continuous cells lines from human and rat BDE cells, as well as bile duct or gallbladder tumour cell lines, have also been successfully developed and investigated at physiological and biological levels[10–12]. Finally bile duct units of different sizes, isolated using enzymatic digestion and microdissection[13] for large ducts (average diameter 100 μm), or mechanical fragmentation and enzymatic digestion of the biliary tree, followed by sequential filtration[14], for small ducts (average diameter 20 μm), have been prepared.

In BDE cells isolated from bile duct-ligated or normal rat liver, the H^+-HCO_3^- transport processes involved in the regulation of intracellular pH (pH_i) have been identified using fluorescent dyes (BCECF)[7–9]. In rat BDE cells two acid extruders, the Na^+/H^+ exchanger (electroneutral) and Na^+/HCO_3^- symporter (electrogenic) driving the recovery of pH_i from acid load, as well as a Na^+-independent Cl^-/HCO_3^- exchanger (electroneutral), responsible for HCO_3^- excretion, have been identified[7–9]. The latter, thought to be the main mechanism of bicarbonate excretion in bicarbonate secretory epithelia, has also been functionally identified in isolated human cholangiocytes[15] and biliary cell lines[11,16], and immunohistochemically in the apical pole of human liver cholangiocytes[17]. In human isolated cholangiocytes and in human biliary cell line[11,15,16], an electroneutral Na^+-dependent Cl^-/HCO_3^- exchanger instead of the electrogenic Na^+/HCO_3^- symport seems to be involved in HCO_3 loading into the cell. Using electrophysiological techniques, channel activity and conductance pathways have been defined. In isolated rat cholangiocytes a low-conductance cAMP-activated Cl^- channel with a linear current–voltage relationship, time-independence and insensitivity to DIDS, has been described[18]. These electrical properties are similar to those associated with the cystic fibrosis transmembrane conductance regulator (CFTR). Immunofluorescence and immunocytochemistry studies identified CFTR in the apical pole of rat cholangiocytes and human cholangiocytes[18,19]. As in other bicarbonate secretory epithelia, a close functional cooperation between CFTR and the Cl^-/HCO_3^- exchanger should play a key role in the regulation of bicarbonate secretion by hormones acting via the cAMP-PKA pathway. A Ca^{2+}-dependent Cl^- conductance showing outward rectification of the current–voltage relation, time-dependence and DIDS sensitivity, as well as K^+ conductance, has been identified in rat cholangiocytes and human biliary cell lines[18,20]. Finally, cAMP and Ca^{2+}-insensitive high-conductance Cl^- channels, inhibited by pertussis toxin-sensitive heterotrimeric GTP-binding proteins, have also been described in isolated rat cholangiocytes although their physiological relevance is still unknown[21,22].

Ductal fluid secretion is under hormonal regulation. Until a few years ago secretin was the only hormone known to target BDE cells. Evidence has very recently been provided showing that different hormones or neuropeptides are involved in the regulation of BDE cell functions, including secretin, somatostatin, gastrin, bombesin, vasoactive intestinal peptide (VIP), and acetylcholine[1–3]. This chapter revises current knowledge on the hormonal regulation of electrolyte transport and secretory processes in BDE cells.

SECRETIN

The choleretic effect of secretin has been known since the beginning of this century[23]. However, only in the 1960s was evidence provided that secretin could exert its choleretic effect by specifically targeting biliary epithelium and inducing bicarbonate excretion followed by osmotically driven water flow[24,25]. A hypothetical Cl^-/HCO_3^- exchange mechanism was suggested in the light of the reciprocal changes in Cl^- and HCO_3^- biliary concentration during secretin administration[25]. These pionering observations were confirmed much later by the finding that in bile duct-ligated rats, with selective proliferation of BDE cells, secretin induces a marked bicarbonate-rich choleresis, an effect proportional with the increase in the biliary epithelium mass, which was almost absent in rats with a normal number of biliary epithelial cells[4]. Definitive evidence of the site of action of secretin was provided in 1993, thanks to the autoradiographic localization of secretin binding sites in cholangiocytes, but not in hepatocytes[26]. Secretin receptors have been detected more recently at the molecular level in cholangiocytes, where they are up-regulated at transcriptional level during BDE cell proliferation, induced either by bile duct obstruction[27] or partial hepatectomy[28]. With regard to the mechanism of action of secretin, it is now well established that cAMP is the intracellular messenger involved, since cAMP, but not Ca^{2+} or cGMP, in response to secretin, increases in isolated rat cholangiocytes[29]. We demonstrated[8], in cholangiocytes isolated from normal rat liver, that secretin induces bicarbonate excretion via a cAMP-mediated stimulation of the Cl^-/HCO_3^- exchanger activity. The same mechanism is active in isolated hepatocyte couplets in response to glucagon, a hormone of the same family[30]. However, stimulation of this anion exchanger by secretin requires a previous activation of cAMP-dependent Cl^- channels, the effect of secretin being blocked by NPPB, a specific inhibitor of these channels. This suggests a link between the opening of cAMP-dependent Cl^- channels (CFTR) and activation of Cl^-/HCO_3^-, although the exact mechanism of this link has not been clarified. It has been postulated[8] that the depolarization induced by the opening of Cl^- channels could enhance HCO_3^- entrance via electrogenic Na^+-HCO_3^- symport. This in turn would activate the Cl^-/HCO_3^- exchanger secondarily at its HCO_3^-- or pH-sensitive sites, as proposed for other cells. An alternative mechanism could be a cAMP-induced apical targeting of CFTR and/or Cl^-/HCO_3^- exchanger. Consistent with this latter mechanism is the observation that secretin, in isolated rat cholangiocytes, increases a cAMP-mediated, colchicine-sensitive unquenching of acridine orange fluorescence, indicative of stimulated exocytosis[29]. The activation of CFTR in intracellular membrane compartments could *per se* regulate the trafficking of membrane and associated membrane proteins by stimulating the acidification of intracellular vesicles[31]. Cystic fibrosis epithelial cells, in which the gene encoding CFTR is defective, exibit defective apical targeting of CFTR as well as defective cAMP regulation of plasma membrane recycling[31]. The involvement of a microtubule-dependent vesicle trafficking in the mechanism of secretin choleresis has been recently questioned following the observation that in the α-naphthyl-isothiocyanate model of BDE cell proliferation, colchicine failed to influence secretin choleresis[32]. As an alternative mechanism of secretin choleresis, it has been proposed that Na^+/H^+ exchanger activity is primarily activated by the hormone, thus inducing intracellular alkalinization and a consequent stimulation of the Cl^-/HCO_3^- exchanger, whose pH/activity relationship is well established. This hypothesis[33], which has been negatively tested in isolated rat cholangiocytes[8], is mainly based on the observation that, in isolated perfused liver from rats with α-naphthyl-isothiocyanate-induced BDE cell hyperplasia, secretin choleresis is blocked by amiloride, an inhibitor of the Na^+/H^+ exchanger[33]. It is, however, important to state that amiloride has a number of aspecific effects, including inhibition of protein kinase C and modification of the pattern of bile salt conjugation (enhanced glucuronidation)[34], both of which markedly influence bile flow.

Mechanisms of segretagogue-induced ductal fluid secretion were further investigated by using the experimental model of isolated rat bile duct units[14]. This model represents the simplest unit of ductal bile formation. The counterpart in hepatic bile formation is the isolated rat hepatocyte couplet. Exposure to specific segretagogues allows direct evaluation of ductal fluid secretion throughout the measurement (video imaging techniques) of changes in the cross-sectional area of a ductal luminal space, delimited by a single layer of polarized cholangiocytes. Luminal pH was also measured by micro-injection of dextran–BCECF in the ductal lumen. In these bile duct units secretin and forskolin induce a significant expansion of luminal space, together with an increase of luminal pH, direct evidence of stimulated alkaline fluid secretion of ductal origin. The Cl^- and HCO_3^- dependence of this secretory process definitively confirmed the role of Cl^-/HCO_3^- exchanger as the main mechanism of the bicarbonate-rich ductal fluid secretion.

To further elucidate the signal transduction pathway activated by secretin, we investigated the role of protein kinase A (PKA) and PKC in secretin-stimulated Cl^-/HCO_3^- exchanger in isolated rat bile duct units[35]. The stimulatory effect of secretin on Cl^-/HCO_3^- exchanger activity was blocked by preincubation and perfusion of IBDU with Rp-cAMPS. This membrane-permeant PKA blocker is a competitive inhibitor for activators of cAMP-mediated signal response transduction. It binds to the regulatory subunit of both type I and II cAMP-dependent protein kinase without dissociating the catalytic subunit. Rp-cAMPS also blocked secretin-induced fluid secretion in the luminal space of isolated rat bile duct units. From these findings it appears that an intact PKA activity is essential for secretin-induced stimulation of the Cl^-/HCO_3^- exchanger and fluid secretion; thus PKA plays a central role in the mechanisms of secretin choleresis. Since the basal activity of the Cl^-/HCO_3^- exchanger was unaffected by PKA blocking (only stimulation by secretin being inhibited), we suggest that phosphorylation of CFTR by PKA is an essential step in the secretin signal transduction pathway. On the other hand, it is well known that the regulatory domain of CFTR contains multiple PKA phosphorylation consensus sequences all of which are essential for CFTR activation or trafficking[31].

SOMATOSTATIN

Somatostatin is a cyclic peptide originally isolated from bovine hypothalamus[36] but now known to be widely distributed throughout the body[37,38]. Other than in the central nervous system, somatostatin is present in the gastrointestinal tract, pancreas, thyroid, adrenal glands and kidney[37,38]. At different levels somatostatin may act as a hormone, paracrine agent and neuropeptide. It inhibits the release of many hormones, including the growth hormone, insulin, glucagon, gastrin, secretin and thyrotropin-stimulating hormone[37,38]. In addition, somatostatin exerts direct inhibitory effects on gastrointestinal exocrine secretions and possesses antiproliferative properties. Five subtypes of high-affinity membrane receptors (SSTR1–SSTR5) for somatostatin have been described in various target tissues[37]. The cloning of somatostatin receptors allowed investigation of SSTR expression at the mRNA level. In the majority of cell types investigated, the five subtypes of somatostatin receptors are G protein-coupled and induce inhibition of adenylate cyclase activity, while the SSTR2 sybtype has also been involved in the regulation of K^+ and Ca^{2+} conductance or channels, as well as Na^+/H^+ exchanger[37,38].

With regard to bile secretion, two pionering studies by Holm *et al.*[39] and Rene *et al.*[40] showed that, in dogs, somatostatin exerts an anticholeretic effect. In the study by Rene *et al.*[40], it was shown that somatostatin decreased bile flow and biliary bicarbonate secretion by a direct mechanism, the effect of somatostatin being unchanged by the anticholinergic agent, pipenzolate. In addition, somatostatin blocked secretin choleresis without affecting secretin release. Since the bile/plasma ratio of erythritol concentration increases during somatostatin infusion, its anticholeretic effect was attributed to enhanced ductular reabsorption, or alternatively to decreased ductular secretion. More recently, Tietz *et al.*[41], using RNase protection assay, detected SSTR2, but not SSTR1 mRNA, exclusively in cholangiocytes of normal rat liver. SSTR2 mRNA expression in cholangiocytes increased 20-fold after bile duct ligation. In the same study somatostatin induced a marked inhibition of basal bile flow and bicarbonate biliary excretion in the bile duct-ligated rat with no appreciable effect in the normal rat. The choleretic effect of secretin was also significantly counteracted by somatostatin. The anticholeretic effect of somatostatin was associated with a marked impairment of secretin-induced cAMP intracellular levels and exocytosis in cholangiocytes isolated from bile duct-ligated rats[41]. From this study it is clear that somatostatin acts directly on cholangiocytes, decreasing basal ductal bicarbonate-rich secretion and counter-regulating secretin choleresis. Somatostatin should bind SSTR2 and counteract the choleretic effect of secretin throughout a G protein-dependent inhibition of adenylate cyclase. Whether somatostatin could directly affect electrolyte transport processes in cholangiocytes has not yet been explored. This, however, appears likely in the light of the evidence that the SSTR2 receptor expression associates, in many different cell types, with a somatostatin regulation of K^+ or Ca^{2+} channels[37,38].

SUBSTANCE P

Substance P is a peptide of 11 amino acids, belonging to the tachykinin family[42]. Substance P-like immunoreactivity has been demonstrated in nerve fibres, located in the myenteric and submucosal plexus of the intestine, suggesting a role of this peptide in the regulation of epithelial cell function[42,43]. Indeed, *in-vivo* and *in-vitro* studies demonstrated marked effects of substance P on intestinal ion transport processes and water secretion[42]. In addition, substance P has been considered to be involved in inflammatory bowel diseases, following observations that, in experimental models of gut inflammation, increased levels of substance P have been found. In isolated pancreatic ducts[43], substance P inhibits basal fluid secretion as well as secretion stimulated by both bombesin and secretin by a mechanism distal to cAMP or Ca^{2+} induction. Very little information is available on the role of substance P in the physiology of biliary epithelium. In isolated rat bile duct units substance P showed no effect on fluid secretion in the ductal lumen or on fluid secretion stimulated by VIP and bombesin[44,45].

We investigated the effect of substance P on H^+-HCO_3^- ion transport processes in isolated rat bile duct units. The activity of the Cl^-/HCO_3^- exchanger was evaluated by measuring pH_i changes induced by acute Cl^- removal/readmission manoeuvre in the presence of bicarbonate in perfusing media. Two sequential Cl^- removal/readmission manoeuvres were performed, the second during superfusion with 0.5 μmol/L substance P (Figure 1). The net pH_i change (0.26 ± 0.06 pHU) and the maximal rate of alkalinization after Cl^- removal (0.141 ± 0.06 pHU/min), as well the maximal rate of pH_i recovery after Cl^- readmission (0.169 ± 0.08 pHU/min), measured during exposure to substance P, were similar in comparison to correspondent control parameters (Cl^- removal = 0.158 ± 0.07 pHU/min; Cl^- readmission= 0.180 ± 0.07 pHU/min; n = 12). Substance P also failed to influence the stimulatory effect of secretin on Cl^-/HCO_3^- exchanger activity. Secretin increased to a similar extent the rates of pH_i changes induced by Cl^- removal/readmission in the presence (n = 10) or absence (n = 12) of substance P (Cl^- removal = 0.232 ± 0.08 vs 0.260 ± 0.08 pHU/min; Cl^- readmission= 0.269 ± 0.07 vs 0.285 ± 0.08 pHU/min; Figure 1). These findings indicate that substance P has no effect on the basal activity of the Cl^-/HCO_3^- exchanger or on the secretin stimulation of this anion exchanger.

The effect of substance P on the activity of the Na^+-HCO_3^- symport was evaluated by measuring the maximal rate of pH_i recovery from an acute acid load in isolated bile duct units perfused with bicarbonate-rich media and with amiloride. When two sequential NH_4Cl^- pulses were performed in these experimental conditions (Figure 1; n = 10), the maximal rate of pH_i recovery was similar in the presence (0.16 ± 0.07 pHU/min) or absence (0.19 ± 0.08 pHU/min) of 0.5 μmol/L substance P, indicating that the Na^+-HCO_3^- symporter was unaffected by this neuropeptide.

Thus, from these data, substance P does not seem to be directly involved in the regulation of electrolyte transport and fluid secretion in biliary epithelium.

GASTRIN

More than 100 different types of gastrin have been isolated in various animal species[46–48]. In humans, that formed by 34 amino acids is the most abundant in plasma. Other than stimulation of acid gastric secretion, gastrin has been reported to influence secretory processes other than motility at different levels of the gastrointestinal tract. In the pancreas, gastrin stimulates enzymic and bicarbonate secretion[46–49]. In gallbladder mucosa, gastrin has been reported to have no effect on bicarbonate and water secretion[50], while in the intestine, reabsorption of water and electrolytes is inhibited by gastrin[46–49]. With regard to biliary epithelium, only one preliminary study has been published so far[51]. In bile duct-ligated rats, gastrin has no significant effect on basal bile flow and bicarbonate biliary excretion, but the secretin-induced bicarbonate-rich choleresis was markedly decreased. This anticholeretic effect of gastrin has been associated with impaired secretin stimulation of cAMP intracellular levels in cholangiocytes isolated from bile duct-ligated but not normal rats[51]. As for somatostatin, G proteins could mediate the inhibition of adenylate cyclase by gastrin, and this merits investigation.

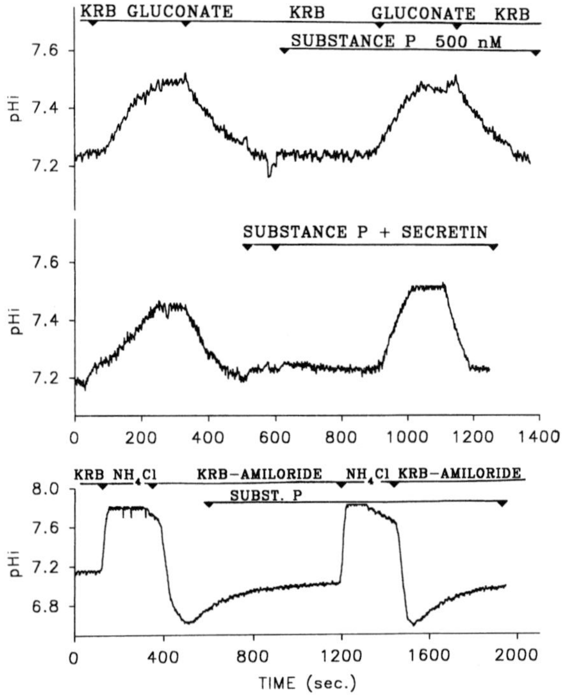

Figure 1 Effect of substance P on Cl^-/HCO_3^- exchanger and Na^+-HCO_3^- symport activity in isolated rat bile duct units (IBDU). *Upper tracing*: two sequential Cl^- removal/ readmission (equimolar substitution of Cl^- with gluconate) manoeuvres were performed in IBDU perfused with KRB (n = 12). After the first control manoeuvre, IBDU were exposed to 500 nmol/L substance P. The net pH_i increase and maximal rate of alkalinization after Cl^- removal, as well as the maximal rate of pH_i recovery after Cl^- readmission, were similar in the absence or presence of substance P, indicating that this peptide has no effect on the basal activity of the Cl^-/HCO_3^- exchanger. *Middle tracing*: two sequential Cl^- removal/readmission manoeuvres were performed in IBDU perfused with KRB. After the first control manoeuvre, IBDU were exposed to 500 nmol/L substance P + secretin 200 nmol/L (n = 10). The net pH_i increase and maximal rate of alkalinization after Cl^- removal, as well as the maximal rate of pH_i recovery after Cl^- readmission, were significantly ($p < 0.02$) higher in the presence of substance P + secretin (second manoeuvre) than corresponding control parameters (first manouevre). However, when compared with paired experiments performed with secretin alone, superfused in correspondence with the second Cl^- removal/ readmission manoeuvre (n = 12, not shown) no significant difference was found. This indicates that substance P does not influence the secretin stimulation of Cl^-/HCO_3^- exchanger activity. *Lower tracing*: two sequential NH_4Cl^- pulses were performed in IBDU perfused with KRB, the second during exposure to 500 nmol/L substance P (p = 10). To exclude the influence of the Na^+/H^+ exchanger on the recovery from the acid load, amiloride (1 mmol/L) was superfused at the moment of NH_4Cl^- withdrawal. The maximal rate of pH_i recovery from the NH_4Cl^-/amiloride pulse was similar either in the absence or presence of substance P, indicating that this peptide has no influence on the activity of the Na^+-HCO_3^- symport

BOMBESIN

Bombesin is a peptide of 14 amino acids predominantly detectable in basal glandular cells of duodenal mucosa[48,49,52,53]. It may be detected by immunocytochemistry at all levels of the gastrointestinal epithelium, other than in submucosal nerve fibres, in the lung and the central nervous system. The release of bombesin precedes that of gastrin reaching comparable plasma levels during the post-prandial phase[48,49,52,53]. Most *in-vivo* effects are due to an interference with the release of other gastrointestinal peptides. However, direct effects of bombesin on gastrointestinal secretory processes and motility have been clearly documented[48,49,52,53]. In pancreatic ducts, bombesin, via intracellular Ca^{2+} increase, stimulates bicarbonate fluid secretion, an effect blocked by substance P[43]. As far as biliary epithelium is concerned, in isolated rat bile duct fragments[44], bombesin stimulates bicarbonate-rich fluid secretion, indicating a direct effect on biliary epithelium. The effect of bombesin is not associated with any modification of cytosolic Ca^{2+} and is not counteracted by substance P[44]. Thus, intracellular messengers and signal transduction pathways involved in the mechanism of action of bombesin on biliary epithelium are still unknown.

VASOACTIVE INTESTINAL POLYPEPTIDE (VIP)

VIP, composed of 28 amino acids, was first isolated in 1970 from proximal intestine of the pig and later detected in the central and periphereal nervous system[54,55]. Many effects have been described, although it remains unknown if these are biological effects or the consequence of pharmacological doses used in experimental studies[54,55]. These effects include vasodilatation, smooth muscle relaxation, stimulation of exocrine pancreas and intestinal secretion, inhibition of gastric secretion and stimulation of the release of somatostatin, insulin, glucagon and prolactin[48,49,54,55]. In most cell types investigated, VIP seems to work via cAMP and the related PKA transduction pathway[48,49,54,55]. In isolated rat bile duct units, preliminary studies showed that VIP induces a bicarbonate-rich fluid secretion by activating the Cl^-/HCO_3^- exchanger, a mechanism partially inhibited by the Cl^- channel blocker NPPB[45,56]. In the bile duct-ligated liver, VIP induced a marked bicarbonate-rich choleresis[45]. These preliminary data indicate that VIP specifically targets biliary epithelium, where it induces a bicarbonate-rich choleresis. However, interference with secretin receptors, as demonstrated in other cell types[57], should be excluded. The intracellular messenger and signal transduction pathways have not yet been elucidated.

ACETYLCHOLINE

The innervation of the biliary tree has been little investigated. In humans, Terada *et al.*[58] identified nerve fibres in the wall of the large, medium and small intrahepatic bile duct, as well as in association with peribiliary glands. Moreover, at a functional level, little information exists on the neuronal control of ductal bile secretion. In the dog[59], vagal stimulation causes a slight increase in bicarbonate biliary output and bile flow, thought to be of ductal origin, only when the enterohepatic circulation was interrupted. In sheep, electrical stimulation of the vagus induces only a slight increase in bicarbonate output[60]. The occurrence of muscarinic receptors has been investigated in isolated rat bile duct units by immunofluorescence and immunoelectron microscopy using antibody against M3 subtype acetylcholine receptors[61]. In this preliminary report, bile ducts of different sizes stained positively with a predominant labelling of basolateral membrane. Nathanson *et al.*[62] investigated the effect of acetylcholine on fluid secretion in isolated rat bile duct units and on bile flow in the isolated perfused rat liver. They found that acetylcholine induces a marked increase in cytosolic Ca^{2+} in cholangiocytes surrounding the lumenal space of bile duct units. Both influx of extracellular Ca^{2+} and mobilization of internal thapsigargin-sensitive Ca^{2+} stores, are responsible for acetylcholine-induced Ca^{2+} increase. However, acetylcholine failed to influence either ductal fluid secretion or paracellular permeability in isolated ducts. In the isolated perfused rat liver, acetylcholine induces a transient decrease of bile flow together with a marked increase in perfusion pressure. Although the inhibitory effect was not abolished by preventing changes in perfusion pressure with vascular active agents, conclusions regarding the effect of acetylcholine on ductal bile secretion are difficult, given the small contribution to total bile flow in the rat.

We investigated, in isolated rat bile duct units, the effect of acetylcholine on basal and secretin-stimulated Cl^-/HCO_3^- exchanger activity. The rationale for studying coordinate regulation of Cl^-/HCO_3^- exchanger by secretin and acetylcholine is that secretin targets BDE cells during parasympathetic predominance. Preliminary data from this study indicate that acetylcholine alone failed to influence the basal activity of the Cl^-/HCO_3^- exchanger. The slope of intracellular alkalinization after Cl^- removal and the slope of pH_i recovery after Cl^- readmission were similar whether or not bile duct units were exposed to acetylcholine. However, when isolated bile duct units were exposed to acetylcholine plus secretin, the stimulatory effect of secretin on the Cl^-/HCO_3^- exchanger was enhanced by approximately 45%. Moreover, we found that the effect of acyetylcholine was not blocked by the PKC antagonist staurosporine. These preliminary data indicate that acetylcholine does not influence the basal activity of the Cl^-/HCO_3^- exchanger, but does enhance the secretin-induced stimulation of the Cl^-/HCO_3^- exchanger by a PKC-insensitive mechanism. Since secretin targets BDE cells during parasympathetic predominance, coordinated regulation of Cl^-/HCO_3^- exchanger and CFTR by cAMP and Ca^{2+} could play a key role in controlling fluid secretion in BDE cells. cAMP and Ca^{2+} could influence fluid secretion not only by regulating activities but also by the recruitment of transporters and channels in the apical membrane. This issue needs extensive investigation in biliary epithelium in the light of studies concerning other bicarbonate secretory epithelia in which a coordinate regulation of CFTR activity and trafficking by Ca^{2+} and cAMP has been demonstrated[63].

Table 1 Hormones and neuropeptides regulating fluid secretion in biliary epithelium cells

Stimulation	*Inhibition*
Secretin	Somatostatin
Bombesin	Gastrin
VIP	
Acetylcholine	

CONCLUSIONS

In conclusion, current data demonstrate that various hormones or neuropeptides are involved in the regulation of fluid secretion in bile ducts or ductules (Table 1). Secretin, bombesin and VIP induce alkaline fluid secretion, acetylcholine enhances the secretin effects while somatostatin and gastrin counterregulate this process. Considerable progress has been made concerning cAMP- and Ca^{2+}-regulated Cl^- conductance, as well as transport processes driving bicarbonate excretion in basal conditions or during hormonal stimulation. The intracellular messengers and signal transduction pathways involved in the hormonal regulation of biliary epithelium function are currently under investigation. While the cAMP–PKA-dependent pathways have been sufficiently clarified, at least for secretin, much work remains to be done with regard to the mechanism of action of the other hormones, and in particular those acting via Ca^{2+}-related pathways. However, considering that research on the physiology and biology of biliary epithelium virtually only began in the 1990s, the mass of work done to date is impressive.

References

1. Alpini G, Phillips IO, LaRusso NF. The biology of biliary epithelia. In: Arias IM, Fausto N, Jacoby WB, Schachter DA, Shafritz DA, editors. The liver: biology and paothobiology. New York: Raven Press; 1984:623–53.
2. Roberts SK, LaRusso N. Pathobiology of biliary epithelia. Curr Opin Gastroenterol. 1994;10:526–33.
3. Boyer JL. Bile duct epithelium: frontiers in transport physiology. Am J Physiol. 1996;270:G1–5.
4. Alpini G, Lenzi R, Sarkozi L, Tavoloni N. Biliary physiology in rats with bile ductular cell hyperplasia. Evidence for a secretory function of proliferated bile ductules. J Clin Invest. 1988;81:569–78.
5. Alpini G, Lenzi R, Zhai WR *et al.* Isolation of a nonparenchymal liver cell fraction enriched in cells with biliary epithelial phenotypes. Gastroenterolgy. 1989;97:1248–60.
6. Ishii M, Vroman B, LaRusso NF. Isolation and morphologic characterization of bile duct epithelial cells from normal rat liver. Gastroenterology. 1989;97:1236–47.
7. Strazzabosco M, Mennone A, Boyer JL. Intracellular pH regulation in isolated rat bile duct epithelial cells. J Clin Invest. 1991;87:1503–12.
8. Alvaro D, Cho WK, Mennone A, Boyer JL. Effect of secretin on intracellular pH regulation in isolated rat bile duct epithelial cells. J Clin Invest. 1993;92:1314–25.
9. Alvaro D, Mennone A, Boyer JL. Effect of ursodeoxycholic acid on intracellular pH regulation in isolated rat bile duct epithelial cells. Am J Physiol. 1993;265:G783–91.

10. Miller SB, Saccomani G, Cihla HP. Purification of cells from liver of carcinogen-treated rats during extrahepatic cholestasis. Cancer Res. 1983;43:4176–9.
11. Grubman SA, Perrone RD, Lee DW *et al.* Regulation of intracellular pH by immortalized human intrahepatic biliary epithelial cell lines. Am J Physiol. 1994;266 (Gastrointest Liver Physiol. 29):G1060–70.
12. Joplin R. Isolation and culture of biliary epithelial cells. Gut. 1994;35:875–8.
13. Roberts SK, Kuntz SM, Gores GJ, LaRusso NF. Regulation of bicarbonate-dependent ductular bile secretion assessed by lumenal micropuncture of isolated rodent intrahepatic bile ducts. Proc Natl Acad Sci USA. 1993;90:9080–4.
14. Mennone A, Alvaro D, Cho W, Boyer JL. Isolation of small polarized bile duct units. Proc Natl Acad Sci USA. 1995;92:6527–31.
15. Strazzabosco M, Joplin R, Zeembery A *et al.* Bicarbonate transport in cultured human intrahepatic bile duct epithelial cells (hBDE) from normal subjects and patients with primary biliary cirrhosis (PBC). Hepatology. 1994;2:404A.
16. Strazzabosco M, Poci C, Spirli' C, Sartori L, Knuth A, Crepaldi G. Effect of ursodeoxycholic acid on intracellular pH in a bile duct epithelium-like cell line. Hepatology. 1994;19:145–54.
17. Martinez-Anso E, Castillo JE, Diez J, Medina JF, Prieto J. Immunohistochemical detection of chloride/bicarbonate anion exchanger in human liver. Hepatology. 1994;19:1400–6.
18. Fitz JG, Basavappa S, McGill J, Melhus O, Cohn JA. Regulation of membrane chloride currents in rat bile duct epithelial cells. J Clin Invest. 1993;91:319–28.
19. Cohn JA, Strong TV, Picciotto MR, Nairn AC, Collins FS, Fitz JG. Localization of the cystic fibrosis transmembrane conductance regulator in human bile duct epithelial cells. Gastroenterology. 1993;105:1857–64.
20. Basavappa S, Middleton J, Mangel AW, McGill JM, Cohn JA, Fitz JG. Cl^- and K^+ transport in human biliary cell lines. Gastroenterology. 1993;104:1796–805.
21. McGill JM, Basavappa S, Fitz JG. Characterization of high-conductance anion channels in rat bile duct epithelial cells. Am J Physiol. 1992;262 (Gastrointest Liver Physiol. 25):G703–10.
22. McGill JM, Gettys W, Basavappa S, Fitz JG. GTP-binding proteins regulate high conductance anion channels in rat bile duct epithelial cells. J Membr Biol. 1993;133:253–61.
23. Bayliss WM, Starling EH. The mechanism of pancreatic secretion. J Physiol Lond. 1902;28:325–63.
24. Wheeler EL, Ramos OL. Role of bile ducts during secretin choleresis in dogs. Am J Physiol. 1966;210:1153–9.
25. Hardison WGM, Norman JC. Electrolyte composition of the secretin fraction of bile from the perfused pig liver. Am J Physiol. 1968;214:758–63.
26. Farouk M, Vigna S, McVey DC, Meyers WC. Localization and characterization of secretin binding sites expressed by rat bile duct epithelium. Gastroenterology. 1992;102:963–8.
27. Alpini G, Ulrich II GD, Phillips JO, Pham LD, Miller LJ, LaRusso NF. Upregulation of secretin receptor gene expression in rat cholangiocytes after bile ligation. Am J Physiol. 1994;266:G922–G928.
28. Gubba S, Glaser S, Robertson W, Lasater J, LeSage J, Alpini G. Compensatory cholangiocyte proliferation in rats with partial hepatectomy is associated with increased ductal secretion. Hepatology. 1995;22:867.
29. Kato A, Gores GJ, LaRusso NF. Secretin stimulates exocytosis in isolated bile duct epithelial cells by a cyclic AMP-mediated mechanism. J Biol Biochem. 1992;267:15523–9.
30. Alvaro D, Della Guardia P, Bini A, *et al.* Effect of glucagon on intracellular pH regulation in isolated rat hepatocyte couplets. J Clin Invest. 1995;96:665–75.
31. Frizzel RA, Morris AP. Chloride conductance of salt-secreting epithelial cells. In: Current topics in membranes. New York: Academic Press; 1994:vol.42:173–214.
32. Dallenbach A, Renner EL. Colchicine does not inhibit secretin-induced choleresis in rats exhibiting hyperplasia of bile ductules: evidence against a pivotal role of exocytic vesicle insertion. J Hepatol. 1995;22:338–48.
33. Renner EL, Heydtmann M. Amiloride, but not DIDS and NPPB, inhibit secretin (SEC)-induced choleresis: evidence for a role of Na^+/H^+, but not Cl^-/HCO_3^- exchanger and Cl^- channles, in ductular bile formation. Hepatology. 1995;22:315A.
34. Lake JR, Renner EL, Scharschmidt BF *et al.* Inhibition of Na^+/H^+ exchange in the rat is associated with decreased ursodeoxycholate hypercholeresis, decreased secretion of unconjugated ursodeoxycholate, and increased ursodeoxycholate glucuronidation. Gastroenterology. 1988;95:454–63.

35. Mennone A, Alvaro D, Boyer JL. Role of proetin kinase A (PKA) and potein kinase C (PKC) on secretin induced fluid secretion and Cl^-/HCO_3^- exchange in small isolated bile duct units (IBDU) from rat liver. Falk Workshop 'Vanishing bile duct syndrome – pathophysiology and treatment', Spoleto, Italy, 1996.
36. Brazeau P, Vale W, Burgus R, Ling N, Butcher M, Rivier J. Guillemin hypothalamic polypeptide that inhibits the secretion of immunoreactive pituitary growth hormone. Science. 1973;179:77–9.
37. Raulf F, Pérez J, Hoyer D, Bruns C. Differential expression of five somatostatin receptors subtypes, SSTR1–5, in the CNS and periphereal tissue. Digestion. 1994;55:46–53.
38. Reichlin S. Somatostatin. N Engl J Med. 1983:309:1495–501, 1556–63.
39. Holm I, Thulin L, Samnegard H, Efendic S, Tyden G. Anticholeretic effect of somatostatin in anesthetized dogs. Acta Physiol Scand. 1978;104:241–3.
40. Rene E, Danzinger RG, Hofmann AF, Nakagaki M. Pharmacologic effect of somatostatin on bile formation in the dog. Gastroenterology. 1983;84:120–9.
41. Tietz PS, Alpini G, Pham LD, LaRusso NF. Somatostatin inhibits secretin-induced ductal hypercholeresis and exocytosis by cholangiocytes. Am J Physiol. 1995;269:G110–18.
42. Sternini C, Dennis SU, Gamp P, Bunnett NW. Cellular sites of expression of the neurokin-1 receptor in the rat gastrointestinal tract. J Comp Neurol. 1995;358:531–40.
43. Ashton N, Argent BE, Green R. Effect of vasoactive intestinal peptide, bombesin and substance P on fluid secretion by isolated rat pancreatic duct. J Physiol. 1990;427:471–82.
44. Cho WK, Mennone A, Boyer JL. Effect of bombesin on secretion in isolated polarized intrahepatic bile ductular units (IBDU). Gastroenretology. 1995;108:A1049(abstract).
45. Cho WK, Mennone A, Rydberg SA, Boyer JL. VIP is a potent stimulus of bicarbonate and fluid secretion in bile ducts. Hepatology. 1995;22:A294(abstract).
46. Rehfeld JF, Larsson LI. The predominant form of antral gastrin and intestinal cholecystokinin corresponds to the common COOH-terminal tetrapeptide. In: Rehfeld JF, Handrup E, editors. Gastrins and vagus. London: Academic Press;1979:85–94.
47. Berson SA, Yalow RS. Nature of immunoreactive gastrin extracted from tissues of gastrointestinal tract. Gastroenterology. 1971;60:215–26.
48. Walsh JH, Mayer EA. Gastrointestinal hormones. In: Sleisenger MH, Fordtran JS, editors. Gastrointestinal disease, 5th edn. Philadelphia: WB Saunders; 1993:18–44.
49. Walsh JH. Gastrointestinal hormones and peptides. In: Johnson LR, editor. Physiology of the gastrointestinal tract. New York: Raven Press;1981:59–144.
50. Svanvik J. Role of gallbladder in modifying hepatic bile composition. In: Tavoloni N, Berk PD, editors. Hepatic transport and bile secretion. Physiology and pathophysiology. New York: Raven Press;1992:607–18.
51. Alpini G, Glaser GG, LeSage G. Gastrin inhibits secretin-induced hypercholeresis by interacting with specific receptors through the cAMP system. Falk Workshop 'Vanishing bile duct syndrome – pathophysiology and treatment', Spoleto, Italy, 1996.
52. Polak JM, Bloom SR. Peptidergin innervation of the gastrointestinal tract. In: Grossman MJ, Speranza V, Basso N, Lezoche E, editors. Gastrointestinal hormones and pathology of the digestive system. New York: Plenum; 1979:27–5.
53. Delle Fave G, Annibale B, De Magistris L *et al.* Bombesin effects on human GI functions. Peptides. 1985;6(Suppl. 3):113–16.
54. Mutt V, Said SI. Structure of the vasoactive intestinal octacosapeptide. The amino acid sequence. Use of kallikrein in its determination. Eur J Biochem. 1974;42:581–3.
55. Bryant MG. Possible dual role for vasoactive intestinal peptide as gastrointestinal hormone and neurotransmitter substance. Lancet. 1976;1:991–993.
56. Cho WK, Mennone A, Rydberg SA, Boyer JL. Characterization of VIP-stimulated bile secretion in rat. Falk Workshop 'Vanishing Bile Duct Syndrome – pathophysiology and treatment', Spoleto, Italy, 1996.
57. Christophe JP, Conlon TP, Gardner JD. Interaction of porcine vasoactive intestinal peptide with dispersed pancreatic acinar cells from the guinea pig: binding of radioiodinated peptide. J Biol Chem. 1976,21;4629–34.
58. Terada T, Nakanuma Y. Innervation of intrahepatic bile ducts and peribiliary glands in normal human livers, extrahepatic biliary obstruction and and hepatolithiasis. An immunohistochemical study. J Hepatol. 1989;9:141–8.
59. Kaminski DL, Dorighi J, Jellinek M. Effect of electrical vagal stimulation on canine hepatic bile flow. Am J Physiol. 1974;227:487–93.

60. Pass M, Heath T. Effect of electrical stimulation of the vagus nerves on bile secretion in anaesthesized sheep. Aust J Biol Sci. 1976;29:351–5.
61. Alvaro D, Jezequel AM, Carli L *et al.* Acetyl-choline regulation of fluid secretion in isolated rat bile duct units (IBDU). Proceedings of the AASLD, Annual Liver Meeting, Chicago, November 1996.
62. Nathanson MH, Burgstahler AD, Mennone A, Boyer JL. Characterization of cytosolic Ca^{2+} signaling in rat bile duct epithelia. Am J Physiol. 1996 (In press).
63. Frizzell RA, Morris AP. Chloride conductances of salt-secreting epithelial cells. In: Current topics in membranes. New York: Academic Press; 1994:vol.42:173–214.

7
Evidence for paracrine regulation of biliary Cl^- secretion by purinergic signalling

J. G. FITZ

INTRODUCTION

Bile formation depends upon complementary interactions between hepatocytes and bile duct epithelial cells, the two primary epithelial cells of the liver[1,2]. Secretion is initiated by hepatocyte transport of bile acids and other solutes into the canalicular space between cells, which generates an osmotic gradient favouring influx of water and electrolytes[3,4]. Subsequently, canalicular bile enters the extensive network of ducts which form the intrahepatic biliary tree. Within these ducts it is alkalinized and diluted as a result of active secretion by cholangiocytes[3,5]. In animal models, experimental manoeuvres which increase the number of bile ductular cells cause parallel increases in bile flow[6,7]. However, the small size (7–10 μm) and intrahepatic location of these cells has limited direct evaluation of the mechanisms responsible for secretion.

Indirect observations indicate that intrahepatic ductular secretion involves transepithelial movement of Cl^- and HCO_3^- ions into the lumen[8]. Application of patch clamp and other techniques to cholangiocytes has identified at least four different Cl^- channel types which might contribute to regulated efflux of Cl^- from the cell into the lumen if they are localized to the apical membrane. One of these, the cystic fibrosis transmembrane conductance regulator (CFTR), which is itself a cAMP-regulated Cl^- channel[9], appears to be responsible for secretin-stimulated Cl^- secretion[10]. Abnormalities of CFTR regulation in the genetic disease cystic fibrosis (CF) contributes to the cholestasis and duct injury observed in some patients[11,12]. Indeed, the presence of duct injury in CF supports the general concept that these channels and Cl^- transport in general contribute importantly to biliary secretion as they do in airway and pancreatic ducts[13–15] where opening of Cl^- channels in the apical membrane has been established as a key point for regulation of secretion[9,16,17].

ROLE OF CFTR IN BILIARY SECRETION

Previous studies of cholangiocytes have focused on the potential roles of CFTR in biliary function because of the importance of secretin in hormonal regulation of duct function. Secretin stimulates an increase in bile flow and biliary HCO_3^- output[3], but there are important species differences in the response. At the cellular level stimulation of secretin receptors increases intracellular cAMP levels, and cAMP-dependent protein phosphorylation[18–20] leads to opening of Cl^- channels[10,21,22], stimulation of Cl^-/HCO_3^- exchange, and net efflux of anions into the lumen (Figure 1). cAMP-stimulated Cl^- currents and/or channels have also been identified in human biliary cell lines[23] and *Necturus* gallbladder[24,25], indicating a widespread distribution in the intrahepatic and extrahepatic biliary system. In cholangiocytes, comparison of the amplitude of unitary currents to whole cell currents suggests that increases in cAMP lead to opening of 500–2000 channels in each cell.

These observations in individual cholangiocytes have been extended by the use of intact duct units isolated from the intrahepatic biliary tree[26,27]. This model shows great promise since intact, polarized bile duct units retain secretory polarity and the lumen is accessible for micropuncture. Shortly after isolation, the

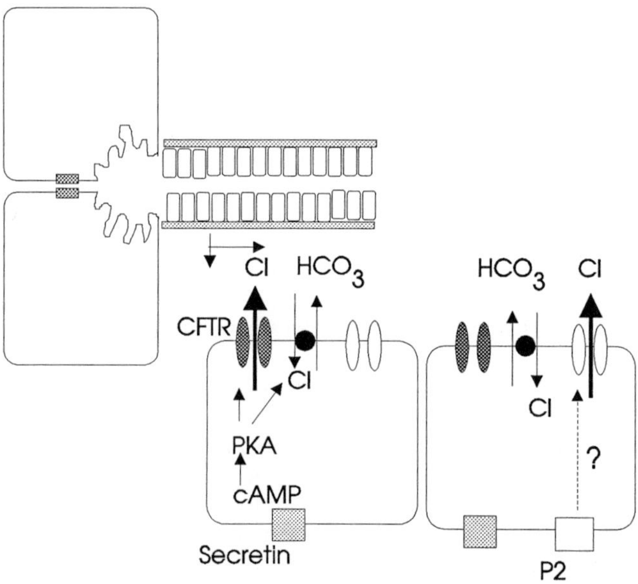

Figure 1 The bile secretory unit, the potential mechanisms for secretion by duct cells. Bile formation is initiated by hepatocyte secretion into the canalicular space. Canalicular bile then enters the lumen of intrahepatic ducts where it is alkalinized and diluted as a result of cholangiocyte secretion. Exposure of duct cells to the hormone secretin increases intracellular cAMP, leading to opening of CFTR-related Cl^- channels and stimulation of Cl^-/HCO_3^- exchange (see text). Since duct cells also express other Cl^- channel types (right), if these are localized to the apical membrane then opening could complement the effects of cAMP to increase the secretory response. P_{2u} receptors are expressed by cholangiocytes, but the cellular localization and the signals which lead to channel opening have not been fully defined

ends of these duct segments seal to form a closed compartment. Stimulation by forskolin causes an increase in lumenal diameter (secretion) as well as alkalinization of the lumenal contents which depends upon the presence of both Cl^- and HCO_3^- ions[20,27]. In addition, secretin stimulates Cl^-/HCO_3^- exchange activity in the apical membrane[28]. These findings support a model analogous to pancreatic ducts, where cAMP-regulated Cl^- channels and Cl^-/HCO_3^- exchangers work in parallel to increase lumenal HCO_3^- concentrations during secretion (Figure 1)[15,29–31].

The biophysical features of cAMP-activated Cl^- channels in cholangiocytes are similar to Cl^- channels associated with expression of CFTR in other tissues. The presence of CFTR has been supported by other techniques which have detected CFTR mRNA by *in situ* hybridization and CFTR protein by immunochemical and immunostaining methods[11,32]. CFTR is localized to the apical (lumenal) membrane of cholangiocytes, but is not detected in other populations of liver cells. This localization is similar to the distribution of the Cl^-/HCO_3^- exchanger[28] and supports the concept that these two ion transport proteins function in parallel at the apical plasma membrane to enable bile duct epithelium to secrete fluid and HCO_3^- in response to cAMP-mediated stimuli (Figure 1).

It is notable that studies in other model systems indicate that CFTR is multifunctional, serving as a cAMP-regulated Cl^- channel[33,34] and also as a regulator of other Cl^- channels[35,36]. In addition, CFTR has been implicated in control of endocytic recycling[37]; protein glycosylation and sulphation[38]; ATP movement across the plasma membrane[36,39]; and regulation of Na^+ channel activity[40]. These diverse roles are not readily explained at the molecular level. Consequently, an important goal of future studies is to clarify the mechanisms and relative contributions of these different functions of CFTR to the pathobiology of cystic fibrosis in biliary and other cell types.

This model of biliary secretion has not been directly validated by measurements of electrogenic Cl^- secretion across intrahepatic ducts. However, it is consistent with the available data, and the fundamental role of regulated Cl^- transport in secretion is supported by clinical involvement of intra- and extrahepatic bile ducts in cystic fibrosis[41,42]. The need for continued validation of this model is apparent.

EVIDENCE FOR ATP AS A SIGNALLING MOLECULE

Biliary disease is an important concern in cystic fibrosis, with intrahepatic and extrahepatic stricture formation, focal cirrhosis, and progression to liver failure in a minority of patients. In general, however, only 20–40% of patients with cystic fibrosis develop these manifestations as compared to 80–90% involvement of lung and pancreatic duct. One potential reason might be the expression by cholangiocytes of alternative Cl^- channels not related to CFTR which are capable of maintaining secretory function (Figure 1, right). In other secretory cells, Cl^- channels which are unrelated to CFTR, and are regulated by intracellular Ca^{2+}, cell volume, or other mechanisms, have been identified[17,43,44]. Indirect support for an important contribution of these channels comes from study of the CFTR 'knockout' mouse (cftr –/–) where there is no detectable cAMP-regulated Cl^- conductance[45]. Tissues from these mice which express Ca^{2+}-activated Cl^- channels are relatively protected from clinical involvement, while tissues that do not express these channels have significantly impaired function[46]. Consequently, studies to evaluate these alternative conductances in biliary cells may provide clues to the presence of cAMP-independent regulatory pathways involved in ductular secretion. In particular, evidence from isolated rat cholangiocytes and biliary cell lines demonstrates that increases in intracellular Ca^{2+} concentration ($[Ca^{2+}]_i$) leads to increases in membrane Cl^- permeability through opening Cl^- channels[22,47]. In view of the important role of Ca^{2+}-dependent regulation of secretion in other cell types[16,17,43,48–50], it seems reasonable to postulate that Ca^{2+}-activated Cl^- channels may operate in parallel with CFTR to modulate secretion by biliary cells.

There is no direct evidence for intracellular Ca^{2+} as a signal for stimulation of secretion in bile duct cells[51]. If Ca^{2+}- or Ca^{2+}-dependent kinases[52,53] do work in this manner, the Ca^{2+}-dependent Cl^- channels would need to be localized to the apical membrane for a role in secretion (Figure 1). Consequently, studies of channels in isolated cells where the Ca^{2+}-activated Cl^- conductance is high may not necessarily reflect the situation in intact monolayers. The availability of models which retain cellular polarity represents an important advance towards addressing these issues[20,27,51].

Extracellular ATP represents one candidate for a secretagogue which might modulate bile ductular transport through Ca^{2+}-dependent signalling. Extracellular ATP modulates a variety of liver transport and metabolic functions through activation of one or more purinergic (P_2) receptor subtypes[54–57]. In rat cholangiocyte[47] and human biliary cell lines[47,58], P_2 receptor stimulation by ATP or UTP mobilizes intracellular Ca^{2+} and increases membrane Cl^- permeability. These findings are consistent with activation of P_{2u} receptors similar to the G-protein coupled receptors recently cloned from the human airway[59]. In airway cells, purinergic receptors are localized to the apical plasma membrane, and stimulation leads to release of Ca^{2+} from intracellular stores, and activation of Cl^- channels through both Ca^{2+}-dependent and Ca^{2+}-independent signalling pathways[16].

The role of purinergic stimulation in biliary secretion is not established. In *Necturus* gallbladder, both the purinergic receptors and the Cl^- conductance can be localized to the apical membrane[60], and ATP is present in human bile in concentrations sufficient to activate P_{2u} receptors[61]. Thus, further evaluation of the potential role of ATP in modulation of biliary secretion will be of interest. The model shown in Figure 1 is speculative, and many questions remain. First, the cellular origins of the ATP in bile have not been established, and the molecular mechanisms involved in movement of ATP out of cells remain controversial[39,62,63]. Second, the cellular localization of P_2 receptors in cholangiocytes has not been established. Findings in *Necturus* gallbladder support an apical (lumenal) localization for both P_2 receptors and Cl^- channels[60], but basolateral receptors may also be present[64]. Finally, purinergic agonists are subject to rapid degradation by nucleotidases on the extracellular surface, representing another potential site for regulation.

We speculate that signalling through ATP might represent an attractive mechanism for autocrine/paracrine regulation of biliary secretory function and for coordinating the separate hepatic and biliary components of bile formation. Further characterization of the channels and receptors involved might provide targets for pharmacological therapy aiming to modulate the volume and composition of bile, and to bypass the Cl^- secretory defect associated with cystic fibrosis. However, full evaluation of the physiological roles of ATP will require development of new experimental models which allow access to the apical and basolateral domains of polarized cell monolayers[65].

Acknowledgements

This chapter is adapted in part from Fitz J. G., Cohn J. A. Biology and pathophysiology of CFTR in biliary epithelial cells. In: Sirica A., Longnecker D., editors. Pathobiology of intrahepatic biliary and pancreatic duct cells. New York: Marcel-Dekker; 1996.

References

1. Nathanson MH, Boyer JL. Mechanisms and regulation of bile secretion. Hepatology. 1991;14:551–66.
2. Boyer JL, Graf J, Meier PJ. Hepatic transport systems regulating pHi, cell volume, and bile secretion. Annu Rev Physiol. 1992;54:415–38.
3. Preisig R, Cooper HL, Wheeler HO. The relationship between taurocholate secretion rate and bile production in the unanesthetized dog during cholinergic blockade and during secretin administration. J Clin Invest. 1962;41:1152–62.
4. Graf J. Canalicular bile salt-independent bile formation: concepts and clues from electrolyte transport in rat liver. Am J Physiol. 1983;244:G233–46.
5. Farouk M, Vigna SR, McVey DC, Meyers WC. Localization and characterization of secretin binding sites expressed by rat bile duct epithelium. Gastroenterology. 1992;102:963–8.
6. Alpini G, Lenzi R, Sarkozi L, Tavoloni N. Biliary physiology in rats with bile ductular cell hyperplasia. J Clin Invest. 1988;81:569–78.
7. Alpini G, Lenzi R, Zhai WR, Slott PA, Sarkozi L, Tavoloni N. Bile secretory function of intrahepatic biliary epithelium in the rat. Am J Physiol. 1989;257:G124–33.
8. Chenderovitch J. Secretory function of the rabbit common bile duct. Am J Physiol. 1972;223:695–706.
9. Anderson MP, Gregory RJ, Thompson S *et al.* Demonstration that CFTR is a chloride channel by alteration of its anion selectivity. Science. 1991;253:202–05.
10. McGill J, Gettys TW, Basavappa S, Fitz JG. Secretin activates Cl channels in bile duct epithelial cells through a cAMP-dependent mechanism. Am J Physiol. 1994;266:G731–6.
11. Cohn JA, Strong TA, Picciotto MA *et al.* Localization of CFTR in human bile duct epithelial cells. Gastroenterology. 1993;105:1857–64.
12. Colombo C, Battezzati PM, Podda M. Hepatobiliary disease in cystic fibrosis. Sem Liv Dis. 1994;14:259–69.
13. Mason SJ, Paradiso AM, Boucher RC. Regulation of transepithelial ion transport and intracellular calcium by extracellular ATP in human normal and cystic fibrosis airway epithelia. Br J Pharmacol. 1991;103:1649–56.
14. Quinton PM. Missing Cl conductance in cystic fibrosis. Am J Physiol. 1986;251:C649–52.
15. Ashton N, Argent BE, Green R. Effect of vasoactive intestinal peptide, bombesin and substance P on fluid secretion by isolated rat pancreatic duct. J Physiol. 1990;427:471–82.
16. Stutts MJ, Fitz JG, Paradiso AM, Boucher RC. Multiple modes of regulation of airway epithelial chloride secretion by extracellular ATP. Am J Physiol. 1994;267:C1442–51.
17. Cliff WH, Frizzell RA. Separate chloride conductances activated by cAMP and Ca2+ in Cl-secreting epithelial cells. Proc Natl Acad Sci USA. 1990;87:4956–60.
18. Lenzen R, Alpini G, Tavoloni N. Secretin stimulates bile ductular secretory activity through the cAMP system. Am J Physiol. 1992;26:G527–32.

19. Kato A, Gores G, LaRusso N. Secretin stimulates exocytosis in isolated bile duct epithelial cells by a cAMP-mediated mechanism. J Biol Chem. 1992;267:15523–9.
20. Roberts SK, Kuntz SM, Gores G, LaRusso N. Regulation of bicarbonate-dependent ductular bile secretion assessed by lumenal micropuncture of isolated rodent intrahepatic bile ducts. Proc Natl Acad Sci USA. 1993;90:9080–4.
21. Hamill OP, Marty A, Neher E, Sakmann B, Sigworth FJ. Improved patch clamp techniques for high resolution recording from cells and cell-free membrane patches. Pfluegers Arch. 1981;391:85–100.
22. Fitz JG, Basavappa S, McGill J, Melhus O, Cohn JA. Regulation of membrane chloride currents in rat bile duct epithelial cells. J Clin Invest. 1993;91:319–28.
23. Basavappa S, Middleton JP, Mangel A, McGill J, Cohn JA, Fitz JG. Cl^- and K^+ transport in human biliary cell lines. Gastroenterology. 1993;104:1796–805.
24. Petersen K-U, Reuss L. Cyclic AMP-induced chloride permeability in the apical membrane of *Necturus* gallbladder epithelium. J Gen Physiol. 1983;81:705–29.
25. Copello J, Heming TA, Segal Y, Reuss L. cAMP-activated apical membrane chloride channels in *Necturus* gallbladder epithelium. J Gen Physiol. 1993;102:177–99.
26. Cornet M, Lambert IH, Hoffmann EK. Relation between cytoskeleton, hypoosmotic treatment and volume regulation in Ehrlich ascites tumor cells. J Membr Biol. 1993;131:55–66.
27. Mennone A, Alvaro D, Cho W, Boyer JL. Isolation of small polarized bile duct units. Proc Natl Acad Sci USA 1995;92:6527–31.
28. Martinez-Anso E, Castillo JE, Diez J, Medina JF, Prieto J. Immunohistochemical detection of chloride/bicarbonate anion exchangers in human liver. Hepatology. 1994;19:1400–6.
29. Gray MA, Plant S, Argent BE. cAMP-regulated whole cell chloride currents in pancreatic duct cells. Am J Physiol. 1993;264:C591–602.
30. Gray MA, Greenwell JR, Argent BE. Secretin-regulated chloride channel on the apical plasma membrane of pancreatic duct cells. J Membr Biol. 1988;105:131–42.
31. Ashton N, Argent BE, Green R. Characteristics of fluid secretion from isolated rat pancreatic ducts stimulated with secretin and bombesin. J Physiol. 1991;435:533–46.
32. Yang Y, Raper SE, Cohn JA, Engelhardt JF, Wilson JM. An approach for treating the hepato-biliary disease of cystic fibrosis by somatic gene transfer. Proc Natl Acad Sci USA. 1993;90:4601–5.
33. O'Riordan CR, Erickson A, Bear CE. Purification and characterization of recombinant cystic fibrosis transmembrane conductance regulator from Chinese hamster ovary and insect cells. J Biol Chem. 1995;270:17033–43.
34. Bear CE, Kartner N, Bridges RJ, Jensen TJ, Ramjeesingh M, Riordan JR. Purification and functional reconstitution of the cystic fibrosis transmembrane conductance regulator (CFTR). Cell. 1992;66:809–18.
35. Gabriel S, Clarke LL, Boucher RC, Stutts MJ. CFTR and outward rectifying chloride channels are distinct proteins with a regulatory relationship. Nature. 1993;363:263–6.
36. Schwiebert EM, Egan ME, Hwang T-H *et al.* CFTR regulates outwardly rectifying chloride channels through an autocrine mechanism involving ATP. Cell. 1995;81:1063–73.
37. Bradbury NA, Lilling T, Berta G, Sorscher EJ, Bridges RJ, Kirk KL. Regulation of plasma membrane recycling by CFTR. Science. 1992;256:530–2.
38. Dosanjh A, Lencer W, Brown D. Heterologous expression of delta-508 CFTR results in decreased sialyation of membrane glycoconjugates. Am J Physiol. 1994;266:C360–6.
39. Reisin IL, Prat AG, Abraham EH *et al.* The cystic fibrosis transmembrane conductance regulator is a dual ATP and chloride channel. J Biol Chem. 1994;269:20584–91.
40. Stutts MJ, Canessa CM, Olsen JC *et al.* CFTR as a cAMP-dependent regulator of sodium channels. Science. 1995;269:847–50.
41. O'Brien S, Keogan M, Casey M *et al.* Biliary complications of cystic fibrosis. Gut. 1992;33:387–91.
42. Colombo C, Petroni ML. Prevention and treatment of liver disease in cystic fibrosis. In: Dodge JA, Brock DJH, Widdicombe JH, editors. Cystic fibrosis: current topics. New York, John Wiley; 1994;327–54.
43. Worrell RT, Frizzell RA. CaMKII mediates stimulation of chloride conductance by calcium in T84 cells. Am J Physiol. 1991;260:C877–82.
44. Worrell RT, Butt AG, Cliff WH, Frizzell RA. A volume-sensitive Cl^- conductance in human colonic cell line T84. Am J Physiol. 1989;256:C1111–19.

45. Snouwaert JN, Brigman KK, Latour AM *et al.* An animal model for cystic fibrosis made by gene targeting. Science. 1992;257:1083–8.
46. Clarke LL, Grubb BR, Yankaskas J, Cotton CU, McKenzie A, Boucher RC. Relationship of a non-cystic fibrosis transmembrane conductance regulator-mediated chloride conductance to organ-level disease in cftr (–/–) mice. Proc Natl Acad Sci USA. 1994;91:479–83.
47. Wolkoff LI, Perrone RD, Grubman SA *et al.* Purinergic Purinoceptor P2u identification and function in human intrahepatic biliary epithelial cell lines. Cell Cal. 1995;17:375–83.
48. Anderson MP, Welsh MJ. Calcium and cAMP activate different chloride channels in the apical membrane of normal and cystic fibrosis epithelia. Proc Natl Acad Sci USA. 1991;88:6003–7.
49. Clancey JP, McCann JD, Li M, Welsh MJ. Calcium-dependent regulation of airway epithelial chloride channels. Am J Physiol. 1990;258:L25–32.
50. Morris AP, Kirk K, Frizzell RA. Simultaneous analysis of cell calcium and calcium-stimulated chloride conductance in colonic epithelial cells (HT-29). Cell Reg. 1990;1:951–63.
51. Nathanson MH, Burgstahler AD, Mennone A, Boyer JL. Characterization of cytosolic Ca^{2+} signalling in rat bile duct epithelia. Am J Physiol 1996 (In press).
52. Kwiatkowski AP, McGill J. Human biliary epithelial cell line Mz-ChA-1 expresses new isoforms of calmodulin-dependent protein kinase II. Gastroenterology. 1995;109:1316–23.
53. McGill J, Yen MS, Basavappa S, Mangel A, Kwiatkowski AP. ATP-activated chloride permeability in biliary epithelial cells is regulated by calmodulin-dependent protein kinase II. Biochem Biophys Res Commun. 1995;208:457–62.
54. Haussinger D, Stehle T, Gerok W. Actions of extracellular ATP and UTP in perfused rat liver. Eur J Biochem. 1987;167:65–71.
55. Vanstapel F, Waebens M, Van Hecke P, Decanniere C, Stalmans W. Modulation of maximal glycogenolysis in perfused rat liver by adenosine and ATP. Biochem J. 1991;277:597–602.
56. Irving HR, Exton JH. Phosphatidylcholine breakdown in rat liver plasma membranes. Roles of guanine nucleotides and P2-purinergic agonists. J Biol Chem. 1987;262:3440–3.
57. Charest R, Blackmore PF, Exton JH. Characterization of responses of isolated rat hepatocytes to ATP and ADP. J Biol Chem. 1985;260:15789–94.
58. McGill J, Basavappa S, Shimokura GH, Middleton JP, Fitz JG. Adenosine triphosphate activates ion permeabilities in biliary epithelial cells. Gastroenterology. 1994;107:236–43.
59. Parr CE, Sullivan DM, Paradiso AM *et al.* Cloning and expression of a human P2u nucleotide receptor, a target for cystic fibrosis pharmacotherapy. Proc Natl Acad Sci USA. 1994;91:3275–9.
60. Cotton CU, Reuss L. Electrophysiologic effects of extracellular ATP on *Necturus* gallbladder epithelium. J Gen Physiol. 1991;97:949–71.
61. Chari RS, Schutz SM, Haebig JA *et al.* Adenosine nucleotides in bile. Am J Physiol. 1996;270:G246–52.
62. Abraham EH, Prat AG, Gerweck L *et al.* The multidrug resistance (mdr1) gene product functions as an ATP channel. Proc Natl Acad Sci USA. 1993;90:312–16.
63. Reddy MM, Quinton PM, Haws C *et al.* Failure of the cystic fibrosis transmembrane conductance regulator to conduct ATP. Science. 1996;271:1876–9.
64. Dho S, Stewart K, Foskett JK. Purinergic receptor activation of Cl-secretion in T84 cells. Am J Physiol. 1992;262:C67–74.
65. Vroman B, LaRusso N. Development and characterization of polarized primary cultures of rat intrahepatic bile duct epithelial cells. Lab Invest. 1996;74:303–13.

8 Transport of non-electrolyte biliary components in cholangiocytes

A. BENEDETTI

PROTEINS

Several lines of evidence have shown that cholangiocytes are involved in the transport and metabolism of different non-electrolyte biliary components[1].

Cholangiocytes actively participate in the transport of proteins from plasma into bile. Specific ductular routes have recently been proposed for the transport of various plasma proteins[2–6]. Epidermal growth factor (EGF) has been shown to be internalized into cholangiocytes by receptor-mediated endocytosis[7]. Other recent studies have been performed to define different steps of highly regulated cellular pathways for the transport of proteins such as horseradish peroxidase (HRP)[8,9]. These studies also provided new insights on cellular membrane traffic and recycling.

The function and physiological role of endocytosis and transcytosis have been well studied in hepatocytes. The development of techniques for isolation of bile duct cells[10,11] or intact polarized intrahepatic biliary ductules[8,12,13] has recently provided new tools for the study of these topics directly in cholangiocytes. Endocytosis has been studied *in vivo* in perfused rat liver and *in vitro* in isolated intrahepatic bile ductules by morphometric quantitative electron microscopy[8]. Endocytic vesicles containing HRP products were seen along the basolateral membrane of cholangiocytes 1–3 min after administration. These vesicles appear either as pinocytic, or large or tubular structures. Fluid-phase endocytosis in our model is largely restricted to the basolateral surface, and appears stimulated by choleretic drugs or bile acids, such as taurocholic acid (TCA) or ursodeoxycholic acid (UDCA). By contrast, it does not appear modified by microtubule inhibitors[8] or by brefeldin A[9], a different inhibitor of the transcytotic vesicular pathway. Furthermore, fluid-phase endocytosis is strongly inhibited by wortmannin, a novel specific inhibitor of phosphatidylinositol 3-kinase (PI3-kinase) activity (Figure 1). Preliminary data from our group suggest that inhibition of endocytic transport by wortmannin is mediated by a specific inhibition of dynamin. This protein has recently been identified as a

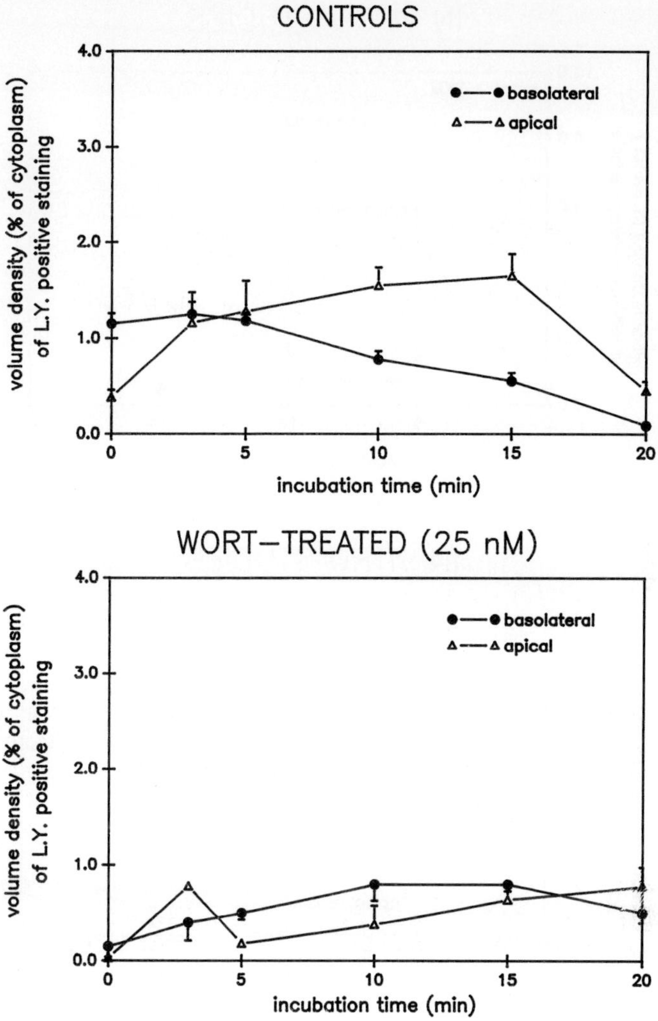

Figure 1 Effect of wortmannin on Lucifer yellow (LY) endocytosis and cellular localization in intrahepatic bile ductules isolated from rat liver. In wortmannin-treated samples (25 nmol/L) vs controls, the serial quantitative image analysis of the uptake and cellular localization of LY showed a significant inhibition of endocytosis (at the time interval: 0 and 3 min) in the basolateral area and a great and significant delay of transport of the fluorescent probe from the basolateral to the apical area (at time interval: 15 and 20 min)

major player in the endocytic pathway[14]. One of the promising candidates activating dynamin GTPase is P85alpha[15], the regulatory subunit of P13-kinase.

Either morphological or morphometric data suggest that a rapid vesicular transcytotic transport of proteins occurs from the cell periphery to the apical domain of bile duct cells[8]. This transport is mediated by microtubules (Figure 2). After their internalization, proteins are rapidly transported either to the apical

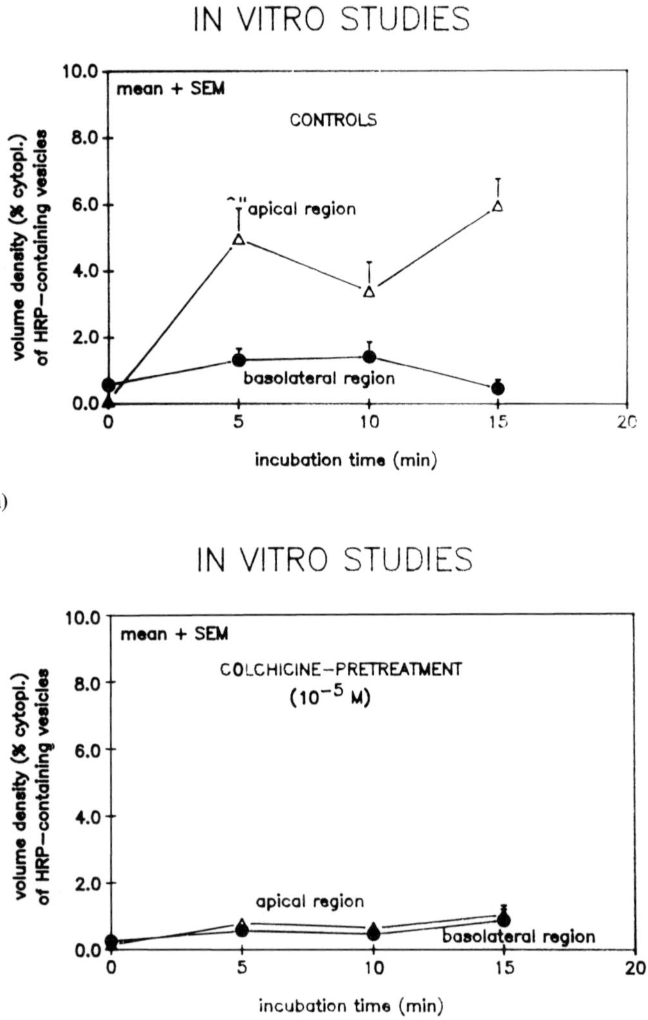

(a) (b)

Figure 2 (**a**) Volume density of HRP-containing structures in basolateral and apical areas of isolated bile ducts at 0, 5, 10, and 15 min after 3 min incubation in HRP-containing medium (time 0). A progressive increase in labelling of the apical region was noted, with a significant difference at 5, 10 and 15 min with respect to time 0. In the basolateral region the volume density progressively decreased with time. (**b**) Effect of 2 h preincubation with colchicine on the volume density of HRP-containing structures in the basolateral and apical areas of isolated bile ducts at 0, 5, 10, and 15 min after 3 min incubation in HRP-containing medium (time 0). The colchicine pretreatment resulted in a significant effect, substantially diminishing the density of HRP-containing structures, especially in the apical region of bile duct cells

domain or to secondary lysosomes or multivesicular bodies where they can be degraded. Similarly to endocytosis, the transbiliary transport of HRP is stimulated by TCA and UDCA which, moreover, increased the transition of vesicles to tubules and the apical targeting of these structures[8].

Brefeldin A (BFA) has recently become a valuable tool to analyse membrane traffic in secretory pathways. Effects of BFA include: (a) retrieval of the Golgi complex to the endoplasmic reticulum[16] through selective inhibition of the binding of beta-clathrin coat protein to Golgi membranes, thus blocking the anterograde transport mediated by these vesicles; (b) induces the trans-Golgi network to fuse with early endosomes; (c) inhibits polymeric IgA receptor-mediated transcytosis; (d) induces an increase of the retrograde traffic and finally (e) inhibits the apical transport of secretory proteins[17–20].

In rat biliary epithelial cells BFA does not interfere with fluid-phase endocytosis but inhibits transcytotic vesicular transport and apical targeting, as shown by the retention of HRP in an extensive tubular network in the Golgi juxtanuclear area (Figure 3)[9]. The morphology of the Golgi apparatus is, however, well preserved, as shown by the preservation of thiamine-pyrophosphatase activity (TPPase), a Golgi enzyme marker[9]. Therefore, structural integrity of the trans-Golgi cisternae coexists with a loss of specific functions involved in vesicle formation[9].

BFA interferes with the apical migration of vesicles inducing a block of the anterograde traffic of proteins by a mechanism different from monensin[21] or cytoskeleton inhibitors such as colchicine[8] or phalloidin[22]. Given the complexity of vesicular transcytotic pathways, these discrepancies may be explained by specific effects on different steps of a more general process.

Wortmannin, a specific novel inhibitor of PI3-kinase, has inhibitory effects on fluid-phase endocytosis in biliary epithelial cells (Figure 1). This drug also has an inhibitory effect on the transcytotic transport of fluid-phase markers to the apical domain in cholangiocytes (Figure 1). PI3-kinase activity has recently been associated with different signalling pathways involved in cell membrane traffic[23–25]. Data obtained in isolated perfused rat liver (IPRL) and in isolated rat hepatocyte couplets (IRHC) have, moreover, demonstrated that wortmannin decreases basal bile flow. This effect is associated with the inhibition of endocytic and transcytotic transport of fluid-phase markers similar to that observed in cholangiocytes, with a pathological dilatation of canalicular lumen and a disorganization of microfilaments, as shown by electron and fluorescence microscopy[26]. These data therefore suggest that PI3-kinase is involved in the regulation of vesicle trafficking and the process of bile formation. A similar disorganization of cytoskeleton has also been observed in isolated cholangiocytes.

In contrast with other cell functions distributed heterogeneously in bile ductules of various sizes[27], a low grade of morphometric heterogeneity is evident for endocytosis and transcytotic transport of fluid-phase markers in intrahepatic bile ductules of different diameter[28].

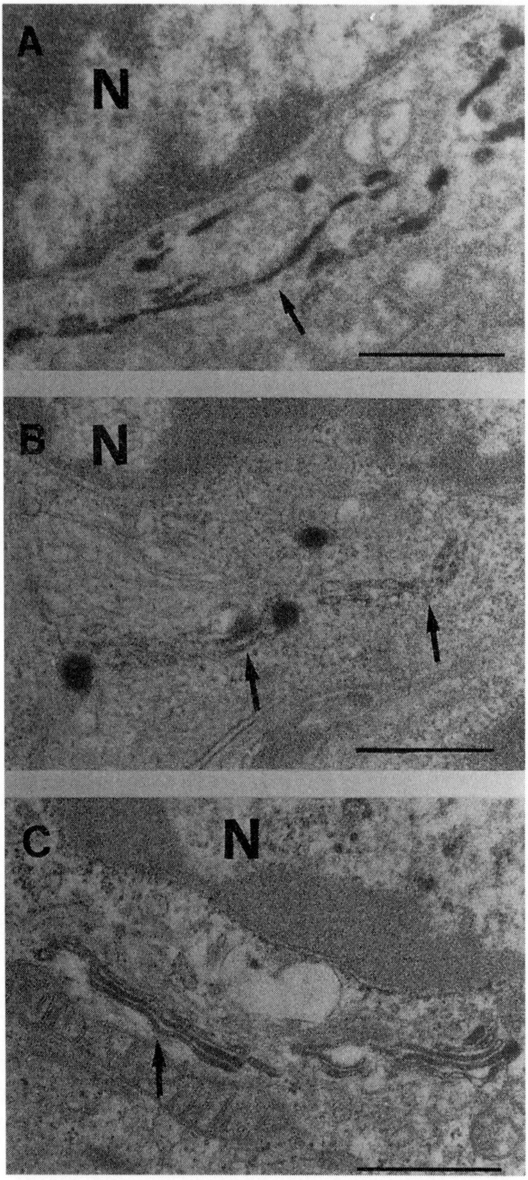

Figure 3 Evidence that the inhibition of exocytosis following exposure to BFA is associated with a retention of HRP at the level of the Golgi apparatus is shown by the similar distribution of HRP in brefeldin A-treated (BFA) ductules (**A**, arrow) and the TPPase activity, a Golgi enzyme marker, whether in untreated ductules (**B**, arrows) or in ductules exposed to BFA for 20 min (**C**, arrow). The morphology of the Golgi apparatus is well preserved in BFA-treated cells, and there is no redistribution of the enzymatic reaction product in the cisternae of the endoplasmic reticulum. Abbreviations: N, nucleus. Bar = 0.5 μm. (From Hepatology, 1995; 22:194–201)

BILE ACIDS

Considerable evidence has been advanced for passive absorption of unconjugated dihydroxy-bile acids by bile ducts under when they are secreted into canalicular bile[29–33]. Under these conditions hypercholeresis may be induced by cholehepatic shunting of bile acids. According to this theory[34], the fraction of bile acids which passively cross the apical membrane of cholangiocytes are conjugated with taurine. Isolated rat biliary ductular cells have been reported to conjugate mono and dihydroxy bile acids with taurine[35]. For a conjugated bile acid to cross the basolateral membrane and reach the plasma in periductular capillary plexus, a carrier mechanism must be present, as conjugated bile acids permeate membranes very slowly at physiological pH unless a transporter is present. Many experiments have been performed to demonstrate carrier-mediated transport of fluorescent conjugated bile acids in the basolateral membranes of polarized preparations of isolated rat biliary ductules[36,37]. Two fluorescent conjugated bile acid analogues were used, a trihydroxy-derivative of cholylglycine (C-NBD-gly) and a dihydroxy-derivative of chenodeoxycholylglycine (CDC-NBD-gly) (Figure 4). A prevalent basolateral staining was observed after 3 min of incubation, while at 10 min the staining was more diffuse in the intracellular space, with major apical localization after 20 min of incubation. Morphometric analysis confirmed these observations for both bile acids with a preferential localization in the basolateral area of biliary epithelium at 1–3 min of incubation (Figure 5). Bile acid movement from the basolateral to apical area appeared to be very rapid and colchicine-independent. No fluorescence was present in the ductular lumen for at least the initial 10–15 min of the experiment. The basolateral uptake was temperature-dependent and was in direct proportion to incubation temperature. It was not decreased by absence of Na^+ in the medium, but was strongly influenced by the composition of anions in the medium. More than 50% inhibition of basolateral uptake was found in

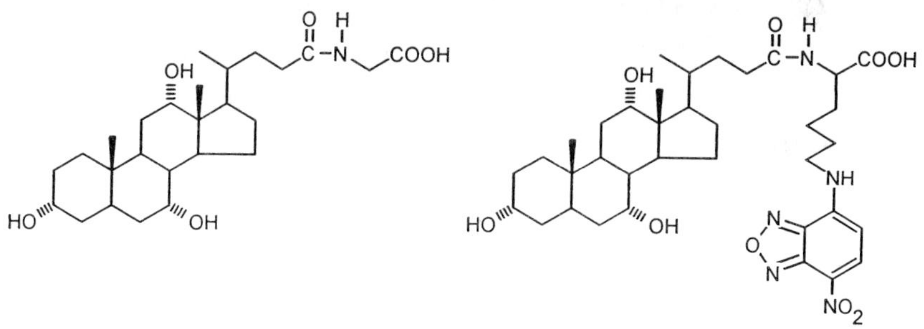

Cholylglycine   Cholyl-NBDAB-gly

Figure 4 Chemical structure of cholylglycine (left), also termed glycocholate, and cholyl-NBDAB-gly (right), one of the two fluorescent bile acids used in this study. In CDC-NBDAB-gly, a chenodeoxycholyl moiety (hydroxy groups at C-3 and C-7) has replaced the cholyl moiety (hydroxy groups at C-3, C-7, and C-12)

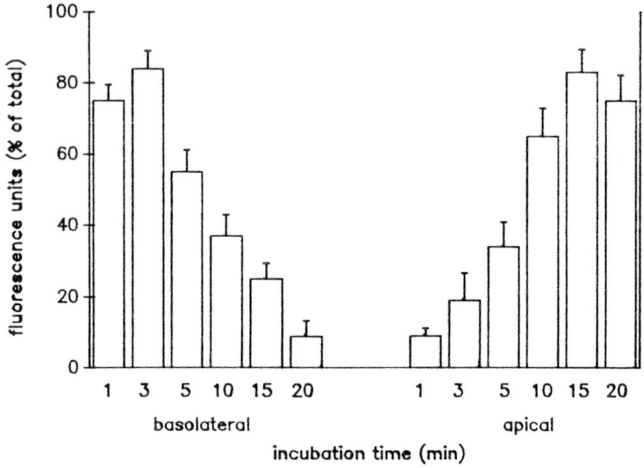

(a)

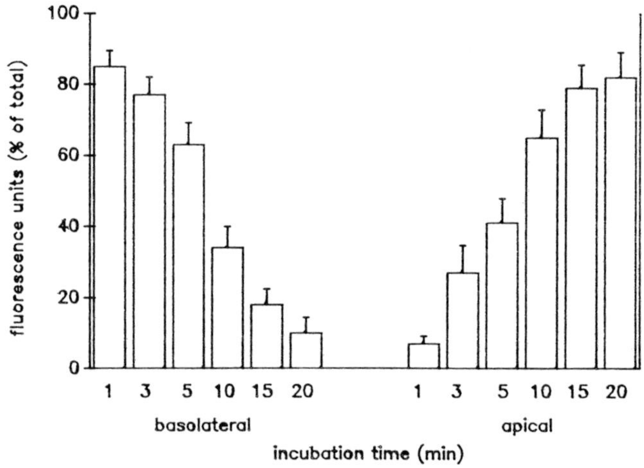

(b)

Figure 5 Time-course of fluorescence, expressed as percentage (M ± SD) of total fluorescence signal in basolateral domains (left) or apical domains (right) using isolated, polarized rat biliary ductules. Data from C-NBDAB-gly are shown in panel **(a)**; those from CDC-NBDAB-gly in panel **(b)**.

samples preincubated in the absence of Cl^- or HCO_3^-. Because 30 min preincubation in the absence of these anions might influence cellular volume, which in turn might cause decreased bile acid uptake, effects of various anion substitutions on the cell volume were evaluated. While bicarbonate substitution did not modify the cell volume up to 1 h, chloride depletion for 30 min induced a cell shrinkage to 77% of control values with almost complete recovery of cell volume at 1 h. Therefore, experiments relating to anion substitution have been repeated after 1 h of chloride depletion, but a similar inhibition of bile acid uptake was observed, thus excluding direct effects of volume modifications on this parameter. Basolateral uptake was also inhibited by addition of DIDS and by coincubation with conjugated and unconjuated bile acids. When bile ductules were preloaded with CDC-NBD-gly, the following administration of external TCA trans-stimulated counter-transport of fluorescent dye out of the cells (Figure 6) with, by contrast, no apparent increase in fluorescence signal into the lumen with respect to controls. At 10 min after administration of TCA, total cell fluorescence decreased to about 60%, compared to about 80% in controls. These data may suggest that carrier transport for conjugated bile acids can function as an anion exchanger, as demonstrated in other epithelial cells.

Uptake was greatly inhibited by BSP and by addition of other organic anions. while it was not modified by preincubation with 10^{-8} mol/L valinomycin, a compound known to depolarize predominantly plasma membrane in intact cells. However, more accurate studies need to explore the exact role of transmembrane potential on bile acid uptake.

Finally, this uptake does not occur in isolated fibroblasts, indicating that this carrier mechanism is not present in all eukaryotic cells.

These studies provide strong evidence for carrier-mediated transport of conjugated bile acids across the basolateral membrane of polarized biliary epithelial cells. Organic anion transport is likely to be another important function of biliary epithelium.

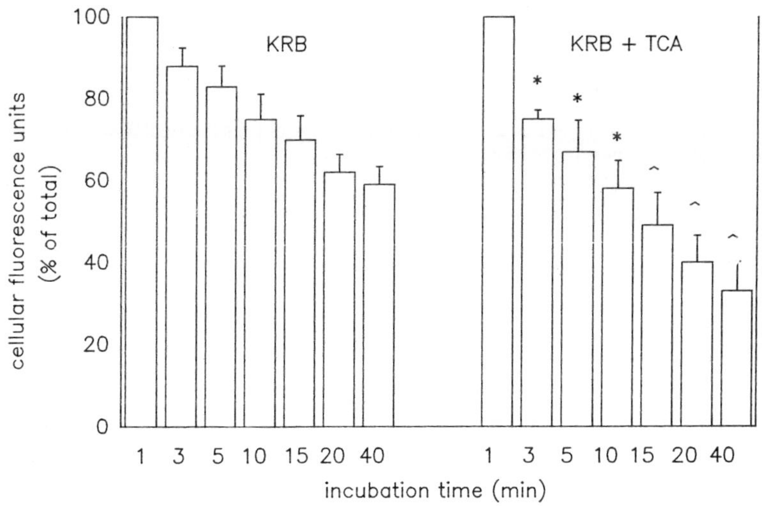

Figure 6 Time-course of total cellular fluorescence signal in the biliary epithelium preloaded with 3 μmol/L CDC-NBDAB-gly for 20 min and perfused with KRB alone (on the left = paired controls) or with KRB + 20 μmol/L TCA (on the right). The fluorescent signal was measured by the quantitative image analysis system when the cells started to be perfused with TCA and up to the following 40 min. * $p < 0.05$ vs corresponding controls; ^ $p < 0.02$ vs corresponding controls

Acknowledgements

We express our most sincere thanks to Professor Anne Marie Jezequel, Professor Francesco Orlandi, and Professor Alan F. Hofmann, for helpful discussions, to Drs Antonio Di Sario, Luca Marucci, Cristina Bassotti, Gianluca Svegliati Baroni, Katia Rapino, Domenico Alvaro, Franco Folli for their excellent cooperation, and to Luciano Trozzi and Antonella Fava for their excellent technical assistance. This work was supported by CNR (Progetto Finalizzato FATMA, 94.00527PF41).

References

1. La Russo NF. Proteins in bile: how they get there and what they do. Am J Physiol. 1984;247:G199–205.
2. Thomas P, Summers JW. The biliary excretion of circulating asialoglycoproteins in the rat. Biochem Biophys Res Commun. 1978;80:335–9.
3. Thomas P, Zamcheck N. Role of the liver in the clearance and excretion of circulating carcinoembryonic antigen (CEA). Dig Dis Sci. 1983;28:216–24.
4. Kressner MS, Stockert RJ, Morell AG, Sternlieb I. Origins of biliary copper. Hepatology. 1984;4:867–70.
5. Sternlieb I, Quintana N. Biliary proteins and ductular ultrastructure. Hepatology. 1985;5:139–43.
6. Ishii M, Vroman BT, La Russo NF. Fluid-phase endocytosis by intrahepatic bile duct epithelial cells isolated from a normal rat liver. J Histochem Cytochem. 1990;38:515–24.
7. Ishii M, Vroman BT, La Russo NF. Morphological demonstration of receptor-mediated endocytosis of epidermal growth factor by isolated bile duct epithelial cells. Gastroenterology. 1990;98:1284–91.
8. Benedetti A, Marucci L, Bassotti C *et al.* Tubulovesicular transcytotic pathway in rat biliary epithelium: a study in perfused liver and in isolated intrahepatic bile duct. Hepatology. 1993;18:422–32.
9. Benedetti A, Marucci L, Bassotti C, Guidarelli C, Jezequel AM. Brefeldin A inhibits the transcytotic vesicular transport of horseradish peroxidase in intrahepatic bile ductules isolated from rat liver. Hepatology. 1995;22:194–201.
10. Ishii M, Vroman BT, La Russo NF. Isolation and morphological characterization of bile duct epithelial cells from normal rat liver. Gastroenterology. 1989;97:1236–47.
11. Alpini G, Lenzi R, Zhai W-R *et al.* Isolation of a nonparenchymal liver cell fraction enriched in cells with biliary epithelial phenotypes. Gastroenterology. 1989;97:1248–60.
12. Roberts SK, Kuntz SM, Gores GJ, La Russo NF. Regulation of bicarbonate-dependent ductular secretion assessed by lumenal micropuncture of isolated rodent intrahepatic intact bile ducts. Proc Natl Acad Sci USA. 1993;90:9080–4.
13. Mennone A, Alvaro D, Cho W, Boyer JL. Isolation of small polarized bile duct units. Proc Natl Acad Sci USA. 1995;92:6527–31.
14. Robinson MS. The role of clathrin, adaptors and dynamin in endocytosis. Curr Opin Cell Biol. 1994;6:538–44.
15. Gout I, Dhand R, Hiles ID *et al.* The GTPase dynamin binds to and is activated by a subset of SH3 domains. Cell. 1993;75:25–36.
16. Tan A, Bolscher J, Feltkamp C, Ploegh H. Retrograde transport from the Golgi region to the endoplasmic reticulum is sensitive to GTPyS. J Cell Biol. 1992;116:1357–67.
17. Pelham HRB. Multiple targets for brefeldin A. Cell. 1991;67:449–51.
18. Hunzinker W, Whitney JA, Mellman I. Selective inhibition of transcytosis by brefeldin A in MDCK cells. Cell. 1991;67:617–27.
19. Low SH, Wong SH, Tang BL, Tan P, Subramanian VN, Hong W. Inhibition by brefeldin A of protein secretion from the apical cell surface of Madin-Darby canine kidney cells. J Biol Chem. 1991;266:17729–32.
20. Miller SG, Carnell L, Moore HPH. Post-Golgi membrane traffic: brefeldin A inhibits export from distal Golgi compartments to the cell surface but not recycling. J Biol Chem. 1992;118:267–83.

21. Reynier MO, Hasieh IA, Crotte C, Carbuccia N, Richard B, Gerolami A. Monensin action on the Golgi complex in perfused rat liver: evidence against bile salt vesicular transport. Gastroenterology. 1992;102:2024–32.
22. DeLisle RC, Williams JA. Regulation of membrane fusion in secretory exocytosis. Annu Rev Physiol. 1986;48:225–38.
23. Okada T, Sakuma L, Fukui Y, Hazeki O, Ui M. Blockage of chemotactic peptide-induced stimulation of neutrophils by wortmannin as a result of selective inhibition of phosphatidylinositol 3-kinase. J Biol Chem. 1994;269:3563–7.
24. Cheatham BC, Vlahos CJ, Cheatham L, Wang L, Blenis J, Kahn CR. Phosphatidylinositol 3-kinase activation is required for insulin stimulation of pp70 S6 kinase, DNA synthesis and glucose transport translocation. Mol Cell Biol. 1994;14:4902–11.
25. Joly M, Kazlauskas A, Fay FS, Corvera S. Disruption of PDGF receptor trafficking by mutation of its P13-kinase binding site. Science. 1994;263:684–7.
26. Folli F, Alvaro D, Gigliozzi A, *et al.* Regulation of endocytic-transcytotic pathways and bile secretion by phosphatidylinositol 3-kinase. J Clin Invest. 1996 (Submitted).
27. Alpini G, Phillips JO, La Russo NF. The biology of biliary epithelia. In: Arias IM, Boyer JL, Fausto N, Jakoby WB, Schachter DA, Shafritz DA, editors. The liver: biology and pathobiology, 3rd edn New York: Raven Press; 1994:623–53.
28. Benedetti A, Bassotti C, Rapino K, Marucci L, Jezequel AM. A morphometric study of the epithelium lining the rat intrahepatic biliary tree. J Hepatol. 1996;24:335–42.
29. Khan M, O'Maille ERL. High biliary HCO_3^- concentration and hypercholeresis induced by hyodeoxycholate in the rat. J Physiol. 1987;386:106.
30. Kinai S, Sato Y, Nokubo M, Kitani K. Hepatic biotransformation and choleretic effect of 7-ketolithocolic acid in the rat. Lipids. 1989;24:859–65.
31. Kitani K, Kanai S. Effect of ursodeoxycholate on the bile flow in the rat. Life Sci. 1982;31:1973–85.
32. Lake JR, Renner EL, Scharschmidt BF *et al.* Inhibition of Na^+/K^+ exchange in the rat is associated with decreased ursodeoxycholate hypercholeresis, decreased secretion of unconjugated ursodeoxycholate, and increased ursodeoxycholate glucuronidation. Gastroenterology. 1988;95:454–63.
33. Lamri Y, Erlinger S, Dumont M, Roda A, Feldmann G. Immunoperoxidase localization of ursodeoxycholic acid in rat biliary epithelial cells. Evidence for a cholehepatic circulation. Liver. 1992;12:351–4.
34. Hofmann AF. The cholehepatic circulation of unconjugated bile acids: an update. In: Paungartner G, Stiehl A, Gerok W, editors. Bile acids and the hepatobiliary system. Boston: Kluwer; 1993:143–60.
35. Hylemon PB, Bohdan PM, Sirica AE, Heuman DM, Vlahcevic ZR. Cholesterol and bile acid metabolism in cultures of primary rat bile ductular epithelial cells. Hepatology. 1990;11:982–6.
36. Benedetti A, Marucci L, Schteingart CD, Ton-Nu H-T, Hofmann AF. Uptake of fluorescent bile acids indicates a basolateral transporter in polarized bile duct epithelial cells. Gastroenterology. 1994;106:A865 (abstract).
37. Benedetti A, Marucci L, Di Sario A *et al.* Serial quantitative image analysis of uptake and transport of fluorescent bile acids in polarized biliary epithelial cells. In: Hofmann AF, Paumgartner G, Stiehl A, editors. Bile acids in gastroenterology: basic and clinical advances. Lancaster: Kluwer; 1995:191–4.

9
Regulation of biliary bicarbonate secretion by bile salts

C. CLERICI, G. GENTILI, A. ERRICO, F. CAMMILLERI, F. BRASACCHIO, R. PELLICCIARI, G. COSTANTINO, L. MATTOLI, D. ANNIBALI and A. MORELLI

INTRODUCTION

The physiological mechanism by which bile acids induce biliary bicarbonate secretion, and how physicochemical parameters of bile acids influence this biological property, is still unclear. Regarding the physiological mechanism of bile acid-induced biliary bicarbonate secretion, one of the first ideas was suggested by Sperber in 1959[1]. He proposed that bile acids are actively pumped into the canalicular space and their osmotic activity causes plasma, water and accompanying solutes to enter the canalicular space through the junctional complex between the hepatocytes. This view continues to be held, but other interesting hypotheses have been proposed.

In recent years two hypotheses, among other possibilities, have attracted interest: The first concerns stimulation of the hepatic sinusoidal Na^+/H^+ exchanger or the Na^+/HCO_3^- cotransporter with increased intracellular bicarbonate and excretion via a canalicular Cl^-/HCO_3^- exchanger. The second concerns cholehepatic recycling due to the reabsorption of unconjugated bile acids from bile in protonated form.

O'Maille and Richards first observed that unconjugated cholic acid (CA) in the dog produced a considerably greater degree of bile flow than that induced by its taurine conjugate[2]. Subsequently Erlinger observed that ursodeoxycholic acid (UDCA), when given at unphysiologically high doses, induces a remarkable bicarbonate-rich hypercholeresis[3]. Studies by Moseley *et al.*[4] and Lake *et al.*[5], using rat liver isolated plasma membrane and isolated perfused rat liver, showed that UDCA can stimulate the hepatic sinusoidal Na^+/H^+ exchanger. This led to the hypothesis that the resulting intracellular alkalinization can stimulate the canalicular Cl^-/HCO_3^- exchanger (Figure 1).

However, studies subsequently carried out by Strazzabosco *et al.*[6] in isolated rat hepatocytes couplets and perfused liver, failed to show the effect of UDCA

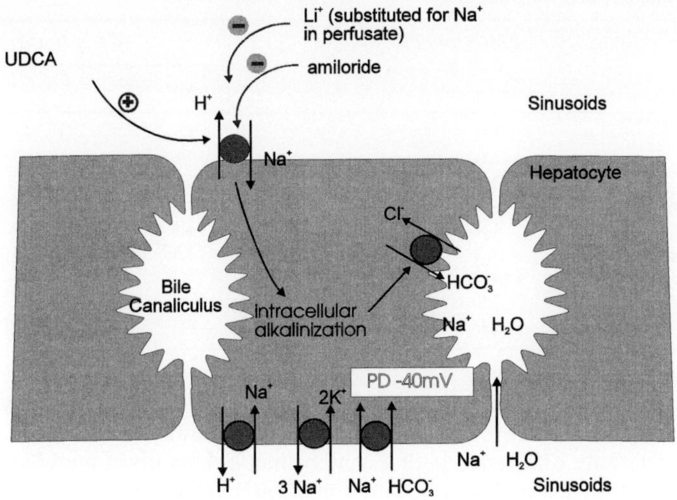

Figure 1 Hypothetical representation of bile acid-induced biliary bicarbonate secretion

on this transporter system. Other studies from Myers *et al.*[7] in isolated perfused rat liver and in rat hepatocytes showed that cyclic GMP (cGMP; guanosine 3′5′-cyclic monophosphate) activated by natriuretic peptides or by *Escherichia coli* heat-stable enterotoxin, is able to increase intracellular pH through activation of the hepatic sinusoidal Na^+/HCO_3^- cotransporter. This, in turn, leads to a stimulation of the canalicular Cl^-/HCO_3^- exchanger. However, neither UDCA nor CA is able to produce a significant increase in intracellular cGMP concentration.

Other studies on the effect of UDCA on intracellular pH regulation in isolated rat bile duct epithelial cells (BDE), carried out by Alvaro *et al.*[8], indicate that UDCA does not stimulate HCO_3^- excretion from isolated rat BDE cells but, as a weak acid, modifies pH in BDE cells. Thus, these data are inconclusive in proving the hypothesis that bile acids stimulate the sinusoidal Na^+/H^+ exchanger, the Na^+/HCO_3^- cotransporter and the Cl^-/HCO_3^- exchanger.

ROLE OF STRUCTURAL FEATURES IN BILE FLOW AND BILIARY BICARBONATE OUTPUT

How can bile acids with different structural features modify the choleresis and the secretion of biliary bicarbonate? As shown in Table 1, natural bile acids with different structures have different physicochemical properties and, in turn, different choleretic activities. Two kinds of structural modification are possible on bile acids: (1) side-chain modification; (2) body modification. Hofmann first described that bile acid derivatives with a shortened side-chain (e.g. nor-UDCA or nor-CDCA[9,10], which are secreted prevalently in unconjugated form and are poorly amidated by glycine or taurine) are able to increase bile flow and biliary bicarbonate secretion.

Table 1 Naturally occurring bile acids

Bile acid	*CMC (mmol/l) 0.15 Na^+*	*ACA ($\mu L/\mu M$)*	
		Rat	*Hamster*
CDCA	4.0	Toxic	20–25
UDCA	7.0	25	20–23
DCA	3.0	9–25	25
CDCA-tau	3.0	—	12
CDCA-gly	1.8	4.1	14
UDCA-tau	2.2	7.1	14
UDCA-gly	4.0	—	10
DCA-tau	2.4	—	11
DCA-gly	2.0	—	14

Semisynthetic bile acids such as nor-UDCA or nor-CDCA are endowed with a physicochemical profile similar to that of the natural derivatives UDCA and CDCA. The only difference is that semisynthetic derivatives are characterized by a higher critical micellar concentration (CMC) value (Table 2).

According to the first hypothesis of Sperber, bile acids characterized by high values of CMC tend to induce more bile flow than do bile acids with lower CMC. However, it should be pointed out that non-micelle-forming bile acids,

Table 2 Comparison of the apparent choleretic activity (ACA) of naturally occurring and side-chain-modified bile acids and their taurine and glycine amidated in the hamster and rat

Bile acid	*ACA ($\mu L/\mu mol$)*		*CMC[d] (mmol/L) 0.15 Na^+*	*Bile Acid*	*ACA ($\mu L/\mu mol$)*		*CMC[d] (mmol/L) 0.15 Na^+*
	Hamster	*Rat*			*Hamster*	*Rat*	
Naturally occurring				**Side-chain modified**			
Unconjugated				*Unconjugated*			
CDCA[a, b]	20–25	Toxic	4	nor-CDCA[b]	108	220	15
UDCA[a, c]	20–23	10–22.5	7	nor-UDCA[c]	67	90.5	22
DCA	25	9–25[g]	3	nor-DCA	40		10
DHC (semisynthetic)	16[i]	13[i]	—	23-MUDCA[e]	110	65[h]	30
Conjugated				*Conjugated*			
CDCA-tau[a]	12		3.0	nor-CDCA-tau[b]	10		15
CDCA-gly[a]	14	4.1[f]	1.8	nor-UDCA-tau[c]	13	8.6	22
UDCA-tau[a]	14	7.1[c]	2.2	nor-UDCA-gly[c]	11		22
UDCA-gly[a]	10		4.0	nor-DCA-tau	8		10
DCA-tau[a]	11		2.4	nor-DCA-gly	8		10
DCA-gly[a]	14		2.0				

[a] Gurantz *et al.* Am J Physiol. 1994:247 G736–48
[b] Palmer, KDR *et al.* Am J Physiol. 1987:252 G219–28
[c] Yoon, YB *et al.* Gastroenterology. 1986:90:837–52
[d] Roda A *et al.* J Biol Chem. 1983:258:6362–70
[e] Clerici C *et al.* Dig Dis Sc. 1992:37:791–9
[f] Rajagopalan N *et al.* Biochem Biophys Acta. 1982:711:66–74
[g] Neoptolemos J *et al.*, Unpublished data
[h] Roda A *et al.* Hepatology. 1988:8:1571–6
[i] O'Maille *et al.* Q J Exp Physiol. 1986:71:475

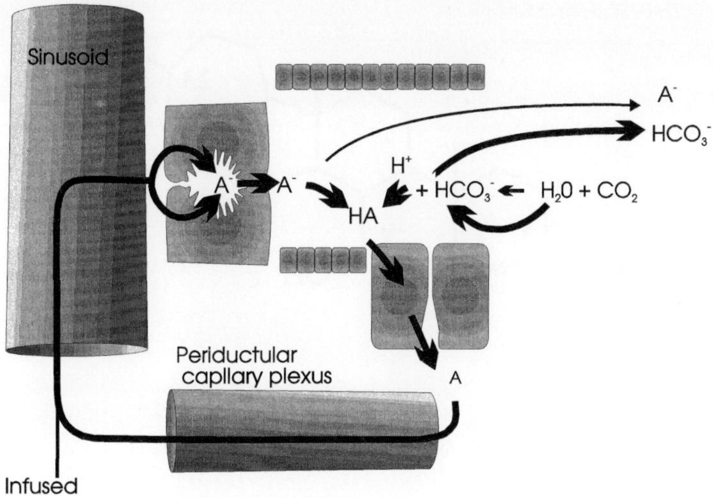

Figure 2 Cholehepatic shunt pathway, according to the hypothesis of A. F. Hofmann

such as dehydrocholic acid (DHC), induce an apparent choleretic activity (ACA) of 13–16 μL/μmol in rat and hamster. Accordingly, the CMC value cannot alone explain the ACA values. This observation leads to Professor Hofmann's hypothesis of the cholehepatic shunt pathway.

According to this hypothesis, unconjugated, lipophilic bile acids secreted from the hepatocytes into the biliary canaliculus in anionic form are protonated by a proton coming from the reaction of the luminal anhydrase and in this form are passively reabsorbed across the lipid domains of the epithelial membranes and enter the periductular capillary plexus. Bile acids then return through the hepatic sinusoid to the liver, where they can be resecreted in anionic form. During this ductular reabsorption the bile acid molecule is replaced by a bicarbonate anion which maintains luminal osmolarity (Figure 2).

The hypothesis of the cholehepatic shunt pathway was also investigated in our laboratory in collaboration with A. Roda's group using a 23-MUDCA[11], a synthetic bile acid in which a C23 methyl group in the side-chain prevents hepatic amidation (Figure 3). Figure 4 shows the effect in hamster (after intraduodenal administration of 23-MUDCA) on rich bicarbonate hypercholeresis. This is compared with that of UDCA, that is dose-dependent.

NEW BODY-MODIFIED BILE ACID

With the aim of broadening the existing structure–activity relationship, we here present preliminary results on bile flow and biliary bicarbonate output induced by a newly synthesized bile acid 3α-7β-fluorocholanoic acid (UPF 652) (Figure 5). This body-modified bile acid is characterized by the replacement of the 7β-hydroxy group with a fluorine atom. This chemical modification is of particular interest because of the peculiar properties of the fluorine atom[12]:

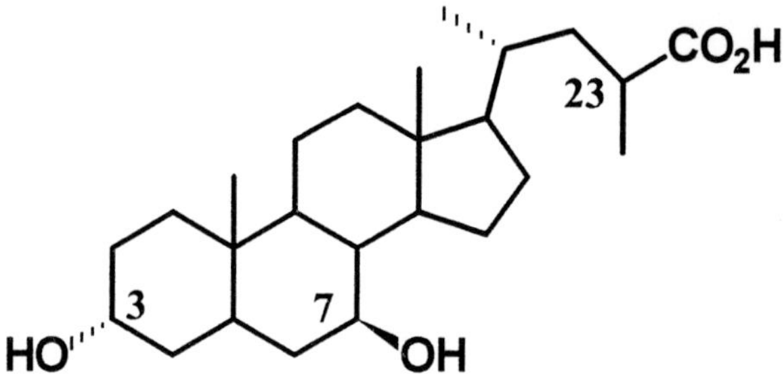

23-MUDCA

Figure 3 23-MUDCA, a bile acid modified in its C23 side-chain position

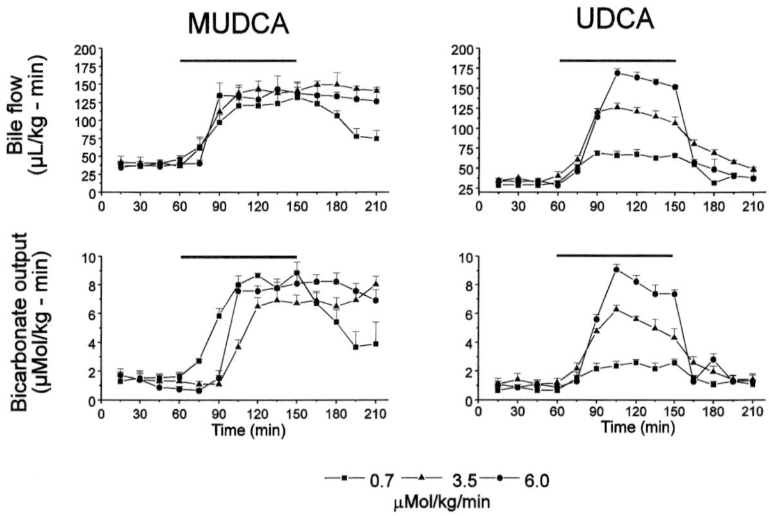

Figure 4 Bile flow and bicarbonate output in hamsters submitted to i.v. infusion (——) with MUDCA or UDCA

1. fluorine is as small as the hydrogen but has a much stronger electronic effect;
2. fluorine is endowed with a peculiar hydrophilic/hydrophobic balance: in particular its hydrophobic character is enhanced in aprotic, lipophilic solvents while the hydrophilic character is amplified in an aqueous environment;
3. different from the hydroxy group, the fluorine atom can only accept and not donate hydrogen bonds;
4. the introduction of the fluorine atom in the 7β-position should have no effect on hepatic amidation.

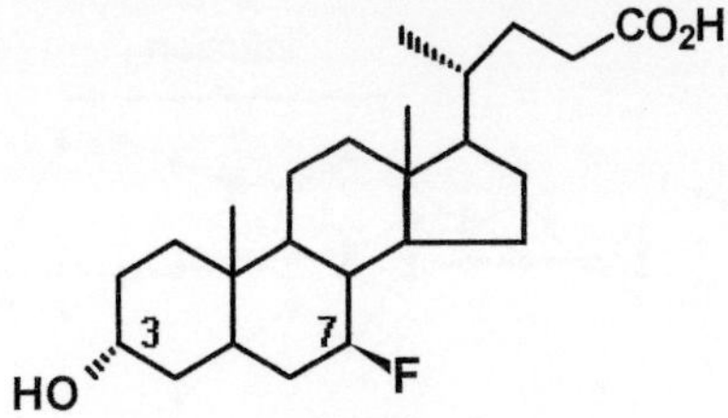

UPF 652

Figure 5 UPF 652, a bile acid with a fluorine substituting the 7β-hydroxy group (from Pellicciari *et al.*, in preparation)

Due to the above properties UPF 652 can be foreseen to have an overall physicochemical profile intermediate between that of UDCA and lithocholic acid (LCA).

METHODS

Experiments were performed on male anaesthetized Sprague-Dawley rats with a biliary fistula. UPF 652, LCA or UDCA was infused intravenously at a dose of 2 μmol/kg per minute. Bile samples were taken from the external biliary fistula every 15 min and weighed in order to determine bile flow. A microgasometric procedure (Micro CO_2 System Harleco, American Hospital Corporation, Gibbstown, New York) was adopted to evaluate biliary bicarbonate concentration. The CMC of UPF 652 was increased as previously described[13].

RESULTS

Figure 6 shows the effect of intravenous administration of UPF 652, UDCA and LCA on bile flow and in biliary bicarbonate output. This is compared with saline infusion in control animals. Figure 7 shows the CMC value of UPF 652, which is intermediate between that of LCA and UDCA.

SUMMARY

1. UPF 652 is a novel body-modified bile acid in which a fluorine atom is present at 7β-position. The fluorine atom intrudes into the hydrophobic back of bile acids. However, its effect is lower than that of a hydroxy group, due to the peculiar hydrophobic/hydrophilic balance. As a result the detergency of UPF 652 is intermediate between that of UDCA and LCA.
2. When administered e.v. in the biliary fistula rat, the effect of UPF 652 on bile flow and biliary bicarbonate output is similar to that in control animals. At the same dose UDCA is more choleretic, while LCA strongly decreases bile flow and biliary bicarbonate output.

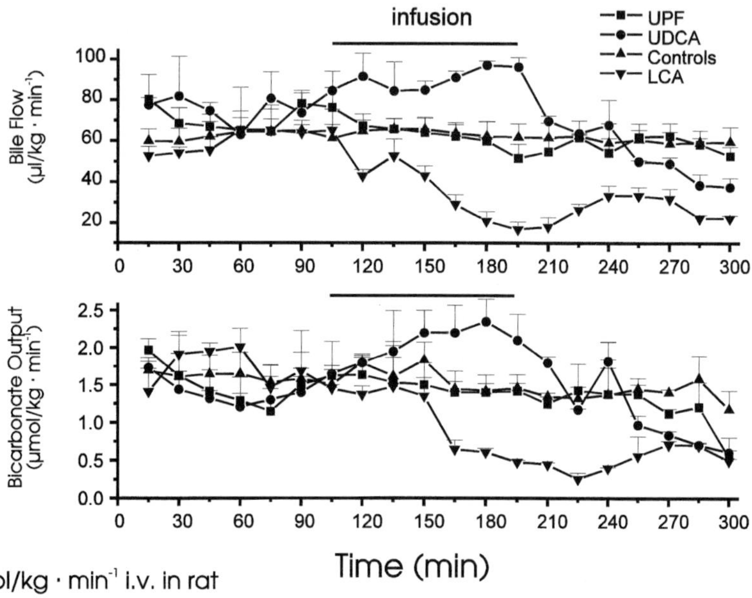

Figure 6 Bile flow and biliary bicarbonate output in rats submitted to i.v. infusion (——) with 2 μmol/kg per minute of UPF, UDCA, LCA or saline

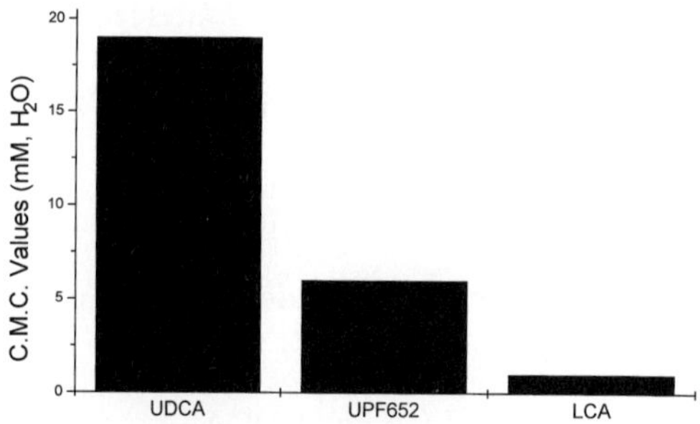

Figure 7 CMC value of UPF 652 compared to that of UDCA and LCA

3. This biological behaviour is in agreement with the physicochemical properties of UPF 652, which are intermediate between those of UDCA and LCA.

References

1. Sperber I. Secretion of organic anions in the formation of urine and bile. Pharmacol Rev. 1959;11:109–34.
2. O'Maille ERL, Richards TG. Possible explanations for the differences in secretory characteristics between conjugated and free bile acids. J Physiol (Lond). 1977;265:855–66.
3. Dumont M, Erlinger S, Uchman S. Hypercholeresis induced by ursodeoxycholic acid and 7-ketolithocholic acid in the rat: possible role of bicarbonate transport. Gastroenterology. 1980;79:82–9.

4. Moseley RH, Ballatori N, Smith DJ, Boyer J. Ursodeoxycholic stimulates Na^+/H^+ exchange in rat liver basolateral plasma membrane vesicles. J Clin Invest. 1987;80:684–90.
5. Lake JR, Van Dike RW, Scharschmidt BF. Effect of Na^+ replacement and amiloride on ursodeoxycholic acid-stimulated choleresis and biliary bicarbonate secretion. Am J Physiol. 1987;252:G163–9.
6. Strazzabosco M, Sakisaka S, Hayakawa T, Boyer J. Effect of UDCA on intracellular and biliary pH in isolated rat hepatocyte couplets and perfused livers. Am J Physiol. 1991;260:G58–69.
7. Myers NC, Grune S, Jameson H, Anwer MS. cGMP stimulates bile acid-independent bile formation and biliary bicarbonate excretion. Am J Physiol. 1996;270:G418–24.
8. Alvaro D, Mennone A, Boyer J. Effect of ursodeoxycholic on intracellular pH regulation in isolated rat bile duct epithelial cells. Am J Physiol. 1993;265:G783–91.
9. Palmer KR, Gurantz D, Hofmann AF. Hypercholeresis induced by norchenodeoxycholate in biliary fistula rodent. Am J Physiol. 1987;252:G219–28.
10. Yoon YB, Hagey LR, Hofmann AF, Gurantz D, Michelotti EL, Steinbach JH. Effect of side-chain shortening on the physiologic properties of bile acids: hepatic transport and effect on biliary secretion of 23-nor-ursodeoxycholate in rodents. Gastroenterology. 1986;90:837–52.
11. Clerici C, Dozzini G, Distrutti E *et al.* Effect of intraduodenal administration of 23-methyl-UDCA diastereoisomers on bile flow in hamsters. Dig Dis Sci. 1992;37:791–8.
12. Roda A, Pellicciari R, Polimeni C *et al.* Metabolism, pharmacokinetics, and activity of a new 6-fluoro analogue of UDCA in rats and hamsters. Gastroenterology. 1995;108:1204–14.
13. Carey MC. Measurement of the physical–chemical properties of bile salt solution. In: Barbara L, Dowling RH, Hofmann AF, Roda E, editors. Bile acids in gastroenterology. Boston MA: MTP; 1982:19–56.

10
The cholehepatic circulation of organic anions: a decade of progress

A. F. HOFMANN, H-Z, YEH, C. D. SCHTEINGART, U. BOLDER, H.-T. TON-NU and L. R. HAGEY

INTRODUCTION

A decade ago our laboratory reported that the synthetic bile acids nor-chenodeoxycholic acid (norCDCA) and nor-ursodeoxycholic acid (norUDCA) induce hypercholeresis in rodents[1,2]. These bile acids differ from their respective, natural C_{24} homologues, in having a side-chain that contains one less methylene group. That the removal of a single methylene group from the side-chain would cause such a remarkable change in physiological properties was unexpected. Because these compounds were recovered in bile partially in unconjugated form, and because unconjugated dihydroxy-bile acids were known from intestinal perfusion studies to pass rapidly across epithelial cell membranes by passive 'non-ionic' diffusion[3–8], we proposed that such hypercholeresis could be explained by cholehepatic shunting of the unconjugated species.

In this scheme, shown in Figure 1, the unconjugated bile acid molecules would be absorbed in protonated form from ductular bile across the apical membrane of the cholangiocyte, would traverse the cytosol and would then pass across the basolateral membrane to enter the plasma of the periductular capillary plexus. This capillary plexus drains into the terminal portal venule, so that molecules being transported from biliary ductules would pass into the hepatic sinusoids without entering the systemic circulation. After extraction from sinusoidal plasma by the hepatocyte, the bile acid molecules would pass through the hepatic cytosol, and be actively transported by canalicular transporters into canalicular bile, once more generating bile acid-dependent flow. The unconjugated bile acid molecule would be reabsorbed once again by the biliary ductular epithelium and repeat this cycle indefinitely. The cycle would stop either when the molecule was biotransformed by hydroxylation or conjugation to a more polar compound that was not absorbed by the biliary ductular epithelium, or when the molecule had passed to a part of the biliary tract from which absorption was negligible, for example, a large bile duct or the gallbladder.

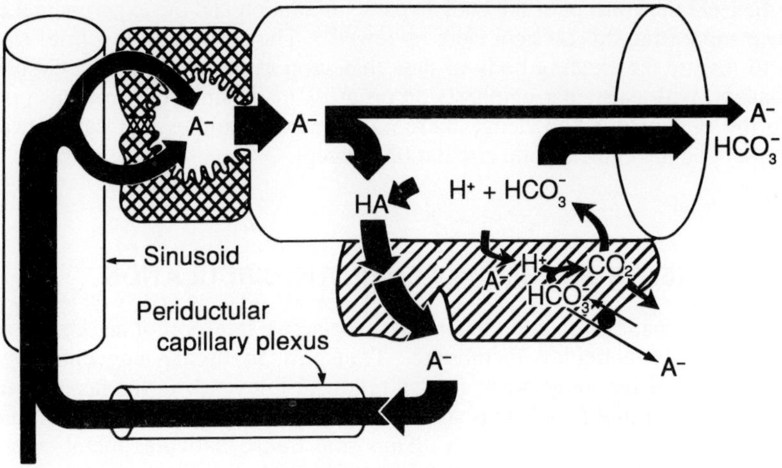

Figure 1 Schematic depiction of the cholehepatic circulation of unconjugated lipophilic bile acids[1]. The types of molecules that participate in such a circulation are summarized in Table 2, and the criteria for molecules engaging in a cholehepatic circulation are given in Table 1. The unconjugated bile acid is secreted actively into the canaliculus, generating bile acid-dependent flow. Biliary lipid secretion may or may not be induced, depending on the surface activity of the bile acid at its concentration in canalicular bile. The bile acid molecule is absorbed passively in protonated form by the biliary ductular epithelium. Removal of the proton from the ductular bile generates a bicarbonate anion, with the result that luminal osmolality remains unchanged. The unconjugated bile acid passes through the cholangiocyte; conjugation of C_{24} bile acids may occur. The bile acid molecule traverses the basolateral membrane by unknown mechanisms, although a carrier molecule is likely to be present[38]. (The carrier molecule may exchange the bile acid molecule for a bicarbonate anion; the bicarbonate anion in the cholangiocyte may combine with the proton liberated from the entering bile acid to form CO_2 and water, catalysed by carbonic anhydrase.) After crossing the basolateral membrane the molecule is transported via the periductular capillary plexus to the terminal portal venule and thence into the sinusoid. Her it is efficiently extracted by the hepatocyte and resecreted into canalicular bile, once more generating bile acid-dependent flow. The cholehepatic cycling continues until the molecule fails to be absorbed by the biliary ductules, or is biotransformed by hydroxylation or conjugation to a more hydrophilic metabolite that is not absorbed by the biliary ductules

Following a suggestion of Dr Edward W. Moore (Medical College of Virginia) the pathway was named the cholehepatic shunt pathway, because molecules traversing this route returned to the liver via a 'shunt' pathway that was much shorter than that of the classical enterohepatic circulation. The circulation was named 'cholehepatic circulation'. The term 'cholehepatic' appeared preferable to 'biliohepatic', as both *chole* and *hepatic* are of Greek origin, whereas *bili* is of Latin origin. Guzelian and Boyer[9] had used the term 'biliohepatic' to characterize the absorption of glucose from the biliary tract, but glucose differs from norCDCA and norUDCA in that it enters bile paracellularly as a secondary solute and does not induce bile flow. In addition, the first-pass extraction of glucose is variable and never as high as that of most bile acids[10], so that a major fraction of the glucose molecules that returned to the liver by the periductular capillary plexus would escape into the systemic circulation and enter peripheral metabolic pools.

In 1993 the concept of the cholehepatic circulation and the experimental evidence supporting this concept were reviewed[11]. The purpose of this brief chapter is to review the existing body of data that support the cholehepatic circulation concept, with particular emphasis on progress made since the previous review. To the best of our knowledge there have been no studies that have seriously challenged the cholehepatic circulation concept.

COMPONENTS OF THE CHOLEHEPATIC CIRCULATION

The cholehepatic circulation begins with the active transport of an organic anion across the canalicular membrane. Transport is highly concentrative, as estimates[12] of the monomeric concentration of bile acids in the hepatocyte are less than 10 μmol/L, whereas the monomeric concentration in bile is likely[13] to be greater than 2000 μmol/L. Thus, the transcanalicular membrane concentration gradient is at least 100-fold in magnitude.

The current view is that most bile acid N-acyl amidates (that is, glycine and taurine conjugated bile acids) are transported by a single canalicular transporter whose major endogenous substrate is conjugated bile acids[14,15]; this carrier is named cBAT (c denotes canalicular; BA denotes bile acid; and T denotes transporter). The cBAT has a greater transport capacity than the other major canalicular anion transporter, termed cMOAT [or cMRP (human) or cMrp (rat)][16]. The $T_{\max}$ for both transporters varies with the substrate, so no exact multiple can be given, but the cBAT transporter is at least five times more powerful. The one caveat is that it remains possible that some natural bile acid amidates are transported by cMOAT. It is possible that the high $T_{\max}$ reported for the bile acid ursodeoxychoyltaurine (tauroursodeoxycholate)[17] indicates that at least some bile acid amidates are transported not only by cBAT but also by cMOAT. Whereas two groups working independently have cloned the cMOAT[18,19], as yet cBAT remains uncloned with certainty, although a well-characterized canalicular ecto-ATPase has been shown to be capable of ATP-stimulated bile acid transport[20].

The active transport of any solute into the canalicular space induces the flow of water and filtrable solutes across the paracellular junctions that separate the canalicular lumen from the space of Disse in response to the osmotic and electrical gradient. The anions that are transported actively, and which generate bile flow, have been termed *primary solutes* to distinguish them from *secondary solutes* which enter the canalicular lumen only as a secondary response to the osmotic gradient induced by the active secretion of primary solutes[21]. Since primary solutes are thought to be impermeable to the paracellular junctions, their molecular weight must be considerably greater than that of secondary solutes. Primary solutes will generally be anions, as the canalicular cation transporter (*mdr1*) has a much lower transport capacity than cBAT and cMOAT.

The exact composition of the filtrable (secondary) solutes that enter the canalicular lumen is not known. Factors to be considered are the effect of size and fixed charges of the functional pores in the paracellular junctions. The classes of secondary solutes will be neutral sugars (glucose, fructose, and other monosaccharides), low molecular weight organic acids (citrate, hydroxy-butyrate, propionate, acetate, phenol, etc), electrolytes (Na^+ K^+, Ca^{2+}, Cl, HCO_3^-), and amino acids[21].

An ultrafiltrate of plasma is nearly isotonic with plasma because most (> 90%) of the osmoles present in plasma are made up of low molecular weight constituents such as electrolytes, urea, glucose, and organic acids[22]. Accordingly dilution of the transiently hypertonic solution by a nearly isotonic filtrate results in canalicular content remaining hypertonic. Secretion of bile into the closed canalicular space, together with contraction of the pericanalicular actin filaments[23], forces canalicular bile through the canals of Hering into the biliary ductules. Here osmotic equilibration is likely to occur, as water flows readily into the biliary ductules, presumably via the paracellular junctions, which are permeable to water, but are sufficiently small to retard the flow of Ca^{2+} ions[24].

In their initial description of hypercholeresis, Dumont *et al.*[25] reported that mannitol clearance (a measure of canalicular bile flow introduced by Wheeler *et al.*[26,27], increased in direct proportion to bile output from the biliary fistula. This observation has been confirmed by others[1,2]. Thus, it is well established that the predominant source of the biliary water secretion occurring during hypercholeresis is at the level of the canaliculus and not at the level of the biliary ductules.

The fate of the different classes of molecules that enter the biliary ductules is dependent on the transport properties of the cholangiocytes. For example, glucose is actively absorbed by Na^+ dependent and independent mechanisms[28]. Organic acids can be absorbed passively. Glutathione is hydrolysed to glutamate and glycine, and both are partially absorbed[29]. Other amino acids are likely to be absorbed by carrier-mediated mechanisms[30]. Conjugated bile acids are not thought to be absorbed in most species. Unconjugated bile acids, however, are likely to be absorbed passively in direct proportion to their lipophilicity, based on studies on intestinal uptake (see below).

The concentration gradient across the biliary ductular epithelium is $[\text{solute}]_{\text{bile}}/[\text{solute}]_{\text{periductular capillary plasma}}$. For secondary solutes the concentration gradient should be directly proportional to the first-pass extraction by hepatocytes. Molecules that are highly cleared by the liver will have a low concentration in the systemic circulation and the periductular capillary plasma, since the periductular capillary plexus has the hepatic artery as its source. For primary solutes the concentration gradient is determined by the magnitude of concentrative canalicular transport, in addition to the first-pass extraction. For example, the concentration of conjugated bile acids in the periductular capillary plexus should be the same as in arterial plasma, that is 3–10 μmol/L total bile acid with < 1 μmol/L in unbound concentration; the concentration of unbound bile acids in ductular bile is likely to be at least 1000 μmol/L.

In the cholehepatic circulation hypothesis, unconjugated bile acids are absorbed passively by the bile duct epithelium. Support for this idea was provided by a number of studies of intestinal absorption of bile acids, all of which indicated that unconjugated bile acids were absorbed by the jejunum in direct relationship to their lipophilicity[3–8]. Unconjugated dihydroxy-bile acids are absorbed rapidly. When compared to the rate of fatty acid absorption, the absorption rate of CDCA was found to be about one-fifteenth as fast[31]. Cholic acid was also absorbed passively at a rate about one-fifth that of CDCA. If these observations for the small intestine applied to the biliary ductules, and if biliary ductules did not contain a bile acid transporter, then unconjugated dihydroxy-bile acids should be absorbed rapidly, and unconjugated trihydroxy-bile acids should be absorbed more slowly.

As yet, direct experimental proof of this assertion has been difficult to obtain. It is likely to become available as new preparations of isolated biliary ductules that retain their polarity are developed[32,33]. If unconjugated bile acids are injected retrograde into the biliary tract of a rat, they are absorbed more rapidly than conjugated bile acids[34], but such experiments can be criticized as artefactual. Using an antibody to unconjugated UDCA, Lamri *et al.* presented immunocytochemical evidence for its being present in the biliary ductular cells during hypercholeresis[35].

Details of events within the cholangiocyte during transport of an unconjugated bile acid are not known. Hylemon *et al.* reported that isolated biliary ductular cells are capable of conjugating C_{24} dihydroxy-bile acids with taurine[36], and this observation has been confirmed by Gebhard and his colleagues in their report at this meeting. However, the C_{23} bile acids form CoA thio esters less than one-tenth as rapidly as the natural C_{24} homologues[37]. Therefore, nor-dihydroxy bile acids might escape conjugation during their transport through the cholangiocytes. It is not known whether cytosolic binding proteins for bile acids are present in cholangiocytes.

Passage of unconjugated nor-dihydroxy bile acids across the basolateral membrane could occur by simple diffusion in response to the concentration gradient between cytosol and the periductular capillary plasma. If reconjugation with taurine (or conjugation with glucuronate) occurred within the cholangiocyte, the resulting conjugated bile acid would require a carrier molecule within the basolateral membrane, as the permeability of conjugated bile acid to cell membranes is quite low. Using fluorescent derivatives of cholylglycine (glycocholate) and CDC-glycine (glycochenodeoxycholate), Benedetti and his colleagues obtained strong evidence for carrier-mediated transport of conjugated bile acids by the basolateral membranes of cholangiocytes[38]. Such transport is Na^+-independent, suggesting that an anion exchange transporter is present on the basolateral membranes of cholangiocytes that is similar to the bile acid transporter reported to be present on the basolateral membranes of ileal enterocytes.

No evidence for an apical membrane transporter for unconjugated bile acids being present in cholangiocytes (of rodents) has been advanced. Were such a carrier to be present, its substrate specificity would be limited to unconjugated dihydroxy-bile acids, which seems unlikely.

Absorption of an organic acid in protonated form transfers a proton from the ductular lumen to the cytosol. Acidification of biliary ductular cells by absorbed unconjugated bile acids has been shown experimentally in the elegant studies of Strazzabosco *et al.*[39]. We proposed that the source of this proton was carbonic acid, this being generated by the continuous diffusion of CO_2 into canalicular bile. Carbonic acid is a relatively strong acid, with a pK_a (of the acid) being well below that of the unconjugated bile acid[40].

If the proposed process is correct the cholangiocyte should be acidified transiently during cholehepatic shunting. The fate of the proton that enters the cholangiocyte is not known. In the enterocyte the proton that enters when a long-chain fatty acid is absorbed is returned to the lumen in exchange for a Na^+ ion, the process being mediated by an apical membrane Na^+/H^+ antiporter[41]. This process simultaneously maintains the acidic microclimate and enhances absorption of water. A process of Na^+/H^+ exchange in the apical membrane of the cholangiocyte cannot be excluded, but seems unlikely because no evidence of ductular absorption during cholehepatic shunting has been observed. (Ductular absorption is readily detected when induced, for example, by somatostatin, as the concentration of a canalicular marker such as erythritol increases[42].) Removal of a proton results in the generation of a bicarbonate anion, and a sign of cholehepatic shunting is an increase in biliary bicarbonate. The idea that absorption of an organic anion in protonated form would generate a lumenal bicarbonate anion did not originate in this laboratory, but was proposed by the Soergel laboratory[43] to explain the increased lumenal bicarbonate observed during the absorption of short-chain fatty acids.

If exiting of the bile acid anion occurs by a $BA^-/[HCO_3]^-$-exchanger, then the basolateral pole of the cholangiocyte would undergo transient alkalinization. The conversion of the proton and bicarbonate anion to CO_2 and H_2O can occur spontaneously, or be catalysed by carbonic anhydrase, which is known to be present in the cholangiocytes of rodents[44]. The bile acid molecule could also exit the cell in protonated form, which would remove a proton in the same way that it entered. Other possibilities for disposition of a proton at the basolateral membrane include Na^+/H^+ exchange, exocytosis of acidic vesicles, or entry of bicarbonate by an inwardly directed Na^+/HCO_3^- symport; all of these seem very unlikely.

CRITERIA FOR CHOLEHEPATIC SHUNTING

In the previous review four requirements for cholehepatic shunting were proposed[11]. These have not changed, and they are summarized in Table 1. In principle, if absorption of the cholehepatic shunting molecule were complete, it would not be present in bile. However, in all of our experiments in which we have induced hypercholeresis we have never failed to detect the presence of the unconjugated lipophilic species in ductal bile during hypercholeresis.

Table 1 Criteria for cholehepatic shunting

Induction of hypercholeresis
Apparent choleretic activity ≥ 25 μl/μmol anion recovered in ductal bile
Increased biliary bicarbonate concentration (≥ 35 mmol/l)
Canalicular secretion of anion in unconjugated form
Presence of unconjugated molecule in ductal bile
Delayed recovery in ductal bile because of cholehepatic shunting
Prolonged hepatobiliary retention
Absence of hypercholeresis when taurine amidate of anion is infused

REQUIREMENTS FOR CHOLEHEPATIC SHUNTING

For cholehepatic shunting to occur, a molecule must have differing properties in its protonated and in its ionized form.

In its ionized form it must be a good substrate for one or both of the canalicular anion transporters; that is, cMOAT, cBAT, or both. To be accessible to cBAT and/or cMOAT it must be transported into the hepatocyte; therefore it must either be a substrate for one or more of the basolateral uptake transporters, or be sufficiently lipophilic to enter the hepatocyte at a rapid rate.

In the biliary ductules the protonated molecule must be sufficiently lipophilic as to pass readily across apical cell membranes. For the ionizing group the data suggest that the pK_a should be $\geqslant 5$. For the remainder of the molecule the lipophilicity should be greater than that of cholic acid. Probably this can be estimated from the n-octanol/buffer distribution ratio at pH 7–8. For norCDCA at pH 8 the distribution ratio is 27; that of norUDCA is 6; and that of cholic acid is 1.2[3,45].

Cholic acid is absorbed from the jejunum, presumably by passive mechanisms, but at a slower rate than dihydroxy-bile acids such as CDCA and DCA. The rate of transmembrane flip-flop in phosphatidylcholine vesicles is also considerably slower for protonated cholic acid molecules than for protonated CDCA or DCA molecules[46]. The minimal hypercholeresis induced by norcholic acid[47] (and by cholic acid under conditions of taurine depletion[48]) suggests that the absorptive site in the biliary ductules for bile acids is quite limited, so that molecules that are not absorbed in this short absorptive segment are also not absorbed in the more distal segments of the biliary tract. It is possible that these more distal segments are rich in CFTR and are secreting bicarbonate, which might decrease passive absorption of a molecule that requires protonation for absorption.

For the anionic form of a weak acid to be presented to the canalicular membrane the molecule must escape conjugation by the hepatocyte. For natural bile acids decreased conjugation occurs when their input into the hepatocyte exceeds its conjugation capacity. Such incomplete conjugation occurs when an unphysiologically high input of the compound is presented to the liver, as is achieved by intravenous infusion. It can occur with a input at a physiological rate if the conjugation capacity of the hepatocyte is diminished. This in turn occurs when there is a deficiency of the enzymes involved in conjugation, of cofactors, or of taurine[49]. (Decreased hepatocyte taurine is readily achieved in the rat by maintaining the animal on a diet enriched in β-alanine, which competitively inhibits hepatocyte uptake of taurine.) For bile acids with modified side-chains (these are usually prepared synthetically), all of the components of the conjugating system are intact, but the molecules are poor substrates for one or more of the conjugating enzymes. Chemical, biological, and physiological requirements for cholehepatic shunting of organic weak acids are summarized in Table 2.

Table 3 lists the bile acids for which cholehepatic shunting has been observed and cites the paper containing the experimental data.

Table 2 Chemical, biological, and physiological requirements for cholehepatic shunting of organic weak acids

I. *Physicochemical requirements*
   A. Lipophilicity: protonated form has high passive permeability across apical and basolateral membranes of cholangiocytes: Octanol/water distribution ratio greater than that of cholic acid
   B. Ionization: molecule present in ionized form within hepatocyte and in protonated form in biliary ductular lumen: $pK_a = 5–6$

II. *Metabolic requirements*
   A. Lack of hydroxylation: molecule does not partition into microsomal compartment and does not undergo hydroxylation
   B. Lack of conjugation: molecule not a substrate for conjugation pathways in hepatocytes or cholangiocytes

III. *Transport requirements*
   A. High first-pass extraction: molecule enters hepatocyte passively and/or is substrate for hepatocyte basolateral uptake proteins
   B. Vigorous canalicular secretion: molecule is substrate for hepatocyte canalicular ATP-energized pumps
   C. Vectorial transport by cholangiocyte by passive or carrier-mediated transport

IV. *Physiological requirements*
   A. Excessive load of unconjugated bile acid to hepatocyte with normal conjugating capacity
   B. Normal load of unconjugated bile acid to hepatocyte with deficient amidation capacity
      1. Taurine deficiency
      2. Inborn deficiency in enzymes required for amidation
   C. Normal load of unconjugated bile acid that is poor substrate form enzymes participating in bile acid amidation

Table 3 Bile acids inducing hypercholeresis

I. *Natural bile acids (C_{24})*
   A. Dihydroxy bile acids
      UDCA[25,49,59–62]
      12-epi-DCA[63]
      Hyodeoxycholic[64]
   B. Hydroxy-oxo bile acids
      7-oxo-lithocholic[25,65]
   C. Trihydroxy-bile acids
      cholic acid[66,67]

II. *Synthetic bile acids*
   A. C_{25} bile acids
      HomoUDCA[68]
      HomoCDCA[69]
      α-methyl-UDCA[70–72]
   B. C_{24} bile acids
      7β-methyl-CDCA[73]
      7α-NBD-LCA[a]
   C. C_{23} bile acids
      norCDCA[2]
      norUDCA[1,54,59]
      norDCA[53]
   D. C_{22} bile acids
      dinorCDCA[74]
      11-oxo-LCA[75]

[a] Unpublished observations from this laboratory; NBD denotes the fluorophore 7-nitrobenzofurazan

MODELLING OF THE CHOLEHEPATIC CIRCULATION

Linear, multicompartmental models have been designed to simulate the metabolism of the major bile acids in man[50–52]. A similar model was developed and used to satisfactorily simulate the cholehepatic circulation of nordeoxycholic acid, by Masa Kurita and one of the authors (A.F.H.). One feature of the cholehepatic circulation is that it should not be present in the retrograde perfused liver because bile acids returning to the liver via the periductular capillary plexus enter the terminal portal vein before it enters the liver. When the liver is perfused retrograde, such molecules are swept away from the sinusoid, precluding a cholehepatic circulation. The model satisfactorily simulated the experimental data derived in the isolated liver perfused in prograde and retrograde fashion with nordeoxycholic acid. We hope to be able to publish this model in the future.

SPECIES DIFFERENCES IN CHOLEHEPATIC SHUNTING OF UNCONJUGATED BILE ACIDS

The cholehepatic circulation predicts that cholehepatic cycling will continue until a molecule is either hydroxylated or conjugated. Hydroxylation and conjugation patterns are highly species-dependent. It would therefore be predicted that if a molecule underwent efficient hydroxylation in one species, it would not be hypercholeretic in that species.

Two examples have been found. Nor-deoxycholic acid (norDC) is hypercholeretic in the rat, a species in which it undergoes relatively little hydroxylation. In the hamster it is efficiently 7-hydroxylated to form norcholic acid, and hypercholeresis is modest[53].

NorUDCA induces vigorous hypercholeresis in rats and hamsters. In a single study in a human volunteer the molecule was found to undergo efficient 23-ester glucuronidation; hypercholeresis occurred, but was extremely transient[54].

HYPERCHOLERESIS AS A PHYSIOLOGICAL EVENT

If natural bile acids were secreted in unconjugated form, and underwent a cholehepatic circulation, they should fulfil the criteria for cholehepatic shunting that have been proposed for synthetic bile acids and which are summarized in Table 1. Candidate animals are those in whom the biliary bicarbonate concentration is much higher than that of plasma. Such animals include the guinea pig, rabbit, and pig. To date, however, no vertebrate animal has been observed that has an appreciable proportion of unconjugated dihydroxy-bile acids in its biliary bile acids. Many animals have an appreciable proportion of unconjugated cholic acid in their bile but, as noted, cholic acid appears to undergo only minimal cholehepatic shunting. The number of species in which the unconjugated bile acid fraction has been examined in detail is quite small.

Hypercholeresis of conjugated bile acids is considered unlikely in most species. Infused taurine conjugates of nor-dihydroxy-bile acids do not induce hypercholeresis. The increased canalicular bile flow induced by dihydroxy-glycine conjugated bile acids in the guinea pig raises the possibility that in this species, whose bile flow is voluminous and bicarbonate rich, cholehepatic shunting of conjugated bile acids occurs. Experiments designed to test this possibility in detail should prove rewarding.

At this meeting, M. Strazzabosco (Padova, Italy) suggested to the author that organic acids might enter bile paracellularly and be absorbed in protonated form, thus generating bicarbonate anions. Short-chain fatty acids have a fairly high first-pass extraction so that paracellular entry should be relatively modest. How short-chain fatty acids are handled by the hepatocyte, and to what extent their entry into bile generates biliary bicarbonate, would appear to be worthy of investigation.

CHOLEHEPATIC SHUNTING OF XENOBIOTICS

Many organic molecules are pumped actively into canalicular bile, presumably mostly by cMOAT. If such molecules are transported into bile in the form of a weak acid, and if the weak acid when protonated is sufficiently lipophilic, then it should undergo a cholehepatic circulation. We examined a series of widely used NSAID, and found that only one – sulindac – fulfilled the criteria for cholehepatic shunting[55]. The molecule had a rather low first-pass extraction so that cholehepatic shunting occurred only when the molecule was continuously infused and plasma concentrations were maintained at a high level. The rate of transport was quite high when compared to other values reported for cMOAT. Subsequent competition experiments suggested that the molecule is a substrate for the basolateral and canalicular bile acid transporters[56].

EPILOGUE: PHYSIOLOGICAL AND CLINICAL SIGNIFICANCE OF THE CHOLEHEPATIC CIRCULATION

In the previous review we noted that the cholehepatic circulation hypothesis helped to clarify the profound effect of conjugation by the hepatocyte for lipophilic molecules that were secreted into bile. The formation of CoA esters by unconjugated bile acids was shown to contribute to the vectorial transport of unconjugated bile acids by preventing their regurgitation from the hepatocyte into sinusoidal plasma.

The formation of glucuronides rather than amidates by nor-dihydroxy bile acids indicated that glucuronidation was an alternative mode of conjugation for molecules that escaped formation of the CoA thio-ester. This observation led to the prediction that an inborn error of bile acid conjugation was not necessarily hazardous for the hepatocyte, as dihydroxy molecules would be glucuronidated instead. Such glucuronidation would not occur with cholic acid, based on studies with nor-cholic acid which is secreted into bile without any biotransformation. We predicted that the effect of a conjugation defect would result in biliary bile acids consisting mostly of unconjugated cholic acid. Cholic acid forms micelles in a manner similar to its taurine conjugate, but differs from its taurine conjugate in being passively absorbed. It also has an appreciably higher critical micellization concentration than dihydroxy conjugates. Because of this we hypothesized that the absence of conjugated bile acids in bile would lead to a deficiency of micelles in the small intestine, that in turn would cause the malabsorption of fat soluble vitamins[57]. This prediction has turned out to be correct, based on the clinical features present in a patient with an inborn deficiency in bile acid conjugation[58].

The cholehepatic circulation also suggests that it should be possible to target drugs to the bile duct epithelium, as bile acids such as norCDCA, norUDCA, and the xenobiotic sulindac, traverse the cholangiocytes on their return to the liver. Whether such molecules could be developed, and whether they would have therapeutic utility, remains to be seen. It might also be possible to design molecules which were totally resistant to hydroxylation and conjugation. Such molecules undergo repeated cholehepatic circulations and induce a continuous flow of bicarbonate-rich bile. Whether such potent choleretics would have clinical utility in conditions in which stasis in the biliary tree occurs also remains to be seen.

In conclusion, it would seem that we have learned a considerable amount of biliary physiology by synthesizing bile acids with one less methylene group in the side-chain. Now the challenge is to translate these physiological advances into therapeutic advances in the treatment of cholangiopathies. Because these diseases are uncommon, there has been little interest by pharmaceutical companies in developing new agents that will be of value in the therapy of these rare diseases.

Acknowledgements

The authors' work is supported in part by the National Institutes of Health (Grant DK 21506) as well as a grant-in-aid from the Falk Foundation eV, Freiburg, Germany. Additional support in the past was received from the Ciba Geigy Company and the Burroughs Wellcome Company. Many associates have contributed to the concepts presented in this chapter, including Kel Palmer MD, Yong-Bum Yoon MD, Devorah Gurantz PhD, Eamonn O'Maille PhD, Linda Clayton DPharm., Enrique Michelotti PhD, Sergio Cecchetti PhD, R. B. Kirkpatrick MD, Kel Lambert MS, John Neoptolomos MD, Salam Zakko MD, A. Schmassmann, MD, and Masahiro Kurita MD, PhD.

References

1. Yoon YB, Hagey LR, Hofmann AF, Gurantz D, Michelotti EL. Steinbach JH. Effect of side-chain shortening on the physiologic properties of bile acids: hepatic transport and effect on biliary secretion of 23-nor-ursodeoxycholate in rodents. Gastroenterology. 1986;90:837–52.
2. Palmer KR, Gurantz D, Hofmann AF, Clayton LM, Hagey LR, Cecchetti S. Hypercholeresis induced by norchenodeoxycholate in biliary fistula rodent. Am J Physiol. 1987;252:G219–28.
3. Wilson FA, Dietschy JM. Characterization of bile acid absorption across the unstirred water layer and brush border of the rat jejunum. J Clin Invest. 1972;51:3015–25.
4. Schiff ER, Small NC, Dietschy JM. Characterization of the kinetics of the passive and active transport mechanisms for bile acid absorption in the small intestine and colon of the rat. J Clin Invest. 1972;51:1351–62.
5. Dupas JL, Hofmann AF. Passive jejunal absorption of bile acids *in vivo*: structure-activity relationships and rate limiting steps. Gastroenterology. 1984;86:1067.

6. Gurantz D, Hofmann AF. Influence of bile acid structure on bile flow and biliary lipid secretion in the hamster. Am J Physiol. 1984;247:G736–48.
7. Krag E, Phillips SF. Active and passive bile acid absorption in man. Perfusion studies of the ileum and jejunum. J Clin Invest. 1974;53:1686–94.
8. van Berge Henegouwen GP, Hofmann AF. Pharmacology of chenodeoxycholic acid. II. Absorption and metabolism. Gastroenterology. 1977;73:300–9.
9. Guzelian P, Boyer JL. Glucose reabsorption from bile – evidence for a biliohepatic circulation. J Clin Invest. 1974;53:526–35.
10. Ludvik B, Nolan BB, Roberts A *et al.* A noninvasive method to measure splanchnic glucose uptake after oral glucose administration. J Clin Invest. 1995;95:2232–8.
11. Hofmann AF. The cholehepatic circulation of unconjugated bile acids: an update. In: Paumgartner G, Stiehl A, Gerok W, editors. Bile acids and the hepatobiliary system. Boston: Kluwer; 1993;143–60.
12. Weinman SA, Maglova LM. Free concentrations of intracellular fluorescent anions determined by cytoplasmic dialysis of isolated hepatocytes. Am J Physiol. 1994;267:G922–31.
13. Donovan JM, Timofeyeva N, Carey MC. Influence of total lipid concentration bile salt/lecithin ratio and cholesterol content on inter mixed micellar/vesicular (non-lecithin associated) bile salt concentrations in model bile. J Lipid Res. 1991;32:1501–12.
14. Meier PJ. Molecular mechanisms of hepatic bile salt transport from sinusoidal blood into bile. Am J Physiol. 1995;269:G801–12.
15. Zimniak P, Awasthi YC. ATP-dependent transport systems for organic anions. Hepatology. 1993;17:330–9.
16. Hofmann AF. Biliary secretion and excretion: the hepatobiliary component of the enterohepatic circulation of bile acids. In: Johnson LR, Alpers DH, Christensen J, Jacobson ED, Walsh JH, editors. Physiology of the gastrointestinal tract. New York: Raven Press; 1994:1555–76.
17. Kitani K, Kanai S, Ohta M, Sato Y. Differing transport maxima values for taurine-conjugated bile salts in rats and hamsters. Am J Physiol. 1986;251:G852–8.
18. Paulusma CC, Bosma PJ, Zaman GJ *et al.* Congenital jaundice in rats with a mutation in a multidrug resistance-associated protein gene. Science. 1996;271:1126–8.
19. Buchler M, Konig J, Brom M *et al.* cDNA cloning of the hepatocyte canalicular isoform of the multidrug resistance protein, cMrp, reveals a novel conjugate export pump deficient in hyperbilirubinemic mutant rats. J Biol Chem. 1996;25:15091–8.
20. Sippel CJ, McCollum MJ, Perlmutter DH. Bile acid transport by the rat liver canalicular bile acid transport/ecto-ATPase protein is dependent on ATP but not on its own ecto-ATPase activity. J Biol Chem. 1994;269:2820–6.
21. Hofmann AF. Overview of bile secretion. In: Schultz SG, editor. Handbook of physiology. Section on the gastrointestinal system. Bethesda: American Physiological Society. 1989;549–66.
22. Issachar D, Holland JF, Sweeley CC. Metabolic profiles of organic acids from human plasma. Anal Chem. 1982;54:29–32.
23. Tsukada N, Ackerley CA, Phillips MJ. The structure and organization of the bile canalicular cytoskeleton with special reference to actin and actin-binding proteins. Hepatology. 1995;21:1106–13.
24. Cummings SA, Hofmann AF. Physiological determinants of biliary calcium secretion in the dog. Gastroenterology. 1984;87:664–73.
25. Dumont M, Erlinger S, Uchman S. Hypercholeresis induced by ursodeoxycholic acid and 7-ketolithocholic acid in the rat. Possible role of bicarbonate transport. Gastroenterology. 1980;79:82–9.
26. Wheeler HO, Ross ED, Bradley SE. Canalicular bile production in dogs. Am J Physiol. 1968;214:866–74.
27. Tavoloni N. Biliary clearance of inert carbohydrates. Expectations and reality. Gastroenterology. 1988;94:217–28.
28. Lira M, Schteingart CD, Steinbach JH, Lambert K, McRoberts JA, Hofmann AF. Sugar absorption by the biliary ductular epithelium of the rat: evidence for two transport systems. Gastroenterology. 1992;102:563–71.
29. Ballatori N, Jacob R, Boyer JL. Intrabiliary glutathione hydrolysis. A source of glutamate in bile. J Biol Chem. 1986;261:7860–5.

30. Moslen MT, Kanz MF, Bhatia J, Smith CV, Rassin DK. Biliary glutathione and some amino acids are markedly diminished when biliary pressure is elevated. Exp Mol Pathol. 1994;61:1–15.
31. Stremmel W, Hofmann AF. Intestinal absorption of unconjugated dihydroxy bile acids: non-mediation by the carrier system involved in long chain fatty acid absorption. Lipids. 1990;25:11–16.
32. Mennone A, Alvaro D, Cho W, Boyer JL. Isolation of small polarized bile duct units. Proc Natl Acad Sci USA. 1995;92:6527–31.
33. Vroman B, LaRusso NF. Development and characterization of polarized primary cultures of rat intrahepatic bile duct epithelial cells. Lab Invest. 1996;74:303–13.
34. Farges O, Corbic M, Dumont M, Maurice M, Erlinger E. Permeability of the rat biliary tree to ursodeoxycholic acid. Am J Physiol. 1989;256:G653–60.
35. Lamri Y, Erlinger S, Dumont M, Roda A, Feldmann G. Immunoperoxidase localization of ursodeoxycholic acid in rat biliary epithelial cells. Evidence for a cholehepatic circulation. Liver. 1992;12:351–4.
36. Hylemon PB, Bohdan PM, Sirica AE, Heuman DMV. Cholesterol and bile acid metabolism in cultures of primary rat bile ductular epithelial cells. Hepatology. 1990;11:982–8.
37. Kirkpatrick RB, Green MD, Hagey LR, Hofmann AF, Tephly TR. Effect of side chain length on bile acid conjugation: glucuronidation, sulfation and coenzyme A formation of nor-bile acids and their natural C24 homologs by human and rat liver fractions. Hepatology. 1988;8:353–7.
38. Benedetti A, Di Sario A, Marucci L *et al.* Evidence for an active transport of conjugated bile acids across the basolateral membrane of biliary epithelial cells. Am J Physiol. 1995 (Submitted).
39. Strazzabosco M, Poci C, Spirli C, Sartori L, Knuth A, Crepaldi G. Effect of ursodeoxycholic acid on intracellular pH in a bile duct epithelium-like cell line. Hepatology. 1994;19:145–54.
40. Edsall JT. Carbon dioxide, carbonic acid, and bicarbonate ion: Physical properties and kinetics of interconversion. In: Forster RE, Edsall JT, Otis AB, Roughton FJW, editors. CO_2: chemical, biochemical, and physiological aspects. Washington, DC: National Aeronautics and Space Administration; 1969:15–27.
41. Schoeller C, Keelan M, Mulvey G, Stremmel W, Thomson AB. Oleic acid uptake into rat and rabbit jejunal brush membrane. Biochim Biophys Acta. 1995;1236:51–64.
42. René E, Danzinger RG, Hofmann AF, Nakagaki M. Pharmacologic effect of somatostatin on bile formation in the dog. Gastroenterology. 1983;84:120–9.
43. Schmitt MG, Jr, Soergel KH, Wood CM. Absorption of short chain fatty acids from the human jejunum. Gastroenterology. 1976;70:211–15.
44. Spicer SS, Ge ZH, Tashian RE, Hazen-Martin DJS. Comparative distribution of carbonic anhydrase isozymes III and II in rodent tissues. Am J Anat. 1990;187:55–64.
45. Roda A, Minutello A, Angellotti MA, Fini A. Bile acid structure–activity relationship: evaluation of bile acid lipophilicity using 1-octanol/water partition coefficient and reverse phase HPLC. J Lipid Res. 1990;31:1433–43.
46. Cabral DJ, Small DM, Lilly HS, Hamilton JA. Transbilayer movement of bile acids in model membranes. Biochemistry. 1987;26:1801–4.
47. O'Maille ER, Kozmary SV, Hofmann AF, Gurantz D. Different effects of norcholate and cholate on bile flow and biliary lipid secretion in the rat. Am J Physiol. 1984;246:G67–71.
48. Anwer MS, Atkinson JM, Zimniak P. Amiloride and taurine inhibit cholate-induced HCO_3-rich choleresis in perfused rat livers. Am J Physiol. 1990;259:G453–61.
49. Kitani K, Kanai S. Ursodeoxycholate-induced choleresis in taurine-deprived and taurine-supplemented rats. Jpn J Physiol. 1985;35:443–62.
50. Hofmann AF, Molino G, Milanese M, Belforte G. Description and simulation of a physiological pharmacokinetic model for the metabolism and enterohepatic circulation of bile acids in man. Cholic acid in healthy man. J Clin Invest. 1983;71:1003–22.
51. Molino G, Hofmann AF, Cravetto C, Belforte G, Bona B. Simulation of the metabolism and enterohepatic circulation of endogenous chenodeoxycholic acid in man using a physiological pharmacokinetic model. Eur J Clin Invest. 1986;16:397–414.
52. Hofmann AF, Cravetto C, Molino G, Belforte G, Bona B. Simulation of the metabolism and enterohepatic circulation of endogenous deoxycholic acid in man using a physiological pharmacokinetic model for bile acid metabolism. Gastroenterology. 1987;93:693–709.
53. Neoptolemos JP, Marassi N, Gurantz D, Hagey LR, Hofmann AF. The unusual physiological properties and unique hepatic biotransformation of nor-deoxycholate. Gastroenterology. 1985;88:1682.

54. Zakko S, Lira M, Clerici C *et al.* Novel metabolism and hypercholeretic effect of nor-ursodeoxycholic acid in man. Gastroenterology. 1987;92:1792.
55. Trang NV, Schteingart CD, Cerrè C, Hofmann AF. Hepatic handling of NSAIDs: evidence for cholehepatic shunting and induction of hypercholeresis by sulindac. Hepatology. 1994;20:A660 (abstract).
56. Bolder U, Schteingart CD, Hagey LR *et al.* Sulindac, a xenobiotic choleretic anion, is transported by bile acid transporters. Gastroenterology. 1995;108:A270 (abstract).
57. Hofmann AF, Strandvik B. Defective bile acid amidation: predicted biochemical and clinical features of a new inborn error of metabolism. Lancet. 1988;2:311–13.
58. Setchell KDR, Heubi JE, O'Connell NC, Hofmann AF, Lavine JE. Absence of bile acid conjugation: a new inborn error in bile acid metabolism. Hepatology. 1996;24:371A (abstract).
59. Gurantz D, Schteingart CD, Hagey LR, Steinbach JH, Grotmol T, Hofmann AF. Hypercholeresis induced by unconjugated bile acid infusion correlates with recovery in bile of unconjugated bile acids. Hepatology. 1991;13:540–50.
60. Kitani K, Kanai S. Effect of ursodeoxycholate on the bile flow in the rat. Life Sci. 1982;31:1973–85.
61. Lake JR, Van Dyke RW, Scharschmidt BF. Effects of Na^+ replacement and amiloride on ursodeoxycholic acid-stimulated choleresis and biliary bicarbonate secretion. Am J Physiol. 1987;252:G163–9.
62. Munoz J, Rege R, Hagey LR, Schteingart CD, Hofmann AF. Novel biotransformation and choleretic activity of ursodeoxycholic acid in the dog. Gastroenterology. 1990;98:A728 (abstract).
63. Schmassmann A, Angellotti MA, Clerici C *et al.* Transport, metabolism, and effect of chronic feeding of lagodeoxycholic acid, a new, natural bile acid. Studies in three rodent species. Gastroenterology. 1990;99:1092–1104.
64. Khan M, O'Maille ERL. High biliary HCO_3^- concentration and hypercholeresis induced by hyodeoxycholate in the rat. J Physiol. 1987;386:106.
65. Erlinger S, Dumont M, Zouboulis-Vafiadis IDC. The importance of conjugation in biliary secretion of ursodeoxycholate and 7-ketolithocholate in the rat. Clin Sci. 1984;66:487–91.
66. O'Maille ERL, Richards TG. Possible explanations for the differences in secretory characteristics between conjugated and free bile acids. J Physiol (Lond). 1977;265:855–66.
67. Paumgartner G, Sauter K, Schwarz HP, Herz R. Hepatic excretory transport maximum for free and conjugated cholate in the rat. In: Paumgartner G, Preisig R, editors. The liver, quantitative aspects of structure and function. Basel: Karger; 1973:337–44.
68. Kuramoto T, Moriwaki S, Kawamoto K, Hoshita T. Intestinal absorption and metabolism of homoursodeoxycholic acid in rats. J Pharmacobio-Dyn. 1987;10:309–16.
69. Miki S, Cohen BI, Mikami T, Mosbach EH. Metabolism and choleretic activity of homochenodeoxycholic acid in the hamster. J Lipid Res. 1993;34:915–21.
70. Zouboulis-Vafiadis I, Dumont M, Erlinger S. Hypercholeretic bile acids. Hepatic metabolism and effect on bile secretion of 23-methyl-ursodeoxycholic acid. In: Paumgartner G, Stiehl A, Gerok W, editors. Bile acids and the liver. Boston: Kluwer; 1986:195–8.
71. Roda A, Aldini R, Grigolo B *et al.* 23-Methyl-3α-7β-dihydroxy-5β-cholan-24-oic acid: dose–response study of biliary secretion in rat. Hepatology. 1988;8:1571–6.
72. Clerici C, Dozzini G, Distrutti E *et al.* Effect of intraduodenal administration of 23-methyl-UDCA diastereoisomers on bile flow in hamsters. Dig Dis Sci. 1992;37:791–8.
73. Yoshii M, Mosbach EH, Schteingart CD *et al.* Chemical synthesis and hepatic biotransformation of 3α,7α-dihydroxy-7β-methyl-24-nor-5β-cholan-23-oic acid, a 7-methyl derivative of norchenodeoxycholic acid: studies in the hamster. J Lipid Res. 1991;32:1729–40.
74. Yeh HZ, Hagey LR, Schteingart CD, Ton-Nu H-T, Hofmann AF. The effect of side chain length – three, four, or five carbons – on the hepatic biotransformation and choleretic properties of bile acids: dinor-, nor-, and chenodeoxycholic acid. Gastroenterology. 1996;110:A1365 (abstract).
75. Ruparelia VA, O'Maille ERL. High biliary bicarbonate concentration and hypercholeresis induced by a bisnor-bile acid derivative in the anaesthetized rat. J Physiol. 1990;424:68P (abstract).

Section II
Pathophysiology

11
Molecular biology of cholestasis

P. J. MEIER

INTRODUCTION

The term *cholestasis* denotes an impairment of bile flow and failure to secrete cholephilic inorganic and organic compounds into bile. As a consequence bile solutes accumulate within hepatocytes and in blood plasma, and induce clinical symptoms such as jaundice and pruritus. Since ongoing canalicular secretion of bile salts is the major driving force for the generation of bile flow within the bile canaliculi, decreased vectorial secretion of bile salts by hepatocytes represents one possible cause of hepatocellular cholestasis. Alternatively, extrahepatic cholestasis (i.e. biliary obstruction) has been shown to alter the physiological bile salt transport polarity of hepatocytes. Hence, decreased expression of sinusoidal (basolateral) and/or canalicular bile salt transporters can represent a primary cause of hepatocellular cholestasis as well as a secondary consequence of extrahepatic obstructive cholestasis. This short overview summarizes the recent evidence for altered expression of hepatocellular bile salt transporters in various forms of cholestatic liver disease. More comprehensive reviews have recently been published regarding the molecular physiology of hepatocellular bile salt secretion[1,2] and the pathobiology of hepatocellular cholestasis[3].

BILE SALT TRANSPORT POLARITY OF HEPATOCYTES

Sinusoidal uptake of bile salts into hepatocytes

Bile salts are taken up into hepatocytes by Na^+-dependent and Na^+-independent pathways[4]. Conjugated bile salts are predominantly taken up by the Na^+-taurocholate cotransporting polypeptide that has been cloned from rat (Ntcp) and human (NTCP) liver (Figure 1)[5,6]. Several properties of the rat liver Ntcp have now been well characterized[2,4] and can be summarized as follows:

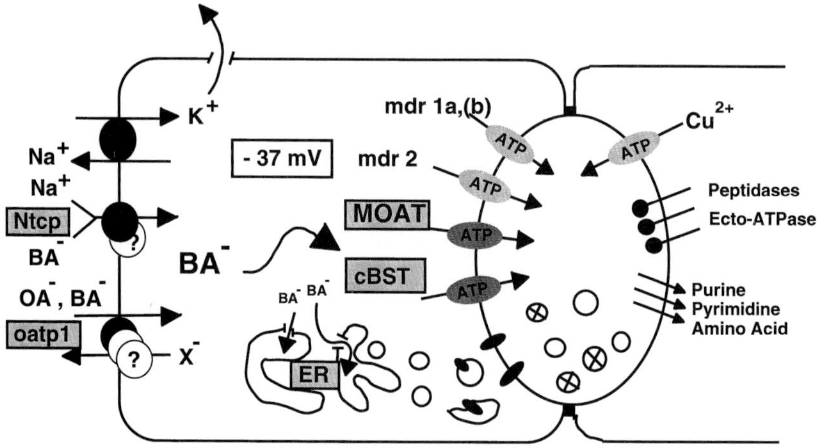

Figure 1 Bile salt transport polarity of rat hepatocytes. Two sinusoidal bile salt uptake systems have been cloned (left): a Na^+/taurocholate cotransporting polypeptide (*Ntcp*) and a Na^+-independent organic anion transporter (*oatpl*). The latter transports a large variety of differently charged substrates and most probably corresponds to the previously suggested 'multispecific bile salt transporter'[2]. While the presence of additional Na^+/bile salt cotransporters is uncertain, additional and probably more specific sinusoidal Na^+-independent organic anion transporters must be present to account for the known physiology of hepatocellular organic anion uptake (*white circles with?*). The endoplasmic reticulum (ER) localizes a potential sensitive taurocholate transport pathway, the molecular nature and exact physiological significance of which are not yet known. Among the known five ATP-dependent canalicular efflux pumps, two are involved in the secretion of bile salts into bile. The 'canalicular bile salt transporter' (*cBST*) mediates secretion of monovalent bile salts, and the 'multispecific organic anion transporter' (*MOAT*) also accepts divalent bile salt-sulphates and -glucuronidates as transport substrates. Parenthetically, the multi-drug resistance gene products mdr1a (or mdr3), mdr 1b and mdr2 mediate canalicular secretion of organic cations (and steroids) and phosphatidylcholine, respectively. In addition to the secretory and excretory mechanisms the canalicular membrane also localizes several Na^+-dependent uptake systems to reabsorb precious cellular constituents including nucleotide precursors and amino acids. *Other abbreviations*: BA^-, monovalent bile salt anions; OA^-, amphipathic organic anions; X^-, unidentified organic anions; ○, intracanalicular lipid vesicles; ⊗, mixed micelles

1. Ntcp represents a seven transmembrane domain glycoprotein with an apparent molecular mass of 51 kDa in isolated basolateral rat liver plasma membrane vesicles[4].
2. Ntcp preferentially mediates Na^+-dependent transport of conjugated bile salts such as taurocholate and, to a lesser degree, unconjugated bile salts such as cholate. In addition, Ntcp can also transport some non-bile acid organic anions such as oestrone-3 sulphates[2,4].
3. Ntcp-mediated Na^+/taurocholate cotransport is electrogenic with a Na^+-taurocholate stoichiometry of 2 : 1 as indicated by a Hill coefficient of 1.9 in *Xenopus laevis* oocytes[4].
4. In all systems the apparent K_m values for Ntcp-mediated taurocholate transport were found to lie between 25 and 42 μmol/L, which is in the same range as the values previously demonstrated for Na^+-dependent taurocholate uptake in isolated hepatocytes[7].

5. Based on Northern blot analysis, Ntcp is present only in differentiated mammalian hepatocytes[8]. Its mRNA is lost to virtually undetectable levels within 72 h in primary cultures of rat heaptocytes[9].
6. Ntcp-mRNA can first be detected between 18 and 21 days of gestation in developing rat liver[8].
7. Hepatic expression of Ntcp is up-regulated in female rats during the postpartum period in a prolactin-dependent manner[10].
8. Multiple factors have recently been identified that potentially regulate the Ntcp-gene promoter including hepatocyte nuclear factor 1 and possibly also bile acids[11].

Na^+-independent bile salt uptake is mediated, at least in part, by an organic anion transporting polypeptide in rat (oatp1) and human (OATP) liver[2,4]. Oatp1 represents a 12 transmembrane domain glycoprotein with an apparent molecular mass of 80 kDa in basolateral rat liver plasma membranes[12]. It is also present in the kidney, where it is localized at the apical plasma membrane of the S3 segment of the proximal tubule of the outer medulla[12]. Oatp1 is a polyspecific and multivalent transport system that accepts a large variety of structurally unrelated and differently charged amphipathic organic substrates including bile salts[13], sulphobromophthalein (BSP)[13], oestrogen conjugates[14,15], ouabain and APD-ajmalinium, a permanently charged quaternary derivative of the antiarrhythmic compound N-propylajmaline[15,16]. Interestingly, an oatp1-cDNA probe reacts with different mRNA size class species in liver and brain, indicating the presence of additional oatp1-related transport systems in these tissues[13]. Recent experiments in rat brain have localized oatp1 as well as an oatp1-related polypeptide of 160 kDa at the apical membrane of the choroid plexus[17]. Another oatp1-related transporter has been cloned and shown to transport prostaglandins[18]. Although the exact driving force for oatp1-mediated substrate transport is not yet known, recent studies in stably transfected HeLa cells indicate that it could mediate bidirectional organic substrate transport across the sinusoidal membrane[14,19]. Hence, oatp1 might also function as a sinusoidal 'overflow' system that could prevent fatal intracellular accumulation of toxic bile salts and other cholephilic compounds in a case of defective canalicular secretion such as occurs during cholestasis.

Intracellular bile salt transport

The mechanisms of intracellular bile salt transport have not been fully elucidated (reviewed in ref. 2). Under normal conditions cytosolic diffusion in association with intracellular binding proteins appears to be the predominant means of transcellular bile salt transport (Figure 1). In contrast, at high bile salt loads canalicular bile flow and bile salt secretion become increasingly dependent on vesicle-mediated transport routes[1]. The exact nature of these bile salt-transporting vesicle pathways is not yet clear, but several observations suggest that they may involve several organelles including smooth endoplasmic reticulum (ER), Golgi complex, transcytotic vesicles and as yet unidentified mechanisms[2]. Interestingly the ER localizes a potential-dependent bile salt diffusion pathway, the exact function of which remains to be elucidated[20].

Canalicular bile salt secretion

The canalicular plasma membrane of rat hepatocytes localizes a variety of ATP-binding cassette (ABC) proteins[21,22]. Among the five ATP-dependent transporters outlined in Figure 1, two are involved in the canalicular secretion of bile salts. The canalicular multiorganic anion transporter (cMOAT) primarily transports divalent organic anions including sulphated and glucuronidated bile salts[23]. cMOAT has recently been cloned and shown to represent a homologue or isoform of the 'multidrug resistance protein' (MRP), now called *mrp2*[22,24] or cMrp[25]. In contrast, the molecular identity of the canalicular transporter for monovalent bile salts (cBST) has not yet been identified[2]. Although the canalicular ecto-ATPase has been suggested to be involved in ATP-dependent bile salt transport[26], a clear separation of immunologically detectable ecto-ATPase and ATP-dependent bile salt transport could be obtained in isolated canalicular plasma membrane vesicles[20]. Hence, it is more likely that the canalicular cBST also belongs to the family of ABC transport proteins.

ALTERED EXPRESSION OF HEPATOCYTIC BILE SALT TRANSPORTERS DURING CHOLESTASIS

Cloning of the sinusoidal hepatocytic bile acid carriers opened the way to study carrier expression in various forms of cholestatic liver disease, including extrahepatic bile duct obstruction as well as oestrogen, endotoxin and drug-induced hepatocellular cholestasis (Table 1).

Extrahepatic obstructive cholestasis

Obstructive cholestasis can be experimentally induced in rat liver by ligation of the common bile duct. This procedure results in the disruption of the structural and functional integrity of hepatocellular tight junctions[27] and in alterations of various intracellular processes including impairment of transcytosis and canalicular exocytosis[28,29]. Moreover, the expression of the canalicular *mdrla* (or *mdr3*) and *mdrlb* gene products (see Figure 1) have been shown to be increased in rat liver during common bile duct ligation (CBDL)[30]. In contrast, CBDL decreased the V_{max} of sinusoidal Na^+-dependent taurocholate uptake by 70% in hepatocytes isolated from the cholestatic livers[31]. In the same study intracellular levels of Ntcp-mRNA and and the expression of Ntcp-protein were decreased by 60% and by more than 90%, respectively, whereas no change in the expression of sinusoidal Na^+/K-ATPase or of the canalicular ecto-ATPase was observed (Table 1). Transcriptional activity as assessed by a nuclear runoff assay was decreased 1 day after CBDL only for Ntcp[31]. Hence, extrahepatic cholestasis results in rapid down-regulation of Na^+-dependent taurocholate uptake and Ntcp-transcription. Furthermore, impaired post-transcriptional regulation also appears to contribute to the overall decrease of Ntcp-protein levels in cholestatic hepatocytes[31]. While the decline of sinusoidal Ntcp may represent a protective feedback mechanism in cholestasis, to diminish uptake of potentially hepatotoxic bile acids, the up-regulation of the canalicular mdr1a-and mdr1b-protein expression[30] further indicates that the canalicular membrane is more resistant to

Table 1 Altered expression of hepatocellular bile salt carriers in various forms of cholestasis in rat liver

	Sinusoidal membrane		*Canalicular membrane*	
Extrahepatic bile duct obstruction[30,31]	Na^+, K, ATPase	normal	ecto-ATPase	normal
	Na^+/TCA uptake	–70%	mdr1a, mdr1b	increased
	Ntcp-mRNA	–60%		
	Ntcp-protein	–90%		
Ethinyloestradiol-induced cholestasis[32,33]	Na^+, K, ATPase, activity	decreased	ecto-ATPase	normal
	Na^+, K, ATPase, protein	normal	cBST-activity	–63%
	Na^+/TCA uptake	–40–87%	cMOAT-activity	decreased
	Ntcp-mRNA	–48%		
	Ntcp-protein	–79%		
	Na^+-indep. TCA uptake	normal		
	oatp-mRNA	–90%		
	oatp-protein	–62%		
Endotoxin-induced cholestasis[37,39]	Na^+, K, ATPase	–50%	ecto-ATPase	normal
	Na^+/TCA uptake	not measurable	cMOAT-activity	decreased
	Ntcp-mRNA	–90%		
	Ntcp-protein	–90%		
Drug-induced cholestasis				
Cyclosporine A[40]	Na^+/TCA uptake	decreased	cBST-activity	decreased
α-Naphthylisothiocyanate[30]			mdr1a, mdr1b	increased

Abbreviations: cBST, canalicular ATP-dependent bile salt carrier; cMOAT (mrp2, cMrp), canalicular multi-organic anion transporter; Ntcp, sinusoidal Na^+/taurocholate cotransporting polypeptide; oatp, sinusoidal organic anion transport protein; TCA, taurocholate

the toxic effects of bile constituents. Further studies with other canalicular transporters are required to elucidate whether up-regulation of canalicular ATP-dependent efflux pumps also represents a general defence mechanism against the intracellular accumulation of toxic bile solutes during extrahepatic obstructive cholestasis.

Ethinyloestradiol-induced cholestasis

Treatment of male rats with ethinyloestradiol (EE; 5 mg/kg per day) for up to 5 days is a well-accepted model to study the pathogenesis of oestrogen-induced cholestasis in women. Studies in isolated plasma membrane vesicles have shown that EE treatment of rats results in a decrease of basolateral Na^+-dependent taurocholate uptake by ~40%, while the V_{max} of canalicular ATP-dependent taurocholate transport (cBST activity, Figure 1) decreased by 63%[32]. In addition, the activity of canalicular MOAT (Figure 1) was also markedly decreased, whereas Na^+-dependent canalicular reabsorption of adenosine and glycine were increased[32]. More recently, Simon *et al.*[33] performed an extensive molecular expression study in rat liver. They demonstrated the following effects of a 5-day EE treatment course in male rats (Table 1):

1. A decreased sinusoidal plasma membrane fluidity causing a decreased Na^+,K,ATPase activity in the presence of a normal Na^+,K,ATPase protein level.
2. A parallel decrease in sinusoidal Na^+-dependent taurocholate uptake (–87%), intracellular levels of Ntcp-mRNA (–48%) and expression of Ntcp protein (–79%). While the decreased Ntcp-mRNA level indicated reduced transcription of the *Ntcp* gene, the quantitative discrepancy between the decrease of Ntcp-mRNA on the one hand, and the impairment of Ntcp activity and protein expression on the other, also indicates additional alterations in the post-transcriptional regulation. However, the perfect quantitative correlation between the reduction of Na^+-dependent taurocholate uptake activity and Ntcp protein lends further support to the concept that Ntcp represents the predominant, if not the only, Na^+-dependent bile salt uptake system in rat liver[2].
3. A virtually normal Na^+-independent taurocholate uptake activity in the presence of reduced oatp1-mRNA (–90%) and oatp1 protein (–62%) levels. These data would clearly indicate that oatp1 does not represent the major Na^+-independent bile salt uptake system in rat liver. However, Na^+-independent taurocholate uptake represents only a minor portion (approximately 10–30%) of total physiological taurocholate uptake in rat hepatocytes, which makes appropriate quantitative detection of a decreased Na^+-independent uptake activity under pathophysiological conditions difficult. Nevertheless, as already outlined above, the existence of additional oatp1-related transport proteins in rat liver is very likely, although their involvement in Na^+-independent taurocholate uptake is uncertain, based on recent antisense oligonucleotide inhibition experiments in *Xenopus laevis* oocytes[34].

4. Expression of the putative canalicular bile salt carrier 'ecto-ATPase' remained unaltered during EE-induced cholestasis. Since canalicular ATP-dependent taurocholate transport was found to be reduced in EE-induced cholestasis[32], the finding of normal ecto-ATPase expression supports the interpretation that the ecto-ATPase does not represent cBST in rat liver[2]. In conclusion, all studies demonstrate that EE-induced cholestasis is associated with marked expressional alterations of hepatocellular bile salt carriers. It remains, however, to be definitely demonstrated whether altered activity and expression of hepatocellular bile salt transporters represent the primary cause of EE-induced cholestasis, or rather a secondary phenomenon of EE-induced liver cell proliferation[32].

Sepsis-induced cholestasis

Sepsis and other severe inflammatory diseases are frequently associated with cholestasis[3]. These conditions are mediated in part by endotoxin and inflammatory cytokines including tumour necrosis factor α (TNFα) and various interleukins. Endotoxin is well known to decrease the hepatocellular transport and biliary excretion of cholephilic compounds including bile acids[3]. More specifically, endotoxin has been shown to inhibit hepatocyte bile salt uptake in a TNFα-dependent manner[35]. Furthermore, in hepatocytes isolated from endotoxaemic livers it could be shown that the inhibition of organic anion (including bilirubin) transport during endotoxaemia is largely due to a reduction in canalicular MOAT activity[36–38]. On the molecular level endotoxin treatment of rats caused gene expression of Ntcp to decrease by more than 90%[39]. As a consequence the activity of Na^+-dependent taurocholate uptake became unmeasurable in isolated basolateral plasma membrane vesicles, indicating again that Ntcp represents the only Na^+-dependent bile salt uptake system in rat liver. The effects of endotoxin on hepatocellular Ntcp expression were mediated by TNFα and IL-1β. Finally, endotoxin also decreased sinusoidal Na^+,K,ATPase activity by 50%, whereas expression of canalicular ecto-ATPase was again not affected (Table 1). Since endotoxin-induced cholestasis represents a frequent and severe complication in patients with sepsis and other inflammatory diseases, the further elucidation of its molecular pathogenesis, including the transcriptional and post-transcriptional regulation of the canalicular bile salt carrier, is very important for the development of new therapeutic strategies.

Drug-induced cholestasis

The molecular pathogenesis of drug-induced cholestasis has so far been investigated in less detail. Studies in isolated plasma membrane vesicles have indicated that cyclosporine A induced cholestasis may primarily result from cyclosporine induced inhibition of the canalicular ATP-dependent bile salt carrier cBST[40]. Although basolateral Na^+-dependent taurocholate uptake was also inhibited by cyclosporine A (Table 1), its IC_{50} value was 15-fold lower for cBST than for the Na^+-dependent taurocholate uptake system. Finally, similar to obstructive cholestasis, α-naphthylisothiocyanate-induced hepatotoxicity has also been shown to be associated with increased canalicular expression of the *mdr1a* and *mdr1b* gene products[30]. Furthermore, induction of hepatic *mdr1* gene expression by the xenobiotic inducer 2-acetylaminofluorene resulted in a marked stimulation of verapamil-sensitive biliary excretion of vinblastine, a classical mdr1 substrate[30]. Parenthetically, P-glycoprotein inhibition or 'knock-out' has been associated with marked alterations in the tissue distribution and pharmacokinetics of dexamethasone, digoxin and cyclosporine[41]. These studies demonstrate the ultimate importance of the hepatocanalicular members of the *ABC*-transporter family for both the molecular pathogenesis of drug-induced cholestasis, as well as for biliary excretion and elimination of xenobiotics from the body.

CONCLUSIONS

The past 15 years of hepatobiliary transport research have led us from carrier identification in basolateral and canalicular rat liver plasma membrane vesicles to the cloning of a rapidly increasing number of polar hepatocellular transport systems[42]. The developed cDNA and antibody probes have already been used by several groups to investigate the molecular pathogenesis and/or consequences of extrahepatic and intrahepatic cholestasis. Although basolateral Na^+-dependent bile salt uptake is not a rate-limiting process in normal hepatocytes, all studies demonstrate a decreased activity and an impaired expression of Ntcp in various forms of cholestasis (Table 1). Intracellular retention of bile constituents, rather than interruption of the enterohepatic circulation itself, appears to be important for down-regulation of Ntcp, since Ntcp protein and steady-state mRNA levels remain unchanged in rats with a complete biliary fistula for up to 7 days[43]. Which specific factors among the numerous possible candidates[11] actually regulate the *Ntcp* gene promoter remains to be investigated. The current picture is less clear with respect to Na^+-independent taurocholate uptake and oatp1 expression in cholestatic liver disease. Although decreased activity and expression is likely in EO-induced cholestasis[33,44] further studies are required to ascertain the exact role of oatp1 for overall Na^+-independent bile salt uptake in rat and human liver. Furthermore, identification and characterization of the repeatedly hypothesized oatp1-related transporters remain to be done. Finally, based on various preliminary observations it can be expected that, at least for many intracellular forms of cholestasis, the real action is occurring at the canalicular membrane. This assumption may especially be true for oestrogen, endotoxin and various drug-induced forms of cholestasis. Since many more canalicular *ABC* transporters are in the process of being cloned in various laboratories, exciting new possibilities will soon be available to further unravel the mystery of cholestatic liver disease. Furthermore, cloning of additional hepatobiliary drug excretory systems will also help to better understand the mechanisms of drug distribution, pharmacokinetics and drug elimination. Hence, it appears that understanding the molecular physiology of hepatobiliary transport will help not only to elucidate the pathophysiology of cholestatic liver disease, but also to better predict drug kinetics in the whole organism and to potentially induce toxic drug elimination from the body[30].

Acknowledgements

This study was supported by the Swiss National Science Foundation (grant 31–45536.95).

References

1. Nathanson MH, Boyer JL. Mechanisms and regulation of bile secretion. Hepatology. 1991;14:551–66.
2. Meier PJ. Molecular mechanisms of hepatic bile salt transport from sinusoidal blood into bile. Am J Physiol. 1995;269:G801–12.
3. Green RM, Crawford JM. Hepatocellular cholestasis: pathobiology and histological outcome. Sem Liver Dis. 1995;15:372–89.
4. Hagenbuch B, Meier PJ. Sinusoidal (basolateral) bile salt uptake systems in hepatocytes. Sem Liver Dis. 1996;16:129–36.
5. Hagenbuch B, Stieger B, Foguet M, Lübbert H, Meier PJ. Functional expression cloning and characterization of the hepatocyte Na^+/bile acid cotransport system. Proc Natl Acad Sci USA. 1991;88:10629–33.
6. Hagenbuch B, Meier PJ. Molecular cloning, chromosomal localization, and functional characterization of a human liver Na^+/bile acid cotransport system. J Clin Invest. 1994;93:1326–31.
7. Boyer JL, Ng OC, Ananthanarayanan M *et al.* Expression and characterization of a functional rat liver Na^+ bile acid cotransport system in COS-7 cells. Am J Physiol. 1994;266:G382–7.
8. Boyer JL, Hagenbuch B, Ananthanarayanan M, Suchy F, Stieger B, Meier PJ. Phylogenic and ontogenic expression of hepatocellular bile acid transport. Proc Natl Acad Sci USA. 1993;90:435–8.
9. Liang D, Hagenbuch B, Stieger B, Meier PJ. Parallel decrease of Na^+-taurocholate contransport and its encoding mRNA in primary cultures of rat heaptocytes. Hepatology. 1993;18:1162–6.
10. Ganguly TC, Liu Y, Hyde JF, Hagenbuch B, Meier PJ, Vore M. Prolactin increases hepatic Na^+/taurocholate co-transport activity and messenger RNA *post partum.* Biochem J. 1994;303:33–6.
11. Karpen SJ, Sun AQ, Kudish B, *et al.* Multiple factors regulate the rat liver basolateral sodium-dependent bile acid contransporter gene promoter. J Biol Chem. 1996;271:15211–21.
12. Bergwerk AJ, Shi B, Ford AC *et al.* Immunologic distribution of an organic anion transport protein in rat liver and kidney. Am J Physiol. 1996, (In press).
13. Jacquemin E, Hagenbuch B, Stieger B, Wolkoff AW, Meier PJ. Expression cloning of a rat liver Na^+-independent organic anion transporter. Proc Natl Acad Sci USA. 1994;91:133–7.
14. Kanai N, Lu R, Bao Y, Wolkoff AW, Vore M, Schuster VL. Estradiol 17β-D-glucuronide is a high-affinity substrate for oatp organic anion transporter. Am J Physiol. 1996;270:F326–31.
15. Bossuyt X, Müller M, Hagenbuch B, Meier PJ. Polyspecific drug and steroid transport by an organic anion transporter of mammalian liver. J Pharmacol Exp Ther. 1996;276:891–6.
16. Kanai N, Lu R, Bao Y, Wolkoff AW, Schuster VL. Transient expression of oatp organic anion transporter in mammalian cells: identification of candidate substrates. Am J Physiol. 1996;270:F319–25.
17. Angeletti RH, Novikoff PM, Juuvadi SR, Fritschy JM, Meier PJ, Wolkoff AW. The choroid plexus epithelium is the site of the organic anion transport protein in the brain. Proc Natl Acad Sci USA. 1996; (Submitted).
18. Kanai N, Lu R, Satriano JA, Bao Y, Wolkoff AW, Schuster VL. Identification and characterization of a prostaglandin transporter. Science. 1995;268:866–9.
19. Shi X, Bai S, Ford AC *et al.* Stable inducible expression of a functional rat liver organic anion transport protein in HeLa cells. J Biol Chem. 1995;270:25591–5.
20. Kast C, Stieger B, Winterhalter KH, Meier PJ. Hepatocellular transport of bile acids. Evidence for distinct subcellular localizations of electrogenic and ATP-dependent taurocholate transport in rat hepatocytes. J Biol Chem. 1994;269:5179–86.
21. Lomri N, Fitz JG, Scharschmidt BF. Hepatocellular transport. Role of ATP-binding cassette proteins. Sem Liver Dis. 1996;16:201–10.
22. Müller M, Roelofsen H, Jansen PLM. Secretion of organic anions by hepatocytes: Involvement of homologues of the multidrug resistance protein. Sem Liver Dis. 1996;16:211–20.

23. Oude Elferink RPJ, Meijer DKF, Kuipers F, Jansen PLM, Groen AK, Groothuis GMM. Hepatobiliary secretion of organic compounds; molecular mechanisms of membrane transport. Biochim Biophys Acta. 1995;1241:215–68.
24. Paulusma CC, Bosma PJ, Zaman GJR *et al.* Congenital jaundice in rats with a mutation in a multidrug resistance-associated protein gene. Science. 1996;271:1126–8.
25. Büchler M, König J, Brom M *et al.* cDNA cloning of the hepatocyte canalicular isoform of the multidrug resistance protein, cMrp, reveals a novel conjugate export pump deficient in hyperbilirubinemic mutant rats. J Biol Chem. 1996;271:15091–8.
26. Sippel CJ, McCollum MJ, Perlmutter DH. Bile acid transport by the rat liver canalicular bile acid transport/ecto-ATPase protein is dependent on ATP but not on its own ecto-ATPase activity. J Biol Chem. 1994;269:2800–26.
27. Rahner C, Stieger B, Landmann L. Structure–function correlation of tight junctional impairment after intrahepatic and extrahepatic cholestasis in rat liver. Gastroenterology. 1996;110:1564–78.
28. Barr VA, Hubbard AL. Newly synthesized hepatocyte plasma membrane proteins are transported in transcytotic vesicles in the bile duct-ligated rat. Gastroenterology. 1993;105:554–71.
29. Sieger B, Meier PJ, Landmann L. Effect of obstructive cholestasis on membrane traffic and domain-specific expression of plasma membrane proteins in rat liver parenchymal cells. Hepatology. 1994;20:201–12.
30. Schrenk D, Gant TW, Preisegger KH, Silverman JA, Marino PA, Thorgeirsson SS. Induction of multidrug resistance gene expression during cholestasis in rats and nonhuman primates. Hepatology. 1993;17:854–60.
31. Gartung C, Ananthanarayanan M, Rahman MA *et al.* Down-regulation of expression and function of the rat liver Na^+/bile acid cotransporter in extrahepatic cholestasis. Gastroenterology. 1996;110:199–200.
32. Bossard R, Stieger B, O'Neill B, Fricker G, Meier PJ. Ethinylestradiol treatment induces multiple canalicular membrane transport alterations in rat liver. J Clin Invest. 1993;91:2714–20.
33. Simon FR, Fortune J, Iwahashi, Gartung C, Wolkoff A, Sutherland E. The early pathogenesis of ethinylestradiol induced cholestasis involves alterations in the expression of liver sinusoidal membrane transporters. Am J Physiol. 1996 (in press).
34. Hagenbuch B, Scharschmidt BF, Meier PJ. Effect of antisense oligonucleotides on the expression of hepatocellular bile acid and organic anion uptake systems in *Xenopus laevis* oocytes. Biochem J. 1996;316:901–4.
35. Whiting JF, Green RM, Rosenbluth AB, Gollan JL. Tumor necrosis factor-α decreases hepatocyte bile salt uptake and mediates endotoxin-induced cholestasis. Hepatology. 1995;22:1273–8.
36. Roelofsen H, Van Der Veere C, Ottenhoff R, Schoemaker B, Jansen PLM, Oude Elferink RPJ. Decreased bilirubin transport in the perfused liver of endotoxemic rats. Gastroenterology. 1994;107:1075–84.
37. Roelofsen H, Schoemaker B, Bakker C *et al.* Impaired hepatocanalicular organic anion transport in endotoxemic rats. Am J Physiol. 1995;32:G427–34.
38. Wettstein M, Noe B, Häussinger D. Metabolism of cysteinyl leukotrienes in the perfused rat liver. The influence of endotoxin pretreatment and the cellular hydration state. Hepatology. 1995;22:235–40.
39. Green RM, Beier D, Gollan JL. Regulation of hepatocyte bile salt transporters by endotoxin and inflammatory cytokines in rodents. Gastroenterology. 1996;111:193–8.
40. Böhme M, Müller M, Leier I, Jedlitschky G, Keppler D. Cholestasis caused by inhibition of the adenosine triphosphate-dependent bile salt transport in rat liver. Gastroenterology. 1994;107:255–65.
41. Schinkel AH, Wagenaar E, van Deemter L, Mol Carla AAM, Borst P. Absence of the mdr1a P-glycoprotein in mice affects tissue distribution and pharmacokinetics of dexamethasone, digoxin and cyclosporine. J Clin Invest. 1995;96:1698–705.
42. Meier PJ. Hepatocellular transport systems: from carrier identification in membrane vesicles to cloned proteins. J Hepatol. 1996;24(Suppl. 1):29–35.
43. Gartung C, Schuele S, Schlosser S, Boyer JL. Expression of the rat liver Na^+/taurocholate cotransporter (*Ntcp*) is regulated *in vivo* by retention of biliary constituents, but not their depletion. Hepatology 1995;22:319A (abstract).
44. Kupferschmidt H, Hagenbuch B, Stieger B, Kraehenbühl St, Meier PJ. Ethinylestradiol induces differential effects on various transporter mRNA and protein levels in rat liver. Hepatology 1994;20:175A (abstract).

12
Pathophysiology of the biliary epithelium

M. STRAZZABOSCO, C. SPIRLÌ, A. ZSEMBERY, A. GRANATO, L. FABRIS, G. M. CAVESTRO, R. M. IEMMOLO, L. OKOLICSANYI and G. CREPALDI

INTRODUCTION

Hepatocytes and cholangiocytes, the two epithelial cell types in the liver, serve different functions, and are affected by different diseases. The intrahepatic bile duct epithelium determines the fluidity and alkalinity of the primary hepatocellular bile from which it reabsorbs fluids, amino acids, glucose and bile acids and secretes water, electrolytes and IgA immunoglobulins[1]. The bile duct epithelium synthesizes and secretes a number of peptides such as interleukin-6 (IL-6)[2], transforming growth factor β (TGFβ)[3], endothelin-1[4], and monocyte chemotactic protein-1 (MCP-1)[5] that probably enable cholangiocytes to communicate extensively with other non-parenchymal liver cells.

The intrahepatic biliary epithelium appears to be a preferred target for immunological aggression to the liver, as in chronic liver transplant rejection, graft-versus-host disease (GVHD), primary biliary cirrhosis (PBC) and autoimmune cholangitis. In addition, a number of toxic, vascular and microbiogical noxae, together with congenital abnormalities, selectively damage the biliary epithelium, resulting in a chronic cholestatic disorder[6,7]. This broad group of cholangiopathies that includes also cystic fibrosis-related focal biliary cirrhosis, primary (PSC) and secondary sclerosing cholangitis and drug-induced ductopenia[8] represents an important cause of morbidity and mortality among young adults. Probably as a result of the known heterogeneity in cholangiocyte function, different portions of the biliary tree appear to be preferentially affected in specific cholangiopathies: while PSC involves both intrahepatic and extrahepatic ducts, PBC damages the interlobular bile ducts and drug-induced ductopenia destroys the smallest ductules (see Chapter 2).

The spectrum of cholangiopathies ranges from conditions in which a normal epithelium is damaged by disordered autoimmunity, infectious agents, toxic compounds or ischaemia, to genetically determined disorders arising from an abnormal bile duct biology, such as cystic fibrosis or biliary atresia. From a pathophysiological point of view, common to all cholangiopathies is the co-existence of *cholangiocyte loss* with *cholangiocyte proliferation* and various degrees of *portal inflammation* and *fibrosis*[6,7,9]. *Cholestasis* is another inherent feature of cholangiopathies and may initiate or worsen the process[6,7,10,11]. Cytokines and proinflammatory mediators released in the portal spaces probably contribute to these processes by activating fibrogenesis, stimulating apoptotic and proliferative responses, damaging the peribiliary circulation, increasing the expression of histocompatibility antigens in cholangiocytes[12] and by altering the transport functions of the epithelium.

Recently the availability of several cultured cholangiocyte models from normal and diseased rodent or human livers has made it possible to begin exploration of cholangiocyte pathobiology in these hiterto little-known syndromes[1,6,7,13]. To date, however, very little is known, and this review is mainly meant to suggest a framework for future research in the field of cholangiopathies. Pathogenetic mechanisms of immune-mediated damage and congenital cholangiopathies will be covered elsewere (see Chapters 2, 14, 15, 16).

CHOLANGIOCYTE LOSS

The hallmark of diseases grouped under the vanishing bile duct syndrome (VBDS) is a decrease in the number of bile ducts per portal tract below 0.9[7]. In PBC, as in several other cholangiopathies, destruction of interlobular bile ducts is associated with the proliferation of marginal ductules. Mechanisms by which cholangiocytes die are not well known, but considerable interest is being expressed in apoptotic phenomena. Cell death occurs either by necrosis or apoptosis. While necrosis is characterized by abrupt loss of plasma membrane integrity followed by release of intracellular contents, apoptosis (a form of programmed cell death) is defined by nuclear and cytoplasmic fragmentation into membrane-bound fragments containing viable organelles. These ‘apoptotic bodies’ are eliminated by phagocytosis; thus the inflammatory reaction is usually limited. Mechanisms of apoptosis in the liver have been reviewed recently[14]; therefore we will summarize only those aspects that may be relevant for cholangiocyte pathophysiology.

Apoptosis is a highly regulated phenomenon that can be initiated by stimulation of a series of receptors, such as the Fas/Apo-1, and the steroid, TGFβ and tumour necrosis factor α (TNFα) receptors. While Fas-mediated cell death may represent a major mechanism of toxicity induced by cytotoxic T lymphocytes (CTL), TGFβ is an ubiquitous growth inhibitor, associated to apoptosis[15]. A number of genes involved in growth control have been shown to block apoptosis. Among them, the *bcl-2* gene blocks apoptosis induced by oxidative damage, but not that mediated by cytotoxic T lymphocytes[16]. In the liver, bcl-2 protein is expressed only in cholangiocytes lining ductules and small interlobular ducts[17]. This observation is in keeping with recent theories on cholangiocyte heterogeneity assigning proliferative capabilities to ductules and secretory capabilities to large bile ducts (see Chapter 5). In cholangiocarcinoma cell lines *bcl-2* is overexpressed and alters the threshold for beauvericin-induced apoptosis[18].

Apoptotic bodies are occasionally seen in the biliary tree[19], and apoptotic cell deletion may play a role in regulating cell turnover in slowly growing tissues, such as the biliary epithelium. A very interesting example indicating the role of thyroid hormones and apoptosis in biliary ontogenesis is the loss of the entire biliary system in the lamprey during metamorphosis from the larval to the adult form[20]. Simultaneously with a sharp decline in thyroid hormones levels, these animals become deeply jaundiced and the bile duct epithelium disappears without inflammation. Apoptosis is also involved in tissue regression after induced hyperplasia[21]. For example in bile duct-ligated rats, apoptotic phenomena lead to the disappearance of proliferated ducts after the relief of the biliary obstruction[22]. Interestingly, proliferated ducts express TGFβ[3], a cytokine that augments apoptosis during regression of mitogen-induced liver hyperplasia.

The role played by apoptosis in the pathogenesis of VBDS is difficult to demonstrate *in vivo*; however, ductopenia can be considered to be the result of bile duct loss prevailing over bile duct proliferation. The anti-apoptotic bcl-2 protein has been shown to be expressed in proliferating ductules at the border of the cirrhotic nodule in PBC, but in ductopenic reactions, ductules expressing bcl-2 were absent[23]. In PBC by *in situ* nick-labelling, DNA fragmentation, one of the hallmarks of the apoptosis, an ultrastructural phenomenon indicating apoptosis, could be detected in interlobular bile ducts[24], an observation that is consistent with the frequent findings of apoptotic bodies in PBC[25]. Apoptosis has also been suggested to play a role in bile duct damage in GVHD and chronic liver transplant rejection[26]. High concentrations of hydrophobic bile acids can cause hepatocellular necrosis. At lower concentrations glycodeoxycholic, glycochenodeoxycholic and chenodeoxycholic acids, but not ursodeoxycholic acid, induced apoptosis in hepatocytes in a manner that was unrelated to bile salt hydrophobicity and was dependent on intracellular endonucleases[27]. Whether bile acids can trigger apoptosis in cholangiocytes is presently unknown, but will clearly need to be investigated in the near future.

CHOLANGIOCYTE PROLIFERATION

Bile duct cells possess latent mitotic capabilities and proliferate following a number of liver injuries, from PBC and PSC, to alcoholic liver disease and drug or viral chronic hepatitis. The putative liver stem cell is probably located in the biliary compartment; an hypothesis that also has great relevance for liver carcinogenesis[16]. Proliferation of phenotypically and functionally normal cholangiocytes (type I hyperplasia) occurs following acute complete biliary obstruction or administration of α-naphthylisothiocyanate. In experimental bile duct ligation (BDL), cholangiocyte DNA synthesis peaks at about 2 weeks after BDL and, by the fifth week, together with a decline in labelling index, there is an increase in apoptotic death of cholangiocytes that further increases after release of BDL[16]. On the other hand, in conditions associated with chronic incomplete biliary obstruction, ductal metaplasia of periportal hepatocytes is thought to support the so-called type II or atypical metaplasia[7]. While type I hyperplasia in chronic cholestasis clearly serves a compensatory function, the role of ductular metaplasia in cholangiopathies is unknown. Failure of cholangiocytes to proliferate leads to ductopenia, the end-stage of a number of bile duct diseases.

Mechanisms responsible for bile duct cell proliferation are not well known and their elucidation is an area of major effort. A number of growth factors (such as epidermal growth factor (EGF), hepatocyte growth factor (HGF) and IL-6 in humans and insulin-like growth factor 1 (IGF-1), EGF and HGF in rats) have been shown to stimulate cholangiocyte growth *in vitro*[2,4,28]. A role for bile acids has been postulated and awaits experimental demonstration. Although not studied in detail, inflammatory mediators and locally released cytokines are clearly involved. Epithelial cells may also be a source of cytokines, for example human cholangiocytes secrete IL-6 following administration of IL-2 and proliferate following IL-6 administration[2].

PORTAL INFLAMMATION AND FIBROSIS

Liver fibrosis and ductular reaction are common pathological changes in most liver injuries. The two entities are frequently concomitant, suggesting a pathogenetic relationship[29]. Liver fibrosis is the result of excessive accumulation of connective tissue in the liver. Fibrosis can be confined to the portal tract, or it may expand into the lobule, bridging with other portal spaces or with the central veins. The fibrotic matrix is composed of collagen type I and III, together with collagen type IV and extracellular matrix glycoproteins such as fibronectin, laminin and undulin[29,30]. These molecules possess signalling properties and thus, in addition to altering the architecture of the organ, they may change the behaviour of the cell. Hepatic stellate cells (HSC) are the main connective tissue-producing cells[30] and respond to a number of autocrine and paracrine stimuli (TGFβ1/β2 and platelet-derived growth factor or PDGF)[29,30]. In chronic liver damage, in response to appropriate signals (such as lipid peroxidation products, nitric oxide, PDGF, interleukin-1 (IL-1) or TGFβ), HSC undergo a switch from the resting fat-storing phenotype to the proliferative myofibroblast-like phenotype that is associated with matrix production and α-smooth muscle actin expression.

In contrast to the liver fibrosis associated with alcoholic liver disease, in chronic cholestatic conditions (such as experimental bile duct ligation) fibrosis involves the portal tracts, where extensive proliferation of cholangiocytes takes place. Most periductular cells express desmin and α-smooth muscle actin, indicating activated HSC[29]. Cholangiocytes may contribute to the synthesis of collagen type IV and laminin[16,29,31,32]. In chronic liver diseases, *in-situ* hybridization shows that mRNA for TGFβ1 and TGFβ2 is expressed in HCS and cholangiocytes, respectively[3], suggesting that TGFβ produced by cholangiocytes may on the one hand stimulate HSC proliferation and matrix production, and on the other hand may modulate cholangiocyte proliferation. TGFβ may have antiproliferative effects in some epithelial cells, where it can also induce apoptosis. A preliminary report showed reduced cell proliferation in a rat cholangiocyte cell line treated with TGFβ[4]. Interestingly IFNγ treatment inhibits collagen deposition and cholangiocyte proliferation in a model of murine cirrhosis[33].

CHOLESTASIS

Given the role of the biliary epithelium in bile production it is clear that impaired fluid secretion by cholangiocytes may contribute to secretory failure and, ultimately, exacerbate the causative disease. 'Ductular cholestasis'[11] may be due to obliteration of bile ducts, to mutations in transport proteins, or to altered secretory responses induced by cell proliferation or inflammatory mediators.

Cystic fibrosis

The role of altered ion transport systems in ductular cholestasis is highlighted by cystic fibrosis, a frequent genetic disease in which a mutation in CFTR, a cAMP-activated Cl^- channel, leads to pulmonary, pancreatic and liver disease[34–37]. Overt liver decompensation affects only about 25% of patients surviving up to 20 years of age; however, bile duct cell damage can also be demonstrated in asymptomatic cases before hepatocellular damage appears[36]; this observation, and the finding that, in the liver, CFTR immunoreactivity is restricted to cholangiocytes, suggests that the primary pathogenetic event is located within the bile duct epithelium[6]. The pathogenesis of liver disease in CF is unclear. It is speculated that, in CF livers, reduced bile fluidity and alkalinity ultimately precipitate a series of events, such as retention of cytotoxic bile acids and production of inflammatory cytokines, that can aggravate and precipitate liver damage[35], ultimately leading to pathognomonic focal biliary cirrhosis.

In normal conditions secretin administration results in increased cellular cAMP levels, activation of CFTR[25], stimulation of bile flow and biliary bicarbonate secretion[1]. Reciprocal changes in biliary Cl^- concentrations indicate that an apical Cl^-/HCO_3^- exchange must be simultaneously activated[1,13,34,38]. It is still unclear how activation of CFTR relates to secretion of bicarbonate in the biliary fluid. In addition, the lower incidence of CF liver disease, with respect to pancreatic damage, suggests that other secretory mechanisms and signals may play a vicarious role in the biliary epithelium.

Based on work done on different epithelia, a number of hypotheses can be formulated to explain how mutated CFTR results in impaired bicarbonate transport. The anion exchange (AE-2) may be driven by the increased out-to-in gradient of Cl^- induced by the outward chloride flux induced by CFTR activation. However, in a human cholangiocyte cell line, AE-2 activity, measured from recovery rates after an intracellular alkali load, increased after administration of agents raising intracellular cAMP concentration, but this effect was not inhibited by pretreatment with the Cl^- channel inhibitor NPPB[39]. In addition, extracellular ATP, a nucleotide known to stimulate Cl^- efflux in cholangiocytes, did not increase AE-2 activity, suggesting that AE-2 is independent of Cl^- efflux mediated by cAMP and ATP-sensitive Cl^- conductances.

Alternatively, CFTR may allow a substantial HCO_3^- conductance, as shown in airways epithelial cells. However, cAMP did not increase HCO_3^- efflux in cells pretreated with DIDS, an inhibitor of AE-2, but not of CFTR. Moreover, neither cAMP nor ATP administration stimulated HCO_3^- influx in acidified, Na^+-depleted cells, indicating that no substantial HCO_3^- conductance is operated by ATP or cAMP-stimulated Cl^- channels[39].

Recent data from nasal and bronchial epithelia suggest that CFTR may function as a dual Cl^- and ATP conductance[40,41], and thus regulate the activity of other ion transporters through an autocrine mechanism involving extracellular ATP. In these cells extracellular ATP activates purinergic receptors, leading to opening of outward rectifying Cl^- channels (ORCC) and inhibition of Na^+ reabsorbtion through Na^+ channels[41]. This hypothesis could provide a link between CFTR activation and apical transport of ions different from Cl^- also in the biliary epithelium. Preliminary data in cholangiocyte cell lines indicate that extracellular ATP induced a P_{2u} receptor-mediated increase in the activity of the Na^+/H^+ exchanger[42]. The shift to the right of Na^+/H^+ exchange set point induced by ATP, caused a secondary increase in Cl^-/HCO_3^- exchange activity. Na^+/H^+ exchange activity was also increased by agents raising cellular cAMP levels, but this effect was inhibited by glybenclamide, a specific CFTR inhibitor that blocks ATP release from CFTR[41] and by the extracellular ATP scavenger hexokinase. Together with a recent preliminary report showing complete abolition of secretin-induced choleresis and bicarbonate secretion by the Na^+/H^+ exchange inhibitor amiloride[43], these data suggest that cAMP may increase Na^+/H^+ exchange through a CFTR-mediated ATP release from the cell. Intracellular pH_i alkalinization increases apical Cl^-/HCO_3^- exchange and further amplifies the secretory response. If confirmed, this model would explain how mutated CFTR results in decreased biliary HCO_3^- secretion. In addition, with ATP being constitutively present in the bile, this pathway would not be completely lost in cystic fibrosis, thus explaining why only a minority of patients develops clinical liver disease.

Extrahepatic cholestasis

Effects of cholestasis on hepatocellular transport systems have been reviewed by Meier (Chapter 11). In contrast to hepatocytes, acid/base transporter activity is not significantly different in cholangiocytes isolated from bile duct-ligated animals, suggesting that chronic cholestasis does not impair ion transport[1]. Rather, in the biliary epthelia, CFTR is more expressed[37,44] and choleretic response to secretin administration is much higher following common bile duct obstruction, partly as a result of an increased expression of the secretin receptor gene[45], findings that might explain the well-known occurrence of colourless, water- and electrolyte-enriched bile after bile duct ligation.

Immune-mediated cholangiopathies

Most primary cholangiopathies recognize an autoimmune pathogenesis. Mechanisms of cholestasis in these syndromes are unclear. Cholestasis may be due to obliteration of bile ducts, but it is usually present well before the onset of ductopenia and can be seen even in the absence of canalicular dilatation and bile plugs[11]. For example, the low sensitivity of PBC to immune-suppressive therapy, the association with secretory failure in other exocrine glands (sicca syndrome) and the beneficial effect of choleretic bile acids, suggest that, in addition to immune regulation, biliary electrolyte transport could also be impaired. A defective expression of the gene coding for the AE-2 apical anion exchanger has been reported in patients with PBC. AE-2 mRNA expression was decreased both in liver biopsies and in peripheral blood monuclear cells from PBC patients, but not in patients with cholestatic chronic liver diseases of different aetiology[46]. Preliminary experiments have shown a decrease in cAMP-stimulated HCO_3^- efflux in cholangiocytes isolated from patients with PBC[47]. These data suggest that alterations in biliary electrolyte transport may contribute to the pathogenesis of cholestasis in primary disorders of bile ducts. As opposed to experimental cholestasis, where inflammation is minimal, most ductopenic syndromes are associated to portal inflammation and the release of a number of cytokines[48]. As in inflammatory bowel disease, these cytokines may have profound effects on epithelial cell function, altering its transport properties[49–51]; it is a common clinical observation that cholestasis may appear during sepsis[52]; endotoxin administration decreases bile flow, an effect that is inhibited by antibodies against TNFα[53]; administration of IL-2 to cancer patients induces a reversible cholestasis[54]. It is known that cytokines may affect epithelial cell transport systems: INFγ has been shown to reduce CFTR expression in T-84 colonic cells[49] and IL-6 decreases the expression of the Na^+-dependent taurocholate transporter in hepatocytes (Ntcp)[55]. Clearly, the field of immune regulation of cholangiocyte function will prove to be very rewarding in the future.

BILE ACIDS AND CHOLANGIOPATHIES

Bile duct cells are exposed to high concentrations of bile acids from the lumenal side. As discussed elsewhere[56], bile acid interactions with the bile duct epithelium are complex. Available information suggests that the bile duct epithelium participates in the cholehepatic circulation of bile acids by passively reabsorbing unconjugated dihydroxy-bile acids that are then glyco- and tauro-conjugated and excreted from the basolateral side to the peribiliary circulation[56]. In addition, unconjugated dihydroxy-bile acids can acidify intracellular pH_i[57] and raise intracellular Ca^{2+} concentration in cholangiocytes[58]. Chronic administration of lithocholate causes bile duct hyperplasia and portal fibrosis in rats; a single oral dose of lithocholate increases DNA synthesis in the mouse biliary epithelium[59].

Recent studies indicate that the presence of cholesterol and phospholipids in the bile protects the biliary epithelium from the unrestrained effects of high monomeric concentrations of bile acids. Mice in which the gene encoding for the hepatocellular mdr-2 P-glycoprotein (a canalicular membrane transporter belonging to the ATP binding cassette superfamily, that acts as a phosphatidylcholine flippase) is disrupted by homologous recombination are characterized by the inability to secrete phospholipids into the bile, and by extensive ductular proliferation, portal inflammation and fibrosis[60] (see Chapter 13). Absence of phospholipids leads to a high monomeric concentration of bile acids into the bile. By changing the hydrophobicity of the bile acid pool through dietary manipulations, development of liver disease can be accelerated, suggesting that bile acids can exert both a damaging effect and a proliferative stimulus on cholangiocytes[30,60,61]. The mechanisms are unknown, and the effects of bile acids on the release of chemotactic inflammatory and paracrine mediators by cholangiocytes will certainly need to be elucidated in the future. Very recently, Deleuze and co-workers described two cases of familial progressive intrahepatic cholestasis associated with high serum γ-glutamyl transferase and ductal proliferation in which biliary phospholipids were remarkably reduced in the bile and mRNA for the *MDR-3* gene, the human homologue of mouse *mdr-2*, could not be detected in the liver[62]. The mdr-2 knock-out mouse will prove to be extremely useful in evaluating these mechanisms at a cellular level.

FROM PATHOPHYSIOLOGY TO THERAPY

The development of effective strategies for the treatment and prevention of liver complications has been included among the priorities to be achieved in cystic fibrosis research[35]. DNA-mediated gene transfer to cholangiocytes has been assessed in preliminary experiments. Adenovirus-mediated strategies have been shown to succesfully transduce reporter genes and CFTR in cultured cholangiocytes from normal and cystic fibrosis livers[63]. Interestingly, retrograde infusion of recombinant adenoviruses carring the CFTR gene resulted in successful gene expression in the biliary tree[64]. We believe that gene transfer approaches will prove to be a very promising strategy, not only to repair monogenic cholangiocyte transport defects, but also to influence the behaviour of cholangiocytes in chronic cholestatic syndromes. Development of genetic or pharmacological agents able to target specific cytokines or chemokines involved in different steps of the inflammatory/fibrotic/cholestatic response will probably provide effective and safe therapeutic strategies[10].

Better understanding of cholangiocyte pathophysiology will help in designing newer pharmacological approaches[65]. Ursodeoxycholic acid (UDCA) has been reported to improve liver function tests in cystic fibrosis patients with liver disease[35,66]. High-dose UDCA increased Ca^{2+} levels in a cholangiocyte cell line, and stimulated Cl^- efflux from the cell[58], an effect that may be helpful in a condition deriving from impaired cAMP-mediated Cl^- efflux, such as cystic fibrosis. UDCA has also been reported to be effective in other cholangiopathies (see chapters by Leuschner and by Podda). Possible mechanisms of action of UDCA in these syndromes are discussed by Calmus and by Beuers (Chapters 17 and 22).

References

1. Strazzabosco M, Zsembery A, Fabris L. Electrolyte transport in bile ductular epithelial cells. J Hepatol. 1996;24(Suppl. 1):78–87.
2. Matsumoto K, Fujii H, Michalopoulos G, Fung JJ, Demetris AJ. Human biliary epithelial cells secrete and respond to cytokines and hepatocyte growth factors *in vitro*: interleukin-6, hepatocyte growth factor and epidermal growth factor promote DNA synthesis *in vitro*. Hepatology. 1994:20:376–82.
3. Milani S, Herbst H, Schuppan D, Stein H, Surrenti C. Transforming growth factors β1 and β2 are differentially expressed in fibrotic liver disease. Am J Pathol. 1991;139:1221–9.
4. De Groen PC, Vroman B, LaRusso NF. Physiologic regulation of cholangiocyte proliferation *in vitro*. Proceedings of Digestive Disease Week, 19–22 May 1996;San Francisco, CA.

5. Marra F, De Franco R, Grappone C *et al.* Expression of monocyte chemotactic protein-1 during active hepatic fibrogenesis in humans. Ital J Gastroenterol. 1996;28:300.
6. Roberts SK, LaRusso NF. Pathobiology of biliary epithelia. Curr Opin Gastroenterol. 1994;10:526–33.
7. Tarsetti F, Lenzen R, Salvi R, Schuler E, Dembitzer R, Tavoloni N. Biology and pathobiology of intrahepatic biliary epithelium. In: Tavoloni N, Berk P, editors. Hepatic transport and bile secretion: physiology and pathophysiology. New York: Raven Press. 1993:619–34.
8. Davies MH, Harrison RF, Elias E, Hübscher SG. Antibiotic-associated acute vanishing bile duct syndrome: a pattern associated with severe, prolonged, intrahepatic cholestasis. J Hepatol. 1994;20:112–16.
9. Woolf GM, Vierling JM. Disappearing intrahepatic bile ducts: the syndromes and their mechanisms. Sem Liver Dis. 1993;13:261–75.
10. Robbins PD, Evans CH. Prospects for treating autoimmune and inflammatory diseases by gene therapy. Gene Therapy. 1996;3:187–9.
11. Popper H. General pathology of the liver: light microscopic aspects serving diagnosis and interpretation. Sem Liver Dis. 1986;6:175–84.
12. Ayres RCS, Neuberger JM, Shaw J, Adams DH. Intercellular adhesion molecule-1 and MHC antigens on human intrahepatic bile duct cells: effect of proinflammatory cytokines. Gut. 1993;34:1245–9.
13. Strazzabosco M, Boyer JL. Use of isolated bile ductular epithelial cells in biliary physiology. In: Muraca M, editor. Methods in biliary research. Boca Raton, FL: CRC Press. 1995;279–91.
14. Patel T, Gores JG. Apoptosis and hepatobiliary disease. Hepatology. 1995;21:1725–41.
15. Oberhammer FA, Pavelka M, Sharma S *et al.* Induction of apoptosis in cultured hepatocytes and in regressing liver by transforming growth factor β1. Proc Natl Acad Sci USA. 1992;85:408–12.
16. Sirica AE, Mathis GA, Sano N, Elmore LW. Isolation, culture, and transplantation of intrahepatic biliary epithelial cells and oval cells. Pathobiology. 1990;58:44–64.
17. Charlotte F, L'Hermine A, Martin N *et al.* Immunohistochemical detection of *bcl-2* protein in normal and pathological human liver. Am J Pathol. 1994;144:460–5.
18. Harnois D, Que F, Gores GJ, Pham LD, Kuntz SM, LaRusso NF. BCL-2 is overexpressed and alters the threshold for apoptosis in a cholangiocarcinoma cell line. Proceedings of the Digestive Disease Week, 19–22 May 1996; San Francisco, CA.
19. Benedetti A, Jezequel AM, Orlandi F. A quantitative evaluation of apoptotic bodies in rat liver. Liver. 1988;8:80–7.
20. Arias IM. State of the art lecture: Do all pathways of cholestasis lead to the canaliculus? In: Reyes HB, Leuschner U, Arias IM, editors. Pregnancy, sex hormones and the liver. Lancaster: Kluwer. 1995;68–76.
21. Terada T, Nakanuma Y. Detection of apoptosis and expression of apoptosis-related protein during human intrahepatic bile duct development. Am J Pathol. 1995;1465:67–74.
22. Bhathal PS, Gall JAM. Deletion of hyperplastic biliary epithelial cells by apoptosis following removal of the proliferative stimulus. Liver. 1985;5:311–25.
23. Koukoulis GK, Shen J, Foster P, Ganger D, Williams J. Immunolocalization of bcl-2 and MET oncoproteins in biliary ductules and ducts of normal liver, cirrhosis and ductopenic rejection. Hepatology. 1995;22:137A (abstract).
24. Koga H, Sakisaka S, Ohishi M, Sata M, Tanikawa K. Nuclear DNA fragmentation in biliary epithelial cells and in hepatocytes in primary biliary cirrhosis. Hepatology. 1995;22:121A (abstract).
25. Mc.Gill JM, Basavappa S, Gettys TW, Fitz JG. Secretin activates Cl^- channels in bile duct epithelial cells through a cAMP-dependent mechanism. Am J Physiol. 1994;266:G731–6.
26. Afford SC, Hubscher S, Strain AJ, Adams DH, Neuberger JM. Apoptosis in the human liver during allograft rejection and end-stage liver disease. J Pathol. 1995;176:373–80.
27. Patel. T, Spivey J, Vadakekalam J, Gores GJ. Apoptosis – an alternative mechanism of bile salt hepatotoxicity. In: Paumgartner G, Beuers U, editors. Bile acids in liver diseases. Lancaster: Kluwer. 1995;88–95.
28. Joplin R, Hishida T, Tsubouchi H *et al.* Human intrahepatic biliary epithelial cells proliferate *in vitro* in response to human hepatocyte growth factor. J Clin Invest. 1992;90:1284–9.
29. Pinzani M, Milani S, Grappone C. Cholestasis and fibrogenesis. In: Gentilini P, *et al.* editors. Cholestasis. Amsterdam: Elsevier. 1994:129–39.
30. Pinzani M. Hepatic stellate (ITO) cells: expanding roles for a liver-specific pericyte. J Hepatol. 1995;22:700–6.

31. Maher JJ, McGuire RF. Extracellular matrix gene expression increases preferentially in rat lipocytes and sinusoidal endothelial cells during hepatic fibrosis *in vivo*. J Clin Invest. 1990;86:1641–8.
32. Milani S, Herbst H, Schuppan D, Riechen EO, Stein H. Cellular localization of laminin gene transcripts in normal and fibrotic human liver. Am J Pathol. 1989;134:1175–82.
33. Elias I, Alpini G, Gubba S *et al.* Antiproliferative effect of γ-interferon in carbon tetrachloride (CCL_4)-induced cirrhosis. Hepatology. 1995;22:277A (abstract).
34. Marino CR, Gorelick FS. Scientific advances in cystic fibrosis. Gastroenterology. 1992;103:681–93.
35. Colombo C, Battezzati PM, Podda M. Hepatobiliary disease in cystic fibrosis. Sem Liver Dis. 1994;14:259–69.
36. Lindblad A, Hultcrantz R, Strandvik B. Bile duct destruction and collagen deposition: a prominent ultrastructural feature of the liver in cystic fibrosis. Hepatology. 1992;16:372–81.
37. Cohn JA, Strong TV, Picciotto MR, Nairn AC, Collins FS, Fitz JG. Localization of the cystic fibrosis transmembrane conductance regulator in human bile duct epithelial cells. Gastroenterology. 1993,105:1857–64.
38. Strazzabosco M, Mennone A, Boyer JL. Intracellular pH_i regulation in isolated rat bile duct epithelial cells. J Clin Invest. 1991;87:1503–12.
39. Zsembery A, Spirli C, Poci C, Okolicsanyi L, Crepaldi G, Strazzabosco M. Cyclic-AMP stimulates bicarbonate efflux in bile duct epithelial cells through Cl^-/HCO_3^- exchange independently of Cl^- conductance activation. Ital J Gastroenterol. 1996;28:306.
40. Reisin IL, Prat AG, Abraham EH *et al.* The cystic fibrosis transmembrane conductance regulator is a dual ATP and chloride channel. J Biol Chem. 1994;32:20584–91.
41. Schwiebert EM, Egan ME, Hwang T-H *et al.* CFTR regulates outwardly rectifying chloride channels through an autocrine mechanism involving ATP. Cell. 1995;81:1063–73.
42. Zembery A, Spirli C, Granato A, Okolicsanyi L, Crepaldi G, Strazzabosco M. Autocrine regulation of transepithelial H^+/HCO_3^- transport through CFTR-mediated ATP release in bile duct cells. Hepatology. 1996(In press) (abstract).
43. Renner EL, Heydtmann M. Amiloride, but not DIDS and NPPB, inhibits secretin-induced choleresis: evidence for a role of Na^+/H^+, but not Cl/HCO_3 exchange and Cl^- channels in ductular bile formation. Hepatology. 1995;22:315A (abstract).
44. Fitz JG, Basavappa S, McGill J, Melhus O, Cohn JA. Regulation of membrane chloride currents in rat bile duct epithelial cells. J Clin Invest. 1993;91:319–28.
45. Alpini G, Ulrich CD II, Phillips JO, Pham LD, Miller JL, LaRusso NF. Upregulation of secretin receptor gene expression in rat cholangiocyte after bile duct ligation. Am J Physiol. 1994;266:G922–8.
46. Prieto J, Qian C, Garcia N, Diez J, Medina JF. Abnormal expression of anion exchanger genes in primary biliary cirrhosis. Gastroenterology. 1993;105:572–8.
47. Strazzabosco M, Joplin R, Zsembery A *et al.* Bicarbonate transport in cultured human intrahepatic bile duct epithelial cells from normal subjects and patients with primary biliary cirrhosis. Hepatology. 1994;20:405A (abstract).
48. Martinez OM, Villanueva JC, Gershwin ME, Krams SM. Cytokine patterns and cytotoxic mediators in primary biliary cirrhosis. Hepatology. 1995;21:113–19.
49. Besançon F, Przewlocki G, Baró I, Hongre A-S, Escande D, Edelman A. Interferon-γ downregulates CFTR gene expression in epithelial cells. Am J Physiol. 1994;267:C1398–404.
50. Balfour Sartor R. Cytokines in intestinal inflammation: pathophysiological and clinical considerations. Gastroenterology. 1994;106:533–9.
51. Perdue MH, McKay DM. Integrative immunophysiology in the intestinal mucosa. Am J Physiol. 1994;267:G151–65.
52. Zimmerman H, Fang M, Utili R, Seef L, Hoofnagle J. Jaundice due to bacterial infections. Gastroenterology. 1979;77:362–74.
53. Whiting J, Rosenbluth A, Narcisso J, Gollan J. Tumor necrosis factor-α inhibits taurocholate uptake by hepatocytes: implications for the pathogenesis of endotoxin-induced cholestasis. Gastroenterology. 1991;100:A811 (abstract).
54. Fisher B, Keenan A, Garra B *et al.* Interleukin-2 induces profound reversible cholestasis: a detailed analysis in treated cancer patients. J Clin Oncol. 1989;7:1852–62.
55. Green RM, Whiting JF, Rosenbluth AB, Beier D, Gollan JL. Interleukin-6 inhibits hepatocyte taurocholate uptake and sodium–potassium–adenosinetriphosphatase activity. Am J Physiol. 1994;267:G1094–1100.

56. Strazzabosco M, Zsembery A, Granato A, Poci C, Rossanese A, Crepaldi G. Effects of bile acids on bile duct epithelial cells. In: Paumgartner G, Beuers U, editors. Bile acids in liver diseases. Lancaster: Kluwer. 1995;113–18.
57. Strazzabosco M, Poci C, Spirli C, Knuth A, Sartori L, Crepaldi G. Effect of ursodeoxycholic acid (UDCA) on intracellular pH in a bile duct epithelium-like cell line. Hepatology. 1994;19:145–54.
58. Shimokura GH, McGill M, Fitz JG. Ursodeoxycholate activates ion permeabilities in biliary epithelial cells. Gastroenterology. 1994;107:236–43.
59. Bagheri SA, Bolt MG, Boyer JL, Palmer RH. Stimulation of thymidine incorporation in mouse liver and biliary tract epithelium by lithocholate and deoxycholate. Gastroenterology. 1978;74:188–92.
60. Smit JJM, Schinkel AH, Oude Elferink RPJ *et al.* Homozygous disruption of the murine mdr-2 p-glycoprotein gene leads to a complete absence of phospholipid from bile and to liver disease. Cell. 1993;75:451–62.
61. Oude Elferink RPJ, Frijters C, Ottenhoff R, Van Wijland M, Groen K. Hepatobiliary cholesterol secretion and the function of mdr-2 P-glycoprotein. In Paumgartner G, Beuers U, editors. Bile acids in liver diseases. Lancaster: Kluwer. 1995:101–5.
62. Deleuze JF, Jacqemin E, Dubuisson C *et al.* Defect of multidrug-resistance 3 gene expression in a subtype of progressive familial intrahepatic cholestasis. Hepatology. 1996,23:904–8.
63. Grubman SH, Fang SL, Mulberg AE *et al.* Correction of the cystic fibrosis defect by gene complementation in human intrahepatic biliary epithelial cell lines. Gastroenterology. 1995;108:584–92.
64. Yang Y, Raper ES, Cohn JA, Engelhardt JF, Wilson JM. An approach for treating the hepatobiliary disease of cystic fibrosis by somatic gene transfer. Proc Natl Acad Sci USA. 1993;90:4601–5.
65. Wagner JA, Chao AC, Gardner P. Molecular strategies for therapy of cystic fibrosis. Annu Rev Pharmacol Toxicol. 1995;35:257–76.
66. Balistreri WF. The liver – the next frontier in the treatment of patients with cystic fibrosis. In: Reyes HB, Leuschner U, Arias IM, editors. Pregnancy, sex hormones and the liver. Lancaster: Kluwer. 1995;114–35.

13
The role of mdr2 P-glycoprotein in lipid secretion and ductular damage

C. VAN NIEUWKERK, M. DE VREE, M. VAN WIJLAND, R. OTTENHOFF, J. G. A. OFFERHAUS, A. K. GROEN and R. P. J. OUDE ELFERINK

INTRODUCTION

Bile salts are cytotoxic compounds. Many studies have demonstrated that incubation of cells with micellar concentrations of bile salts leads to rapid lysis. It is the aggregated, micellar state which is the lytic component, as it is clearly observed that cytotoxicity increases steeply when the critical micellar concentration (CMC) is reached[1–3]. Therefore there is a clear correlation between the degree of cytotoxicity and hydrophobicity. The cytotoxicity of bile salt solutions can be drastically reduced by the addition of phospholipid[1,3]. This leads to the formation of mixed micelles, which are much less capable of extracting phospholipids from cellular membranes than simple micelles. When cholesterol is also added toxicity decreases further. It was therefore hypothesized that one of the main functions of biliary lipid secretion is to reduce the cytotoxic action of the high concentrations of bile salts that prevail in the biliary tree. Indeed, concentrations of bile salts measured in hepatic bile are far above the CMC, and a mechanism must therefore exist to protect cells lining the biliary tree. So far studies into the protective effect of phospholipid and cholesterol have been performed only in acute experimental systems with model cells or membranes, and it it still not clear what role biliary lipids play in the protection against bile salts *in vivo*. For this purpose the *mdr2* (–/–) knockout mouse represents an interesting model[4]. These animals do not secrete phospholipid into bile as it has been shown that mdr2 P-glycoprotein is a phosphatidylcholine translocator[5,6]. Cholesterol and phosphatidylcholine secretion are coupled under most conditions; therefore these animals also have virtually no cholesterol secretion[7]. Interestingly, these animals develop progressive liver disease which can best be described as inflammatory non-suppurative cholangitis. Portal inflammation, bile duct proliferation and fibrosis are the hallmarks of this pathological pattern[8]. On the basis of the studies mentioned above it was hypothesized that this pathology was induced by the cytotoxicity of bile salts in the absence of lipids.

The endogenous bile salt pool of mice is very hydrophilic, i.e. consists of bile salts with a relatively high CMC. About 70% of the murine bile salt pool consists of tauromuricholate, the remainder being taurocholate. In order to test the role of bile salts in the induction of the pathology we have fed *mdr2* (–/–) mice diets to which either cholate or ursodeoxycholate was added. This feeding regime rendered the bile salt pool more hydrophobic or hydrophilic, respectively. Progression of the liver disease was monitored by measurement of liver enzymes in serum and by semiquantitative scoring of liver histology. The severity of the pathological process could be related to the hydrophobicity of the bile salt pool. In addition a difference was observed in the severity of liver disease between male and female *mdr2* (–/–) and this correlated with a more hydrophobic bile salt composition of female mice.

METHODS

Directly upon weaning, *mdr2* (–/–) mice and wild-type (+/+) mice were divided into three groups receiving either control purified diet or the same diet to which 0.1% cholate or 0.5% ursodeoxycholate was added. After 22 weeks on this diet serum was collected and the liver was excised for histological examination. Liver histology was semiquantitatively scored for five histopathological parameters in four grades of severity (0–3): mitotic activity, portal inflammation, ductular proliferation, Councilman bodies and fibrosis. This scoring system is the same as described previously[8].

RESULTS

Female *mdr2* (–/–) mice had an almost two-fold higher content of taurocholate in their bile than male *mdr2* (–/–) mice (34 ± 4% vs 18 ± 2%); the remainder being tauromuricholate (Figure 1). Tauromuricholate was efficiently replaced by taurocholate after feeding 0.1% cholate-supplemented diet in both male and female mice. On the other hand, when the mice were fed an ursodeoxycholate-supplemented diet the bile salt pool was largely replaced by tauroursodeoxycholate (75% and 78% in male and female mice respectively), the remainder being tauromuricholate.

The mean total histological score for male and female *mdr2* (–/–) mice on the various diets is given in Figure 2. Female (–/–) mice on a purified control diet showed significantly higher histopathological scores than male (–/–) mice. Portal inflammation and ductular proliferation especially contributed to this higher score, and were mainly responsible for the difference. Mice that had been fed a cholate-containing diet for 22 weeks had a very severe pathology, consisting of portal inflammation, ductular proliferation and severe fibrosis. As this picture gave an almost maximal score in both male and female (–/–) mice, there was no longer a gender difference. Mice fed an ursodeoxycholate-containing diet had an overall decrease in histopathological score and here, too, no difference was observed between male and female animals.

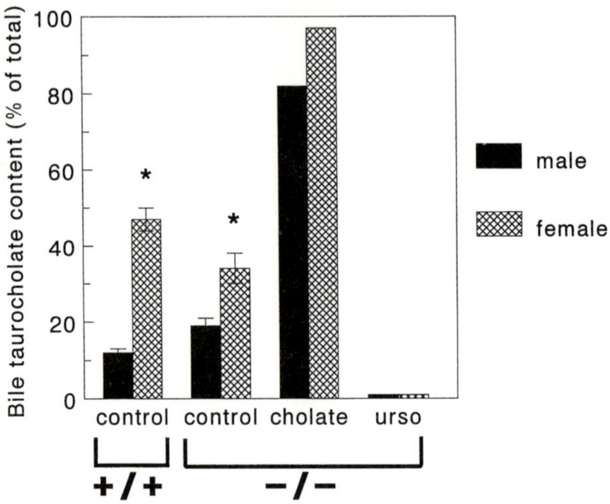

Figure 1 Biliary bile salt composition of *mdr2* (+/+) and (–/–) mice on various diets. Mice were fed for 22 weeks with a purified diet to which either nothing (control) or 0.1% cholate (cholate) or 0.5% ursodeoxycholate (urso) was added. Subsequently, bile was sampled and bile salt composition analysed. The figure indicates the taurocholate content as a percentage of total bile salts. On control diet and cholate-supplemented diet the remainder of the bile salts consisted of tauromuricholate. On an ursodeoxycholate-supplemented diet 78% ± consisted of tauroursodeoxycholate, the remainder being tauromuricholate. This content was identical in male and female *mdr2* (+/+) and (–/–) mice

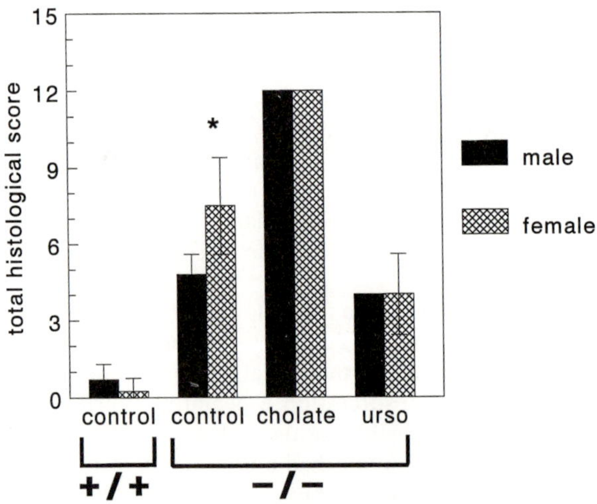

Figure 2 Mean histological score of *mdr2* (+/+) and (–/–) mice on various diets. Mice were fed for 22 weeks with a purified control diet to which either nothing (control) or 0.1% cholate (cholate) or 0.5% ursodeoxycholate (urso) was added. Subsequently the livers were excised and scored histologically as described in Methods. Mean histological scores of *mdr2* (+/+) mice on cholate- and ursodeoxycholate-supplemented diets were not different from the indicated scores on control diet

DISCUSSION

The liver pathology in *mdr2* (–/–) mice is characterized by a gradually progressive picture that affects mainly the portal triads. The main features are ductular proliferation and portal inflammation with relatively little hepatic damage and only weak fibrosis. The nature of the bile salt species in bile of the *mdr2* (–/–) mouse clearly determines the course and outcome of this pathological process. The majority of the endogenous murine bile salt pool consists of tauromuricholate, which is a relatively hydrophilic bile salt. When the bile salt pool is largely replaced by taurocholate, which is more hydrophobic than tauromuricholate, a more rapid and severe progression of the liver disease is observed. Under these conditions extreme proliferation of bile ducts is observed, accompanied by heavy inflammation of the portal fields together with striking fibrosis. In addition, pathology was more severe in female than in male *mdr2* (–/–) mice when fed a purified control diet. This correlated with a higher taurocholate content of female bile compared to male bile. The reason for the difference in bile salt composition is unclear, but may relate to a different expression of the enzymes in the bile salt synthetic route between the two genders. The difference in bile salt composition is independent from the *mdr2* (–/–) phenotype, as the same difference was observed in *mdr2* (+/+) mice. The difference in the total pathology score between male and female mice disappeared when the animals were fed cholate or ursodeoxycholate and this correlated with the fact that the bile salt pool became similar in both sexes, i.e. mainly taurocholate or tauroursodeoxycholate respectively. In conclusion our data show that subtle changes in bile salt composition of *mdr2* (–/–) already have a profound influence on the development of pathology. This suggests that a complete phospholipid secretion defect in humans would most probably lead to severe liver damage, because the bile salt composition in humans is much more hydrophobic than in mice. This, however, does not exclude the possibility that in humans a partial defect in phospholipid secretion may lead to inflammatory non-suppurative destruction of bile ducts. The two most important entities in which this morphology is the predominating characteristic are primary biliary cirrhosis (PBC) and primary sclerosing cholangitis (PSC). The aetiology and pathophysiological mechanism of these two disorders are not understood, but immunological, cytotoxic and infectious noxes may be important factors. So far, no aberrations in bile composition, including phospholipid content, have been reported for these patient groups. It could, however, be that a (small) subgroup of patients exists in which the disease is caused or promoted by a partial defect in the phospholipid secretion capacity.

References

1. Sagawa H, Tazuma S, Kajiyama G. Protection against hydrophobic bile salt-induced cell membrane damage by liposomes and hydrophilic bile salts. Am J Physiol. 1993;264:G835–9.
2. Heuman DM. Hepatoprotective properties of ursodeoxycholic acid. Gastroenterology. 1993;104:1865–70.
3. Velardi ALM, Groen AK, Oude Elferink RPJ, van der Meer R, Palasciano G, Tytgat GNJ. Cell type-dependent effect of phospholipid and cholesterol on bile salt cytotoxicity. Gastroenterology 1991;101:457–64.

4. Smit JJM, Schinkel AH, Oude Elferink RPJ *et al.* L, Homozygous disruption of the murine mdr2 P-glycoprotein gene leads to a complete absence of phospholipid from bile and to liver disease. Cell. 1993;75:451–62.
5. Smith AJ, Timmermans-Hereijgers JLPM, Roelofsen B *et al.* The human MDR3 P-glycoprotein promotes translocation of phosphatidylcholine through the plasma membrane of fibroblasts from transgenic mice. FEBS Lett. 1994;354:263–6.
6. Ruetz S, Gros P. Phosphatidylcholine translocase: a physiological role for the mdr2 gene. Cell. 1994;77:1071–82.
7. Oude Elferink RPJ, Ottenhoff R, van Wijland M, Frijters CMG, van Nieuwkerk C, Groen AK. Uncoupling of biliary phospholipid and cholesterol secretion in mice with reduced expression of mdr2 P-glycoprotein. J Lipid Res. 1996 (In press).
8. Mauad TH, van Nieuwkerk CMJ, Dingemans KP *et al.* Mice with homozygous disruption of the mdr2 P-glycoprotein gene: a novel animal model for studies of nonsuppurative inflammatory cholangitis and hepatocarcinogenesis. Am J Pathol. 1994;145:1237–45.

14
Pathogenesis of non-suppurative destructive cholangitis

R. JOPLIN and J. NEUBERGER

INTRODUCTION

The term 'non-suppurative destructive cholangitis' (NSDC) defines the bile duct pathology associated with the condition more commonly referred to as primary biliary cirrhosis (PBC)[1]. PBC can be considered as a systemic condition characterized by a wide range of symptoms in addition to the liver pathology, and including pruritus, elevated serum immunoglobulins, circulating autoantibodies and a generalized 'dry gland' syndrome[2]. Despite the presence of these other features which collectively contribute to the diagnosis of PBC the overriding clinical manifestation of PBC is NSDC. The NSDC associated with PBC is chronic and characterized by inflammatory lesions specifically in the intrahepatic biliary tree[3]; extrahepatic biliary tracts appear unaffected by the disease process. Progressive damage to intrahepatic biliary ducts leads to fibrotic replacement of portions of biliary tree and protracted intrahepatic cholestasis ensues, followed ultimately by liver failure, for which liver transplantation is the only viable therapeutic option. The histological progression of NSDC is defined by four grades of disease severity termed histological stages I–IV[2]. These stages range from inflammation and damage of small to medium-sized interlobular bile ducts (stage I), through progressive loss of interlobular ducts with fibrosis and accompanying compensatory ductular proliferation (stages II and III), to cirrhosis (stage IV). Despite the generalizations in staging it is well recognized that there is lack of uniformity with respect to both distribution and extent of disease within the biliary tree; even in end-stage disease, and in the presence of extensive cirrhosis, some portal tracts remain in which continuing inflammatory activity is present, while still others may appear relatively uninvolved by the disease process[3].

The pathogenesis of NSDC remains unknown. Studies into possible pathogenetic mechanisms are complicated because of the protracted duration of the condition; the intitiating event may be temporally far removed from onset of symptoms. In addition, study of the target tissue for NSDC, the intrahepatic biliary ducts and biliary epithelium has, historically, been difficult. In the absence of a convincing animal model for PBC, studies of NSDC have been limited to observations of histological sections of patients' liver obtained either from post-mortem tissue, diagnostic biopsy or, in recent years, end-stage tissue from hepatectomy specimens. The histological characteristics of such tissues may have little relevance to the original lesion or initiating event. Many recent developments have concentrated on immunological aspects of PBC, partly because of the relatively easier access to immunological cells and molecules, and a large body of evidence has accumulated in support of autoimmune aetiological mechanisms.

HYPOTHETICAL MECHANISMS FOR THE PATHOGENESIS OF NON-SUPPURATIVE DESTRUCTIVE CHOLANGITIS

The close association of inflammatory infiltrates in the portal regions composed predominantly of T lymphocytes of both CD4 and CD8 phenotypes is only one of several lines of evidence to suggest an autoimmunological pathogenesis for PBC. Patients may also show a number of other features commonly associated with autoimmune diseases. The biliary epithelium of patients with PBC has been shown aberrantly to express HLA class II antigens[4] and intercellular adhesion molecule I[5]; both factors important in lymphocyte recognition of antigen in target cells. Other features include association with other autoimmune diseases[6], female preponderance (approximately 10 : 1 female to male ratio)[7] and weak association with specific HLA profiles[8]. Additionally, patients with PBC have highly specific circulating autoantibodies which recognize mitochondrial antigens, and which are virtually diagnostic of the condition[9]. Despite much circumstantial evidence implicating autoimmunological pathogenetic mechanisms there are a number of features which suggest that other factors are also involved. Environmental factors may be important, as geographical clustering has been reported[10] and there have been reports of transmissibility between non-genetically linked individuals[11]. In addition, patients with PBC do not respond to conventional immunosuppresive therapy. Finally, the HLA associations are weak and no clear-cut strong HLA associations have emerged. Thus it remains unclear whether the appearance of autoimmunological features is of aetiological significance, or whether these features arise as a consequence of pathology, and several hypotheses as to other potential aetiological factors and mechanisms for disease progression have been proposed.

Olomu *et al.* reported that patients with PBC had reduced capacity for *in vivo* sulphoxidation of *S*-carboxy-methyl-cysteine[12]. Some agents depend on sulphation in the liver for detoxification prior to excretion. The alternatives to sulphated forms are potent cholestatic glucuronides. Hypothetical alteration in the balance of sulphated oestrogens to hepatotoxic glucuronides was proposed as a pathogenetic mechanism for generation of the biliary lesions in NSDC, citing involvement of impaired sulphation as a mechanism of predisposition of PBC for menopausal females. However, despite its initial attractiveness this hypothesis has subsequently been refuted.

More recently involvement of chloride–bicarbonate anion exchangers, a family of proteins thought to participate in intracellular pH regulation and generation of hydroionic fluxes into secretions, has been implicated. Decreased levels of mRNA for the AE2 anion exchanger were reported for liver from patients with PBC[13]. AE2 was localized to the canaliculi and lumenal membrane of interlobular bile ducts, but in PBC the ductular expression of AE2 as judged by immunohistochemistry was significantly reduced relative to controls[14]. Thus the results of both molecular biological and immunohistochemical studies suggested some deficit in ductular AE2, leading to the hypothesis that AE2 expression might be involved in the pathogenesis of NSDC.

Other investigators have proposed that some of the immunological features of PBC are consistent with the expected response to an infectious agent. A wide range of infectious agents have been identified which have antigens in common with mitochondria, and it has been suggested that patients' antimitochondrial antibodies (AMA) could arise by cross-reactivity with a microbial species. If the infectious agent carried antigens cross-reactive with biliary tree components, chronic autoreactivity towards the biliary tract could ensue. Evidence implicating mutant R forms of *Escherichia coli*[15] and *Mycobacterium gordonae*[16] have been reported with the suggestion that the observed autoimmune reaction ensues as the result of cross-reaction between the infectious agent and patients' own antigens.

MITOCHONDRIAL AUTOANTIBODIES AND ANTIGENS

An important advance in the study of PBC was identification of the autoimmune targets for AMA as components of the 2-oxo-acid dehydrogenase (2-OAD) complexes. These complexes are high molecular weight assemblies of multiple copies of several enzymes, and occupy key positions in cellular respiration. The major antigenic component of these functionally related enzymes has a molecular weight of approximately 70 kDa and has been identified as a sequence within the inner lipoyl domain of the dihydrolipoamide acetyltransferase (E2) component of pyruvate dehydrogenase complex (PDC)[17–19]. Mammalian PDC is composed of multiple copies of four separate enzymes termed E1 (pyruvate decarboxylase), E2, E3 (dihydrolipoamide dehydrogenase) and component X, which promote oxidative decarboxylation of pyruvate with production of acetyl-CoA and NADH[20]. Sixty separate E2 subunits form an oligomeric 'core' to which E1 (20–30 molecules), E3 (six molecules) and component X (12 molecules) are attached. The other four antigens recognized by patients' antibodies are the E2 components of branched chain oxo-acid dehydrogenase (BCOADC) and 2-oxoglutarate dehydrogenase complex (OGDC) and E1 and component X of PDC. Sera from more than 95% of patients with PBC contain antibodies which recognize both PDC-E2 and PDC-X, and approximately 50% of patients' sera recognize E2 components of all three 2-oxo-acid dehydrogenase complexes. Only 5% recognize BCOADC-E2 and OGDC-E2 but not PDC-E2. Three per cent of patients' sera have no detectable reaction with any of the five antigens (AMA negative)[21].

ROLE OF MITOCHONDRIAL AUTOANTIBODIES AND ANTIGENS IN THE PATHOGENESIS OF NSDC

The 2-OAD complexes are associated with the mitochondrial inner membrane where they catalyse key reactions of intermediary metabolism. They are present in all aerobic cells, but are particularly abundant in tissues with high energy requirement, such as muscle. Historically, the involvement of either mitochondrial autoantibodies or antigens in the pathogenesis of PBC has been uncertain. The biliary epithelial cell targets have a relative paucity of mitochondria and form a minority population in liver, yet the damage in NSDC shows extraordinary specificity for biliary epithelium. Thus the autoantibodies and antigens were considered as probably irrelevant or secondary features to the induction or progress of the disease. However, there are now increasing lines of evidence that involvement of PDC-E2 may be of more significance than originally thought. First, lymphocytes from patients with PBC but not controls have been shown to be stimulated by PDC-E2 but not the other components of PDC[22,23]. Secondly, the major autoantigen, PDC-E2, shows atypical distribution in target tissue (biliary epithelium), specifically in patients with primary biliary cirrhosis[24–26].

Autoantibodies

In order to speculate about the possible aetiological significance of autoantibodies and antigens in PBC, studies should be undertaken very early in the natural history of disease progression; before the onset of clinical symptoms if possible. Serological studies by Mitchison *et al.* have demonstrated that elevated titre of antimitochondrial antibody precedes development of histological NSDC[27]. The serum of 29 subjects with normal serum bilirubin, alkaline phosphatase and transaminase, and who had no symptoms of liver disease, were found to be positive for AMA. During follow-up of 16 of these individuals, symptoms associated with PBC developed, including NSDC. The AMA reactivity in these subjects was in the same IgG subclass as a control group of 23 patients with clinically, biochemically and histologically advanced PBC. As the presence of the AMA pre-dated development of clinical manifestations of NSDC these data suggest that antimitochondrial antibodies may have a role other than as a secondary feature of tissue damage.

Autoantigens

As a key enzyme of the respiratory chain the major mitochondrial antigen, PDC-E2, has very widespread distribution in tissue and is present in all aerobic cell types. Patients' antimitochondrial antibodies show typical particulate staining of kidney (routinely used in diagnosis of PBC) corresponding to the distribution of mitochondria in kidney cells. Recent studies of the distribution of PDC-E2 in human tissues using a variety of antibodies, including antibodies raised in rabbit[24], mouse monoclonals[25] and human monoclonals and combinatorial antibodies[26] have revealed characteristic mitochondrial staining of most cells in

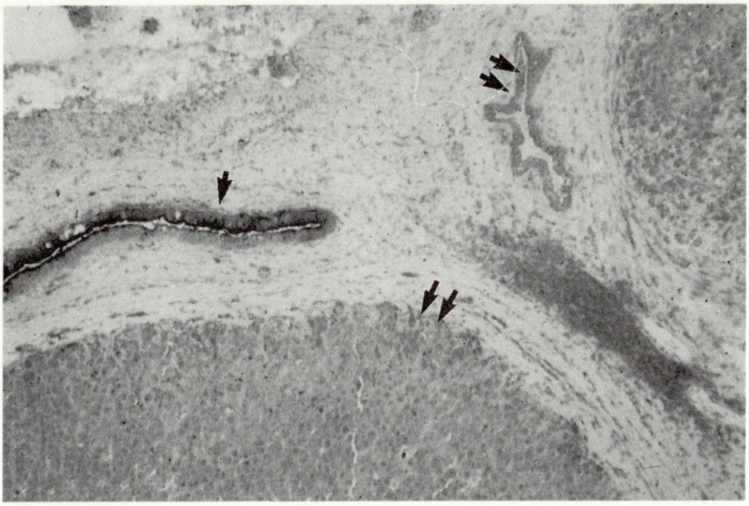

Figure 1 Micrograph of the distribution of binding of rabbit anti-PDC-E2 antibody to a section of PBC liver. One bile duct shows high intensity of antibody binding (single arrow) relative to another duct and to hepatocytes (double arrows) (from ref. 24)

human tissues. However, high-intensity diffuse staining was seen on the biliary epithelium, specifically in patients with PBC, when rabbit, human and some mouse antibodies were used (Figure 1). In our own experiments we have used immunohistochemistry to compare the intensity of PDC-E2 in biliary epithelium in PBC liver with that of E1 and E3 components of PDC. The results, summarized in Figure 2, indicate increased intensity of E2 relative to E1 and E3 and other mitochondrial enzymes, citrate synthase, monoamine oxidase and mitochondrial inner membrane antigen, MCA151A[28]. Previous studies had shown the mitochondria of biliary epithelial cells in PBC liver to be variably enlarged and/or increased in number[29,30]. Thus the higher intensity of PDC-E2 in biliary epithelium could have been due to mitochondrial metaplasia. However, double-labelling studies demonstrated that in the biliary epithelium of PBC liver, but not hepatocytes or other cell types, the atypical distribution of PDC-E2 was not related to the distribution of mitochondria. Further confocal microscopic and electron microscopic studies by Gershwin and co-workers indicated that antigen was concentrated at the lumenal surface of bile ducts, associated with the apical membrane of biliary epithelial cells[31,32].

Gershwin and co-workers also demonstrated increased intensity and atypical distribution of PDC-E2 on biliary epithelium very early in the ontogeny of PBC. Elevated intensity of PDC-E2 in biliary epithelial cells preceded detection of class II expression or the T cell co-stimulatory factor BB1/B7[33]. Thus one of the earliest events in the pathogenesis of NSDC may be over-expression of PDC-E2 or a PDC-E2-like molecule by the biliary epithelial cell targets. A high level of intracellular antigen would lead to association with MHC class I molecules with consequent presentation on the biliary ductular surface. This could then render

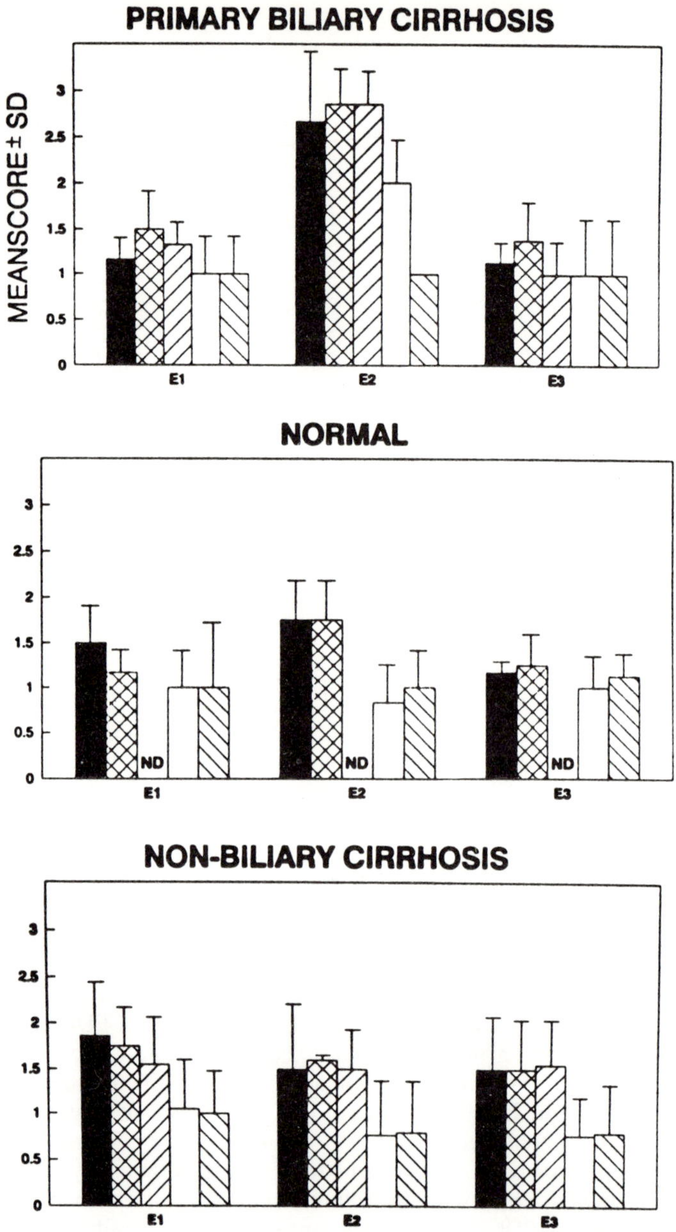

(a)

(b)

(c)

Figure 2 Intensity of binding of rabbit anti-PDC-E1, E2 and E3 to biliary epithelium and hepatocytes in the liver of patients with PBC **(a)**, normal **(b)** and other liver disease controls **(c)**. Intensity was expressed semiquantitatively on a scale of increasing intensity from 0 to 3. Bar key (left to right): filled, septal ducts; cross-hatch, interlobular ducts; diagonal shade, atypical biliary ductules; open, periportal hepatocytes; diagonal shade, perivenular hepatocytes. ND = none detected. (from ref. 24)

the biliary epithelial cells targets for CD8+ cytotoxic lymphocytes, and generate an immune cascade including differentiation of plasma cells and secretion of autoantibody.

Our understanding of the T cell response in PBC may be further enhanced by identification of the biliary epithelial cell antigens recognized by cytotoxic T cells and by anti-PDC-E2 antibodies. However, there are a number of problems to confront when attempting to undertake studies to elucidate the nature of biliary epithelial cell antigens. First, the biliary epithelial cell lining of the biliary tract represents a minority population of cells in the liver. The problem is exacerbated in PBC as the biliary epithelial cell population is depleted by the disease process. A further problem relates to the heterogeneity in distribution of the disease within an individual liver, in that when only relatively small fragments of tissue are available for study there may be difficulties in achieving adequate representative sampling of ducts involved in the disease. Finally, use of whole tissue to study a minority cell population is limiting in terms of the resolution available. Because of the widespread tissue distribution of E2, when whole tissue is used, large amounts of data may be generated, and it may be difficult to differentiate between results pertaining to the disease process and normal expression of E2. Recently, advances in the purification of biliary epithelial cells from human cholestatic diseased liver have permitted the development of focused approaches to study human biliary epithelium. Sampling efficiency of biliary epithelial cells is improved if the cells are isolated from a larger volume of liver than is possible using tissue sections. In addition, the ability to focus on the target cells of the disease minimizes the contribution of irrelevant data to the results generated.

PURIFICATION OF INTRAHEPATIC BILIARY EPITHELIAL CELLS

Intrahepatic biliary epithelial cells represent only about 3–5% of total cells in normal liver[34], presenting problems with isolating adequate cell numbers for *in-vitro* studies. In animal models, induction of compensatory proliferated ductules by bile duct ligation can expand the biliary epithelial cell population by up to 100-fold, and this has been used extensively to generate sufficient cells for study[35]. However, it is debatable whether the hyperplastic cells represent an acceptable model of normal biliary epithelial cells. Preparations of hyperplastic biliary epithelial cells will contain a relatively decreased population of cells from the original ducts. This could be an important factor if the property of interest is differentially expressed on the unproliferated epithelial cells of larger ducts. In addition, animal models may not accurately reflect normal or pathobiological processes in humans. Indeed, differences in anion exchange mechanisms have been reported between biliary epithelial cells derived from the liver of rats and humans[36], and expression of phenotypic markers may differ between humans and animals[37].

Several techniques have been described for physically separating intrahepatic biliary epithelial cells from other cell types in the liver of rodents. Almost all techniques described rely on initial dissociation of the liver tissue with digestive enzymes. This process generates a heterogeneous mixture of cell types which requires further purification to enrich the proportion of biliary epithelial cells. Improvements in the purity of the isolated cells can be achieved in a number of ways, including differential density centrifugation, centrifugal elutriation, fluorescence-activated cell sorting and immunological selection procedures, used either singly or in combination[38]. Adaptations of some of these methods to permit isolation of human intrahepatic biliary epithelial cells from normal[39–41] and diseased[40,42] human liver have been described.

In our own laboratories we have devised a method to isolate intrahepatic biliary epithelial cells from normal and end-stage diseased human liver, based on the positive selection of cells expressing the biliary epithelial cell surface antigen egp34[43]. Following collagenase digestion of liver, biliary epithelial cells are semipurified by differential density centrifugation on a 1.04/1.09 mg/ml Percoll gradient (Figure 3). This yields a non-parenchymal cell fraction at the 1.04/1.09 mg/ml Percoll interphase, of which biliary epithelial cells constitute approximately 10%. Biliary epithelial cells are further purified from this fraction by immunomagnetic separation of cells expressing egp34 which is recognized by the monoclonal antibody HEA125[39,42]. HEA125 positive cells, which fractionate differentially because of altered buoyant density, may also be extracted from other parts of the Percoll gradient. HEA125 positive cells from the pre-biliary epithelial cell Percoll fraction (1.04 mg/ml Percoll; Figure 3) are less than 95% viable and extensive cellular damage can be demonstrated ultrastructurally (Figure 4). HEA125 positive cells immunopurified from the post-biliary epithelial cell fraction (1.09 mg/ml Percoll; Figure 3) are small, non-polar cells

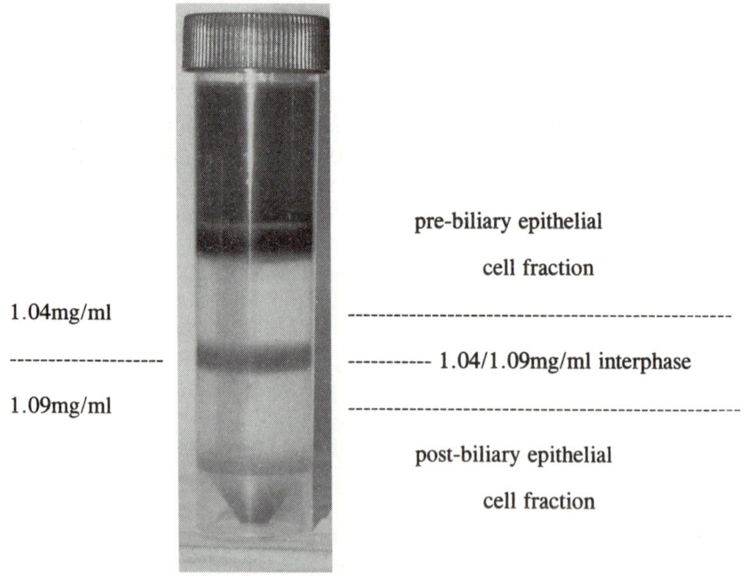

Figure 3 Differential density centrifugation of liver digests on Percoll

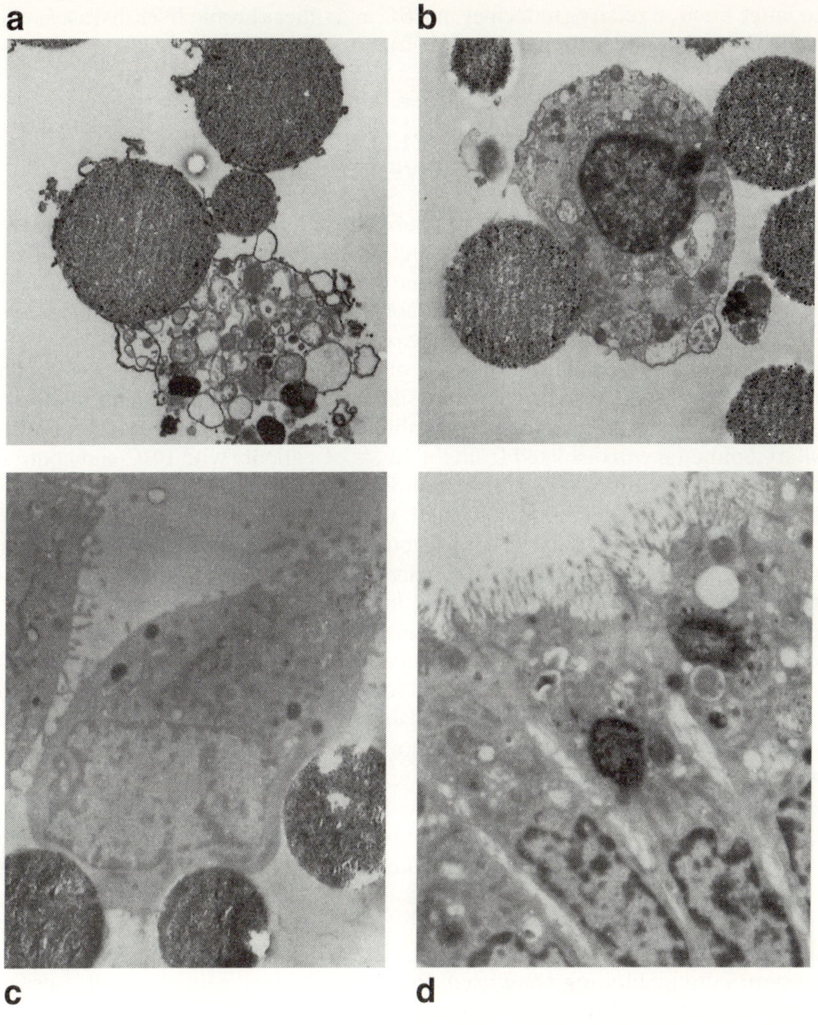

Figure 4 Transmission electron micrographs of cells isolated from the pre-biliary epithelial cell fraction **(a)**, post-biliary epithelial cell fraction **(b)**, and the Percoll interphase **(c, d)**

with a high nucleus to cytoplasm ratio (Figure 4). Characterization studies indicate that the biliary epithelial cell population isolated from the 1.09/1.04 mg/ml Percoll interphase exhibits features associated with normal biliary epithelial cell phenotype and morphology, while cells from the post-biliary epithelial cell fraction (1.09 mg/ml Percoll) show features associated with atypical proliferative ductular cells. The relative yield of the biliary epithelial cell and atypical ductular cell populations varies according to the type of tissue used. The ratio of cells isolated from the 1.04/1.09 mg/ml Percoll interphase and post-biliary epithelial cell (1.09 mg/ml Percoll) fractions indicates increased proportion of cells from the latter fraction relative to former in PBC and other chronic liver diseases relative to normal controls (unpublished data).

PURIFIED BILIARY EPITHELIAL CELLS IN THE STUDY OF NON-SUPPURATIVE DESTRUCTIVE CHOLANGITIS

We have used our isolated biliary epithelial cells to initiate a number of studies to analyse the subcellular distribution and biochemical nature of autoantigens in biliary epithelial cells in PBC. For this work we used biliary epithelial cells derived from the 1.04/1.09 mg/ml Percoll interphase, and thus excluded cells derived from atypical ductular hyperplasia.

To study the subcellular distribution of PDC-E2 in isolated biliary epithelial cells differential immunocytochemical staining was used, based on the property of viable cells to exclude antibody. Viable (unfixed) and permeabilized (fixed) biliary epithelial cells isolated from the livers of patients with PBC and controls were incubated with human anti-human-PDC antibodies, affinity-purified from the serum of patients with PBC and with antibodies raised in rabbits by immunization with PDC-E2. The distribution of antibody binding to cells was examined by high-resolution microscopy using laser scanning confocal microscopy and transmission electron microscopy. For confocal microscopy cells were analysed in a series of 0.5 μm optical sections in the *Z*-axis. In fixed cells intense diffuse staining was seen in cells isolated from PBC liver, while in controls staining was particulate and compatible with the distribution of mitochondria. Because unfixed cells were viable when incubated with antibody they excluded antibody from the cell interior. Thus only binding of antibodies to target molecules associated with the external surface of the cells was possible. Surface staining was identified specifically in cells isolated from the liver of patients with PBC and not controls (Figure 5). The data suggest that in PBC and not controls a biliary epithelial cell membrane antigen recognized by antibodies to PDC-E2 is present[44,45].

To identify those biliary epithelial cell antigens recognized by anti-PDC-E2 antibodies biochemically, polyacrylamide gel electrophoresis (PAGE) and Western immunoblotting were used. Proteins in biliary epithelial cells purified from PBC and control livers were separated by polyacrylamide gel electrophoresis (PAGE). After transfer to nitrocellulose by Western blotting, those antigens recognized by human anti-human-PDC were determined by immunostaining of blots using human antibodies affinity-purified from patients' serum. Two protein bands were detected which co-migrated with E2 and X components of purified human heart PDC (Figure 6). Novel cross-reactive, non-PDC antigens or breakdown products of PDC-E2 or PDC-X were not detected[46].

There is compelling evidence to suggest that the antigen which is atypically distributed in the biliary epithelial cells of patients with PBC is not PDC-E2 but a cross-reactive molecule. Gershwin and co-workers demonstrated that, out of eight mouse monoclonal antibodies that reacted with PDC-E2, only one showed atypical distribution on biliary epithelial cells in PBC liver[31]. These data were interpreted as evidence that only a single epitope of PDC-E2 is responsible for the atypical reaction with biliary epithelium, and the presence of a cross-reactive

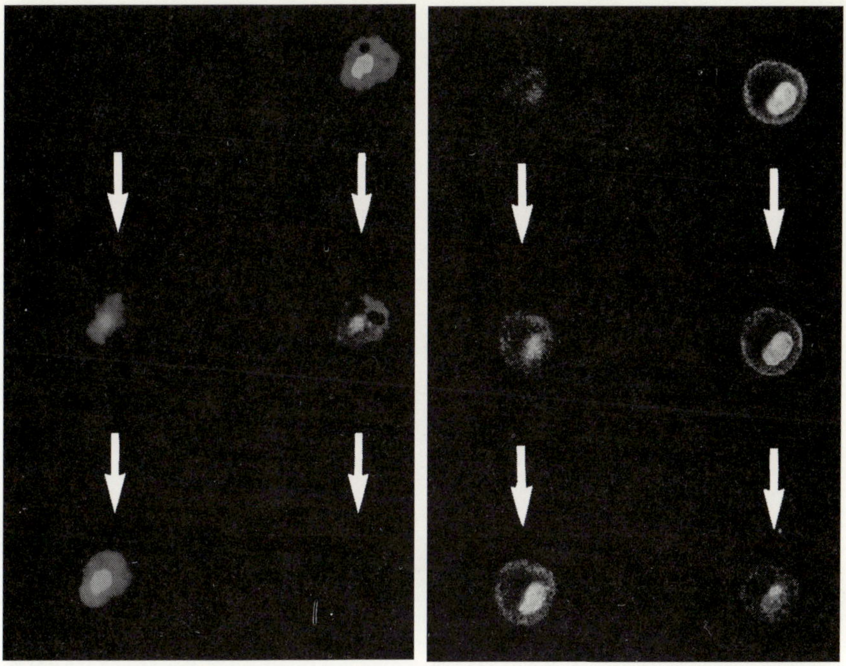

(a) (b)

Figure 5 Laser scanning confocal micrographs showing the distribution of human anti-human-PDC to fixed (**a**) and unfixed (**b**) biliary epithelial cells from a patient with PBC. Each image in the *Z*-axis represents antibody binding to serial optical sections at increments of 1 μm through an individual cell, as indicated by arrows. Nuclei were visualized using propidium iodide counterstain

epitope on an unrelated molecule was suggested as a possible explanation. However, our own immunoblotting experiments have failed to reveal any different, cross-reactive antigens in biliary epithelial cells from patients with PBC, as only PDC-E2 and PDC-X were detected. Immunohistochemistry using antibody raised specifically against PDC-X showed high intensity of anti-X binding to biliary epithelium in PBC liver. Furthermore, confocal microscopy showed that anti-PDC-X binding was stronger towards the lumenal pole of the cells[47], similar to the distribution previously reported for PDC-E2[31]. This suggests that the cross-reactive antigen recognized by antibodies to PDC-E2 could be PDC-X.

Less is known about PDC-X than about the other components of PDC. In contrast to E1 and E3, protein X remains tightly associated with the E2 core assembly after treatment with high salt or high pH and, through ^{14}C-acetylation studies, the single lipoyl domain of protein X has been shown to be capable of all E2-type reactions. In addition, following selective proteolysis or gene deletion of the lipoyl domains of E2, protein X can substitute for E2[48]. This functional homology is reflected in considerable structural homology between the lipoyl domains of E2 and X, and antibodies which recognize the lipoyl domains of E2 usually cross-react with the lipoyl domain of X. Thus extensive structural

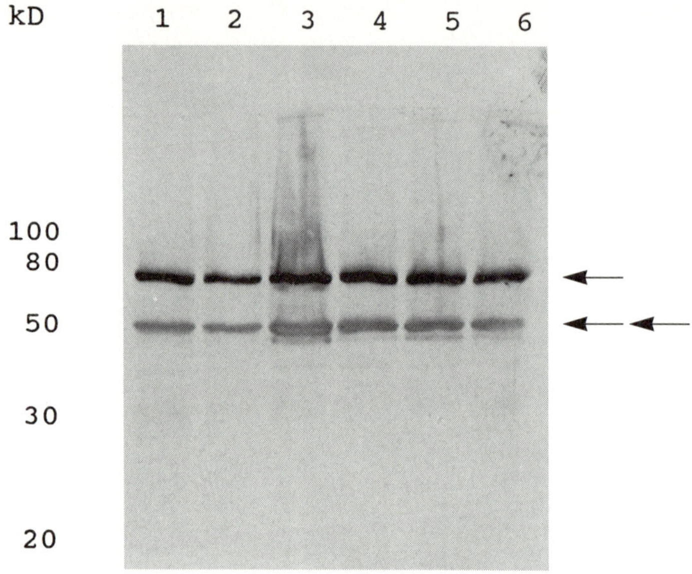

Figure 6 Western blot of proteins from 10^5 biliary epithelial cells, immunostained using human anti-human-PDC antibodies. Biliary epithelial cells were isolated from PBC liver (lanes 1, 3, and 5) and normal controls (lanes 2, 4, and 6) and cultured for 2–3 weeks before preparation for PAGE. Two major bands were identified in all samples which migrated with molecular weights of 70 kDa (PDC-E2, single arrow) and 50 kDa (PDC-X, double arrow)

and functional homology exists between the lipoyl domains of the two autoantigens. These data indicate that the higher intensity of antibody binding to biliary epithelium of patients with PBC could be as a result of PDC-X. The availability of purified biliary epithelial cell isolates will enable further studies to characterize the mitochondrial antigens.

HYPOTHETICAL MECHANISMS OF IMMUNE-MEDIATED DAMAGE TO BILIARY EPITHELIUM IN NON-SUPPURATIVE DESTRUCTIVE CHOLANGITIS

A number of cytotoxic mechanisms could bring about the destruction of bile ducts in NSDC, including T cell-mediated cytotoxicity, antibody-dependent cytotoxicity and complement-mediated damage.

Complement-mediated damage

The complement system has been shown to be activated in PBC[49]. Circulating immune complexes containing AMA and biliary antigens could activate complement, which could lead to complement-mediated lysis of biliary epithelial cells[50]. Alternatively antibody binding to cell surface antigen could activate complement. However, such immune complexes have been identified only in a minority of patients with PBC.

Antibody-dependent cell cytotoxicity

Antibody-dependent cell cytotoxicity (ADCC) depends on binding of an effector cell with receptors for the Fc portion of immunoglobulin to antibody on target cells. The finding of autoantigen associated with the plasma membrane of biliary epithelial cells in PBC suggests that cell lysis could occur through ADCC. ADCC as a mechanism of damage in PBC has not been demonstrated, but decreased activity of the natural killer effector cells which mediate ADCC has been reported for peripheral blood cells[51]. Thus it seems unlikely that ADCC is an important mechanism of cell damage *in vivo*.

T lymphocyte-mediated cytotoxicity

A number of observations suggest involvement of T lymphocyte cytotoxicity in damage to biliary epithelium in PBC. Cytotoxic T cells are present in intimate contact with damaged biliary epithelial cells in histological sections of PBC liver[52,53]. This appears to be most marked in specimens obtained from patients with stage I PBC, suggesting a primary involvement in aetiological mechanisms rather than a secondary response in tissue damage[54]. The nature of the biliary epithelial cell antigens recognized by cytotoxic T lymphocytes is unknown, but evidence from two groups has demonstrated the ability of patients' T cells to respond to the mitochondrial antigen PDC-E2. Jones *et al.* demonstrated that peripheral blood T cells from patients with PBC showed significantly higher proliferative responses to PDC-E2/X than lymphocytes from control patients[22]. No difference between PBC and controls was observed when responses to E1 and E3 components were studied. Van de Water *et al.* demonstrated the ability to generate PDC-E2 specific T lymphocyte clones from T cells sequestered in the liver of patients with PBC but not controls[23,25]. Thus specificity of the autoantibody response is reflected at the level of T cell responses also.

Jones *et al.* proposed that the immune response in PBC is initiated by the interaction of T lymphocytes with either biliary epithelial cells or a professional antigen-presenting cell[50] (Figure 7). T lymphocyte recognition of specific antigen depends critically on interaction between major histocompatibility complex (MHC) antigen complexed with specific antigen, adhesion molecules and other co-stimulatory co-factors on target cells. Numerous studies have now demonstrated that biliary epithelial cells are, in certain circumstances, immunologically active. In PBC (and a range of other liver diseases) biliary epithelial cells show aberrant expression of MHC class II antigens, increased expression of MHC class I[4,33,55], expression of the T cell co-stimulatory factor BB1/B7[33] and expression of lymphocyte adhesion molecules[5,56,57]. Despite variation in estimates regarding the extent of up-regulation of certain of these molecules the data demonstrate that the immunological molecules which are a prerequisite of immune recognition and damage to cells are all in place in the biliary epithelial cell targets in PBC. In addition several studies of biliary epithelial cells *in vitro* have demonstrated the inducibility of these molecules in response to certain cytokines[58,59]. However, the role of expression of MHC, adhesion and co-stimulatory factors in induction of PBC is uncertain, as data regarding the extent of expression of these molecules and their relationship to the progression of PBC are conflicting.

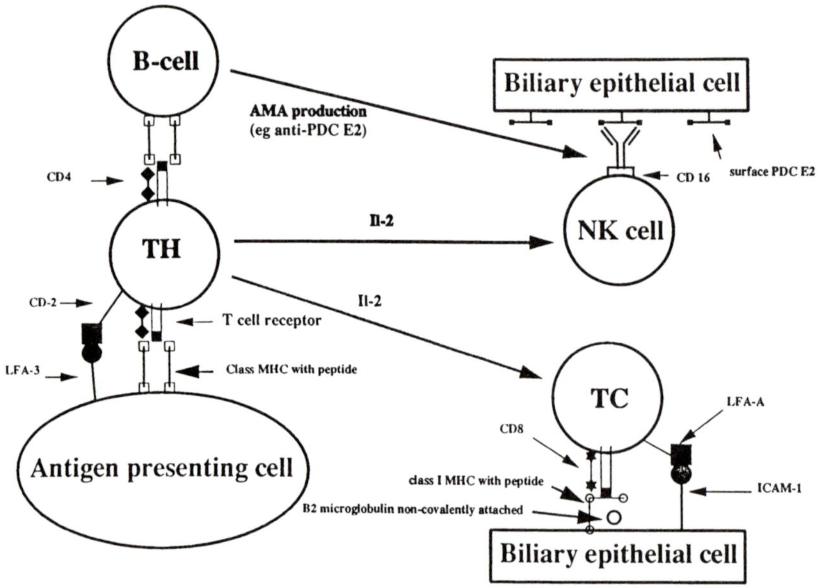

Figure 7 Proposed model of cell interactions in the autoimmune response to biliary epithelial cells in PBC (from Jones *et al.* 1994[50])

Biliary epithelial cell cytotoxicity in vitro

Study of potential cytotoxic mechanisms in PBC has been limited due to the inavailability of the targets for *in-vitro* studies. Some studies were undertaken using hepatocytes to study ADCC, but no increase in cytotoxicity could be demonstrated[60]. However, hepatocytes are not the primary target cell in PBC. Another potential application of isolated biliary epithelial cells is to address the question of mechanisms for cytolytic damage of biliary epithelial cells. In our own laboratories we have developed and validated a sensitive LDH release assay for assessing lymphocyte-mediated damage to biliary epithelial cells. Our preliminary studies indicate that biliary epithelial cells are potent stimulators of cytotoxic T cell activation and toxicity (Figure 8). A strong cytolytic response can be generated by incubating lymphocytes with biliary epithelial cells. This response is enhanced if the lymphocytes are pre-incubated with biliary epithelial cells and re-challenged after 3 days. The data suggest that PBC biliary epithelial cells express antigens which are able to induce a strong cytolytic reaction (unpublished data).

CONCLUSIONS

The precise mechanisms in the pathogenesis of non-suppurative destructive cholangitis remain to be determined. New technologies are enabling study of the importance of biliary epithelial cell antigens in the development of NSDC.

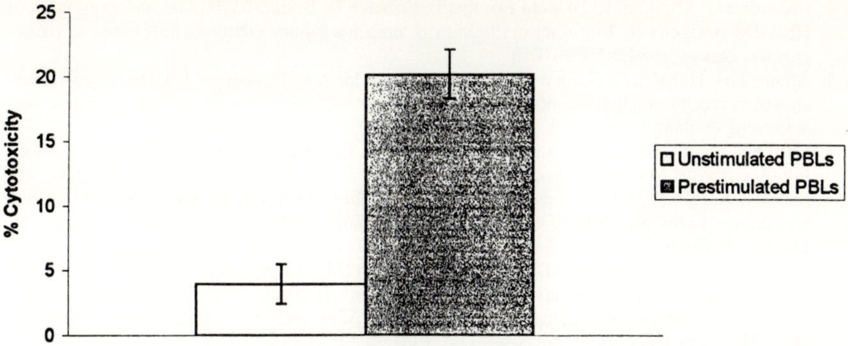

Figure 8 Percentage cytotoxicity of lymphocytes towards biliary epithelial cells. Biliary epithelial cells were incubated with prestimulated (previously exposed to the biliary epithelial cells) or unstimulated peripheral blood lymphocytes (PBL) at a ratio of 100 : 1 effectors to targets for 4 h. Prestimulated lymphocytes showed significantly more toxicity towards allogeneic biliary epithelial cells than did unstimulated lymphocytes. Mean of five experiments ± SEM

The data derived from our studies of biliary epithelial cells *in vitro* tend to support the concept of autoimmunological mechanisms in PBC. PDC-E2 or a PDC-E2-like antigen was detected associated with the plasma membrane of biliary epithelial cells specifically in PBC. Characterization of the biliary epithelial cell autoantigens by PAGE and Western blotting indicated that only native PDC-E2 and PDC-X was recognized by anti-PDC-E2 antibodies; cross-reactive, non-PDC antigens were not detected in biliary epithelial cells from patients with PBC. In addition, biliary epithelial cells from patients with PBC evoked a strong cytolytic reaction from lymphocytes. The rationale of using end-stage diseased liver to study the role of target cells in the pathogenesis of PBC has been the subject of some valid criticism. The argument assumes that disease-specific cells will have been destroyed by the disease process, and the isolated cells will merely represent a population of cells which are unaffected by the disease process. However, abnormalities both in autoantibody and antigen which have been demonstrated in end-stage PBC have also been reported during early disease. Although it could be argued that the biliary epithelial cells isolated from end-stage tissue must represent those which had escaped damage during progression of the disease, it should be remembered that, even in late-stage disease, portal tracts are involved with continuing inflammatory activity, suggesting that stimulation by antigen is still occurring. However, the precise role of biliary ductular expression of PDC molecules as aetiological factors in NSDC remains uncertain.

References

1. Rubin E, Schaffner F, Popper H. Primary biliary cirrhosis: chronic non-suppurative destructive cholangitis. Am J Pathol. 1965;46:387–407.
2. Schaffner F, Popper H. Clinical–pathologic relations in primary biliary cirrhosis. In: Popper H, Schaffner F, editors. Progress in liver disease. New York; Grune & Stratton. 1982:529–54.
3. Nakanuma Y, Ohta G. Histometric and serial observations of intrahepatic bile ducts in primary biliary cirrhosis. Gastroenterology. 1979;76:1326–32.

4. Ballardini G, Mirakian R, Bianchi FB, Pisi E, Doniach D, Bottazzo GF. Aberrant expression of HLA-DR antigens on bile duct epithelium in primary biliary cirrhosis: relevance to pathogenesis. Lancet. 1984;2:1009–1013.
5. Adams DH, Hubscher SG, Shaw J, Johnson GD, Rothlien R, Neuberger JM. Increased expression of intercellular adhesion molecule 1 (ICAM-1) on bile ducts in primary biliary cirrhosis and sclerosing cholangitis. Hepatology. 1991;14:426–31.
6. Culp KS, Fleming RC, Duffy J, Baldus WP, Dickson ER. Autoimmune associations in primary biliary cirrhosis. Mayo Clin Proc. 1982;57:365–70.
7. Sherlock S. Primary biliary cirrhosis. In: Wright R, Millward-Sadler G, Alberti KGMM, Karran S, editors. Liver and biliary disease, pathophysiology, diagnosis, management. 2nd edn. London: Bailliere Tindal WB Saunders; 1985;861–79.
8. Gores GJ, Moore SB, Fisher LD, Powell EC, Dickson ER. Primary biliary cirrhosis: association with class II major histocompatibility complex antigens. Hepatology. 1987;7:889–92.
9. Munoz LE, Thomas HC, Scheuer PJ, Doniach D, Sherlock S. Is mitochondrial antibody diagnostic of primary biliary cirrhosis? Gut. 1981;22:136–40.
10. Triger DR. Primary biliary cirrhosis: an epidemiological study. Br Med J. 1980;28:772–75.
11. Douglas JG, Finlayson NDC. Are increased individual susceptibility and environmental factors both necessary for the development of primary biliary cirrhosis. Br J Med. 1979;2:419–20.
12. Olomu AB, Vickers CR, Waring RH *et al.* High incidence of poor sulfoxidiation in patients with primary biliary cirrhosis. N Engl J Med. 1988;318:1089–92.
13. Prieto J, Qian C, Garcia N, Diez J, Medina JF. Abnormal expression of anion exchanger genes in primary biliary cirrhosis. Gastroenterology. 1993;105:572–8.
14. Medina JF, Martinez-Anso E, Vasquez JJ, Prieto J. Reduced AE2 immunoreactivity in the liver in primary biliary cirrhosis (PBC) and in salivary glands from PBC patients with sicca syndrome (SS). J Hepatol. 1995;23:71.
15. Hopf U, Stemeromicz R, Rodloff A *et al.* Relation between *Escherichia coli* R (rough)-forms in gut, lipid A in liver and primary biliary cirrhosis. Lancet. 1989;2:1421–2.
16. Vilagut L, Vila J, Pares A *et al. Mycobacterium gordonae* DNA in liver tissue of patients with primary biliary cirrhosis. J Hepatol. 1994;21:S87.
17. Gershwin ME, Mackay IR, Sturgess A, Coppel RL. Identification and specificity of a cDNA encoding the 70kD mitochondrial antigen recognized in primary biliary cirrhosis. J Immunol. 1987;138:3525–31.
18. Coppel RL, McNeilage J, Surh CD *et al.* Primary structure of the human M2 mitochondrial autoantigen of PBC: dihydrolipoamide acetyltransferase Proc Natl Acad Sci USA. 1988;85:7317–21.
19. Fussey SPM, Guest JR, James OFW, Bassendine MF, Yeaman SJ. Identification and analysis of the major M2 autoantigens in PBC. Proc Natl Acad Sci USA. 1988;85:8654–8.
20. Yeaman SJ. The 2-oxo acid dehydrogenase complexes: recent advances. Biochem J. 1989;257:625–32.
21. Bassendine MF, Fussey SPM, Mutimer DJ, James OFW, Yeaman SJ. Identification and characterisation of four M2 mitochondrial autoantigens in primary biliary cirrhosis. Semin Liver Dis. 1989;9:124–31.
22. Jones DEJ, Palmer JM, James OFW, Yeaman SJ, Bassendine MF, Diamond AG. T cell responses to the components of the pyruvate dehydrogenase complex in primary biliary cirrhosis. Hepatology. 1995;21:995–1002.
23. Van de Water J, Ansari A, Prindiville T *et al.* Heterogeneity of autoreactive T cell clones specific for the E2 component of pyruvate dehydrogenase complex in primary biliary cirrhosis. J Exp Med. 1995;181:723–33.
24. Joplin R, Lindsay JG, Hubscher SG *et al.* Distribution of dihydrolipoamide acetyltransferase (E2) in the liver and portal lymph nodes of patients with primary biliary cirrhosis: an immunohistochemical study. Hepatology. 1991;14:442–7.
25. Van de Water J, Ansari AA, Surh CD *et al.* Evidence for the targeting by 2-oxo-dehydrogenase enzymes in the T cell response of primary biliary cirrhosis. J Immunol. 1991;146:89–94.
26. Cha S, Leung PSC, Gershwin ME, Fletcher MP, Ansari AA, Coppel RL. Use of a combinatorial immunoglobulin library to generate antibodies to pyruvate dehydrogenase complex (PDC-E2), the major autoantigen of primary biliary cirrhosis. Proc Natl Acad Sci USA. 1993;90:2527–31.
27. Mitchison HC, Bassendine MF, Hendrick A *et al.* Positive antimitochondrial antibody but normal liver function tests: is this primary biliary cirrhosis? Hepatology. 1986;6:1279–84.

28. Joplin RE, Johnson GD, Matthews JB *et al.* Distribution of pyruvate dehydrogenase dihydrolipoamide acetyltransferase (PDC-E2) and another mitochondrial marker in salivary gland and biliary epithelium from patients with primary biliary cirrhosis. Hepatology. 1994:19:1375–80.
29. Berneau D, Feldmann G, Degott C, Gisselbrecht C. Ultrastructural lesions of bile ducts in primary biliary cirrhosis. Human Pathol. 1981;12:782–93.
30. Tobe K. Electron microscopy of liver lesions in primary biliary cirrhosis. Acta Pathol Jpn. 1982;32:57–70.
31. Van de Water J, Turchany J, Leung PSC *et al.* Molecular mimicry in primary biliary cirrhosis. Evidence for biliary epithelial cell expression of a molecule cross-reactive with pyruvate dehydrogenase complex-E2. J Clin Invest. 1993;91:2653–64.
32. Nakanuma Y, Tsuneyama K, Kono N, Hoso M, Van de Water J, Gershwin ME. Biliary epithelial expression of the pyruvate dehydrogenase complex in primary biliary cirrhosis: an immunohistochemical and immunoelectron microscopic study. Human Pathol. 1995;26:92–8.
33. Tsuneyama K, Van de Water, Leung PSC *et al.* Abnormal expression of PDC-E2 on the luminal surface of biliary epithelium occurs before MHC class II and BB1/B7 expression. Hepatology. 1995;21:1031–7.
34. Sternlieb I. Functional implications of human portal and bile ductular ultrastructure. Gastroenterology. 1972;63:321–7.
35. Sirica AE, Mathis HA, Sano N, Elmore LW. Isolation, culture and transplantation of intrahepatic biliary epithelial cells and oval cells. Pathobiology. 1990;58:44–64.
36. Strazzabosco M, Joplin R, Szembery A, *et al.* Bicarbonate transport in cultured human intrahepatic bile duct epithelial cells (hBDE) from normal subjects and patients with primary biliary cirrhosis (PBC). Hepatology. 1994;20:405A.
37. Paradis K, Sharp HL. *In vitro* duct-like structure formation after isolation of bile ductular cells from a murine model. J Lab Clin Med. 1989;113:689–94.
38. Joplin R. Isolation and culture of biliary epithelial cells Gut. 1994;35:875–8.
39. Joplin R, Strain AJ, Neuberger JM. Immuno-isolation and culture of biliary epithelial cells from normal human liver. In Vitro Cell Dev Biol. 1989;25:1189–92.
40. Strain AJ, Wallace LL, Joplin R *et al.* Characterization of biliary epithelial cells isolated from needle biopsies of human liver in the presence of hepatocyte growth factor. Am J Pathol. 1995;146:537–45.
41. Demitris AJ, Markus B, Saidman S, *et al.* Isolation and primary cultures of human intrahepatic bile ductular epithelium. In Vitro Cell Dev Biol. 1988;24:464–70.
42. Joplin R, Strain AJ, Neuberger JM. Biliary epithelial cells from the liver of patients with primary biliary cirrhosis: isolation characterization, and short-term culture. J Pathol. 1990;162:255–60.
43. Momburg F, Moldenhauer G, Hammerling GH: Immunohistochemical study of the surface expression of a M_r 34,000 human epithelium-specific glycoprotein in normal and malignant tissues. Cancer Res. 1987;47:2883–91.
44. Joplin RE, Lindsay JG, Johnson GD, Strain AJ, Neuberger JM. Membrane dihydrolipoamide acetyltransferase (E2) on human biliary epithelial cells in primary biliary cirrhosis. Lancet. 1992;339:93–4.
45. Joplin R, Wallace LL, Johnson GD, *et al.* Subcellular localization of pyruvate dehydrogenase dihydrolipoamide acetyltransferase in human intrahepatic biliary epithelial cells. J Pathol. 1995;176:381–90.
46. Joplin R, Wallace LL, Palmer JM, Yeaman SJ, Neuberger JM. Reaction of anti-pyruvate dehydrogenase antibodies with biliary epithelial cell antigens in primary biliary cirrhosis. J Hepatol. 1995;23:164.
47. Joplin R, Wallace LL, Johnson GD, Lindsay JG, Strain AJ, Neuberger JM. Distribution of component X of pyruvate dehydrogenase complex (PDC-X) in liver and salivary gland of patients with primary biliary cirrhosis (PBC) and controls. Hepatology. 1994;20:150A.
48. Neagle J, de Marcucci O, Dumbar B, Lindsay JG. Component X of mammalian pyruvate dehydrogenase complex: structural and functional relationship to the lipoamide acetyltransferase (E2) component. FEBS Lett. 1989;253:11–15.
49. Wands JR, Dienstag JL, Bhan AK, Feller ER, Isselbacher KJ. Circulating immune complexes and complement activation in primary biliary cirrhosis. N Engl J Med. 1978;298:233–7.
50. Jones DEJ, Gregory WL, Bassendine MF. Primary biliary cirrhosis. In: Thomas HC, and Waters I, editors Immunology of liver diseases. Dordrecht: Kluwer; 1994:121–43.

51. James SP, Hoofnagle JH, Strober W, Jones EA. Primary biliary cirrhosis – a model autoimmune disease. Ann Intern Med. 1983;99:500–12.
52. Yamada G, Hyodo I, Tobe K *et al.* Ultrastructural immunocytochemical analysis of lymphocytes infiltrating bile duct epithelia in primary biliary cirrhosis. Hepatology. 1986;6:385–91.
53. Aizawa Y, Toda G. Primary biliary cirrhosis (PBC): concept, pathogenesis and classification. Jpn J Clin Med. 1994;52:240–56.
54. Miller KB, Elta GH, Rudders RA, Kaplan MM. Lymphocyte subsets in primary biliary cirrhosis. Ann Intern Med. 1984;100:385–7.
55. Broome U, Hultcrantz R, Scheynius A. Lack of concomitant expression of ICAM-1 and HLA-DR on bile duct cells from patients with primary sclerosing cholangitis and primary biliary cirrhosis. Scand J Gastroenterol. 1993;28:126–30.
56. Bloom S, Fleming K, Chapman R. Adhesion molecule expression in primary sclerosing cholangitis and primary biliary cirrhosis. Gut. 1995;36:604–9.
57. Yasoshima M, Nakanuma Y, Tsuneyama K, Van de Water J, Gershwin ME. Immunohistochemical analysis of adhesion molecules in the micro-environment of portal tracts in relation to aberrant expression of PDC-E2 and HLA-Dr on the bile ducts in primary biliary cirrhosis. J Pathol. 1995;175:319–25.
58. Saidman SL, Duquesnoy RJ, Zeevi A, Fung JJ, Starzl TE, Demetris AJ. Recognition of major histocompatibility complex antigens on cultured human biliary epithelial cells by alloreactive lymphocytes. Hepatology. 1991;13:239–46.
59. Ayres RCS, Neuberger JM, Shaw J, Joplin R, Adams DH. Intercellular adhesion molecule-1 and MHC antigens on human intrahepatic bile duct cells: effect of pro-inflammatory cytokines. Gut. 1993;34:1245–9.
60. Vierling JM, Nelson DL, Strober W, Bundy BM, Jones EA. *In vitro* cell-mediated cytotoxicity in primary biliary cirrhosis and chronic hepatitis. J Clin Invest. 1977;60:1116–28.

15 Immunological mechanisms of cholangiocyte injury

J. M. VIERLING

INTRODUCTION

Multiple diseases and congenital–developmental abnormalities result in immunological injury of cholangiocytes and destruction of bile ducts[1,2]. Collectively, those processes resulting in ductopenia have been referred to as 'vanishing bile duct syndromes'[3]. Although immunological mechanisms may be involved in cholangiocyte and bile duct injury observed in many diseases[1,2], several diseases appear to have a primary autoimmune or alloimmune basis (Table 1)[1–6]. The principal autoimmune diseases include primary biliary cirrhosis (PBC), autoimmune cholangitis (AIC or alternatively antimitochondrial antibody-negative PBC) and primary sclerosing cholangitis (PSC)[1,2–4]. The major alloimmune diseases causing ductopenia are chronic graft versus host disease (CGVHD)[1,2,3,5] and hepatic allograft rejection (AR)[1,2,6].

Theoretically, loss of intrahepatic bile ducts could result from the destruction of cholangiocytes, the endothelial cells of hepatic arteries or arterioles (ischaemic atrophy) or the endothelial cells of the peribiliary capillary plexi[1–4,6]. Recent data indicate that cholangiocyte gene expression varies along the branching segments of the intrahepatic bile ducts[7,8] and that cytokines produced by local inflammation (e.g. IFNγ, IL-1β, IL-2, TNFα) stimulate increased expression of Class I MHC molecules and aberrant expression of Class II MHC, as

Table 1 Classification of immunological diseases of bile ducts

Autoimmune	*Alloimmune*	*Other*
Primary biliary cirrhosis (PBC)	Chronic graft versus host disease (CGVHD)	Hepatitis C virus infection Chronic hepatitis Recurrence after liver transplantation
Autoimmune cholangitis (AIC)	Hepatic allograft rejection	Lymphoma
Primary sclerosing cholangitis (PSC)		

well as adhesion molecules on cholangiocytes[2,9–12]. Cholangiocytes in biopsies of patients with PBC also express the co-stimulatory molecules B71/B72[12]. Human cholangiocytes can also express Fas, a cell-surface receptor mediating apoptosis induced by cytokines or cytotoxic T lymphocytes (CTL) expressing Fas-ligand[13,14]. Similarly, cytokines also induce expression of adhesion molecules on the endothelial cells of arteries and portal veins that promote leucocyte adhesion and trans-endothelial migration of inflammatory cells into the portal tracts and peribiliary space[2,15,16]. Collectively, the phenotypic changes make both cholangiocytes and peribiliary endothelial cells potential target cells for CD8 and CD4 CTL, and confer antigen-presenting cell (APC) capacity[2,17]. The portal inflammatory milieu may also generate additional antigenic peptides through proteolysis that are capable of exogenous binding to Class II MHC molecules for presentation to CD4 T cells[17].

Three primary mechanisms (Figure 1) may result in immunological bile duct destruction: (a) direct and/or indirect (e.g. cytokine-mediated) cytotoxicity of cholangiocytes; (b) ischaemic necrosis of cholangiocytes; (c) obliterative peribiliary fibrosis of bile ducts[2]. In addition, injury induced by lymph stasis may occur, but has not been adequately studied. Individual mechanisms of bile duct injury may be perpetuated by multiple immunological effector mechanisms (e.g. antibodies, antigen-specific and antigen-non-specific effector cells or cytokines). In specific ductopenic diseases it is probable that several immunopathogenic mechanisms may act concurrently or sequentially[1,2].

NON-SUPPURATIVE DESTRUCTIVE CHOLANGITIS

Non-suppurative destructive cholangitis (NSDC) is defined as a histopathological process that is characterized by the segmental inflammation of interlobular and septal bile ducts by T cells that results in destruction of cholangiocytes and ultimate disappearance of intrahepatic bile ducts of a restricted calibre[1–3]. Although first described in PBC, NSDC is now recognized as the primary histological process in AIC[18], CGVHD[1–3,5] and AR[2,3,6]. The occurrence of NSDC in alloimmune diseases such as CGVHD and AR has provided important opportunities for the development of animal models[2,4,6]. We and others have primarily used murine models of GVHD to study the effector mechanisms of NSDC.

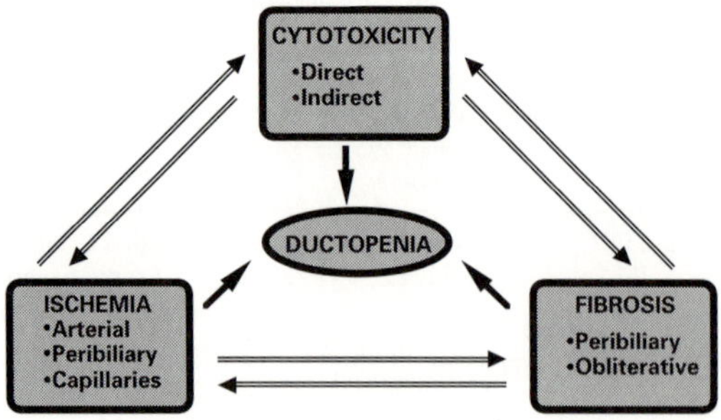

Figure 1 Potential interdependent mechanisms of cholangiocyte and bile duct injury

MURINE MODELS OF CHRONIC GVHD

GVHD results from donor T cell responses against allogeneic histocompatibility antigens of the recipient[2,5]. There are three obligatory requirements for GVHD: (a) engraftment of viable T cells; (b) histoincompatibility between the graft donor and host; and (c) inability of the host to destroy the donor T cells. The latter requirement is often fulfilled in animal models by immunosuppression of the recipient, or by injecting donor T cells from a parental strain animal into an F_1 hybrid offspring (product of mating two allogeneic strains). Thus, the F_1 hybrid recognizes the parental donor strain T cells as self, while the donor strain T cells recognize allogeneic major histocompatibility complex (MHC) molecules of the other parental strain expressed in the F_1 offspring.

In both humans and rodents, GVHD results in preferential injury of three target organs: liver, skin, and intestine[2,5]. Within the liver the alloreaction is primarily against interlobular bile ducts. This curious restriction suggests that the alloantigens recognized by engrafted T cells are not ubiquitously expressed throughout the body, but preferentially or exclusively expressed by cells within the target organs. Indeed, recent studies of alloimmune T cell receptor (TCR) recognition indicate that the majority of allogeneic TCR may be directed against peptide antigens in the antigen-binding grooves of allogeneic molecules, rather than the allogeneic MHC molecules themselves[6,19–23]. These data suggest that expression of cholangiocyte-specific peptide antigens in the antigen-binding groves of self- or allogeneic-MHC molecules may explain target cell specificity of autoimmune and alloimmune mechanisms of NSDC, respectively[2,4,6].

Several murine models result in NSDC of interlobular bile ducts. The role of Class I and II MHC and minor histocompatibility antigen mismatching in the development of NSDC has been studied in F_1 hybrid models. Substantial NSDC occurs in Class I and combined Class I and II MHC mismatching[24]. In contrast, Class II MHC mismatching results in variable outcomes, ranging from portal inflammation without NSDC[24] to NSDC with granulomas[25]. The reason for these differences remains unclear. Models matched for MHC molecules, but mismatched for non-MHC encoded minor histocompatibility antigens, also exhibit NSDC[24]. Selective depletion of CD8 cytotoxic precursors did not prevent NSDC in F_1 hybrid studies[24]. However, depletion of both CD4 and CD8 cytotoxic precursor cells from the grafts reduced NSDC on day 21 but did not prevent NSDC on day 42[24]. In contrast, elimination of CD4 cytotoxic precursors significantly decreased inflammation and prevented NSDC.

We have studied the murine model of CGVHD B10.D2 ($H\text{-}2^d$, Mls^{1b2b}) $\rightarrow$ BALB/c ($H\text{-}2^d$, Mls^{1b2a})[26]. In this model unfractionated spleen cells are intravenously injected into BALB/c recipients who are sublethally radiated (600 r) to prevent rejection of the spleen-cell grafts. Despite Mls (minor lymphocyte stimulatory) histoincompatibility, neither strain produces a mixed lymphocyte response (MLR) against the other *in vitro*, even using activated spleen cells from mice with established CGVHD. Thus, the response of the grafted splenic T cells is against undefined minor histocompatibility antigen(s) that are not expressed on leucocytes, and is similar to the situation of an HLA-identical, MLR-nonreactive bone marrow transplant.

The B10.D2 → BALB/c murine model is associated with reproducible evolution of non-suppurative destructive cholangitis[26]. Uniformly, from day 39 onwards, bile duct injury is observed and is characterized by NSDC and segmental destruction of cholangiocytes. From day 39 through day 130 there was progressive increase in ductopenia. As is also characteristic of NSDC in human diseases, the degree of bile duct injury varied along the course of the individual interlobular duct.

EFFECTOR CELLS OF NSDC

The working hypothesis in our model is that NSDC results from an alloimmune response of Class II MHC-restricted donor CD4 T cells to recipient antigen(s) expressed preferentially or exclusively by intrahepatic cholangiocytes. Therefore, we assessed the ability of donor spleen cell subsets to mediate NSDC[27]. Using immunomagnetic bead purification we prepared B10.D2 grafts of unfractionated spleen cells (positive controls), non-T cells (negative controls), CD4 T and non-T cells and CD8 T and non-T cells. As anticipated, there was an increase in the inflammatory bile duct injury score between day 21 and day 42 using unfractionated spleen cell grafts. In accordance with the requirement for T cells to produce CGVHD, non-T cell grafts did not mediate bile duct injury on either day 21 or 42. In contrast, grafts composed of CD4 T and non-T cells mediated substantial NSDC, characterized by cholangiocyte injury and interlobular bile duct destruction on both days 21 and 42. However, grafts composed of CD8 T cells caused minimal periductular inflammation and neither inflammatory destruction of epithelia nor ductopenia was observed. Immunocytochemical studies of CGVHD livers[28] showed that engraftment with CD4 T and non-T cells resulted in aberrant expression of Class II MHC (I-A^d; mouse analogue of HLA DQ) on the basolateral membranes of the cholangiocytes. In addition, ICAM-1 expression was induced on the basolateral membranes of the cholangiocytes in the presence of grafts containing CD4 T and non-T cells. Moreover, CD4 T cells were identified infiltrating the bile duct epithelia. Thus, a graft containing CD4 T cells was an obligatory requirement for NSDC. Indeed, NSDC appeared to be mediated by the CD4 cells, and their putative cytokine production was the most likely stimulus for the aberrant expression of Class II MHC and ICAM-1 necessary for effective interaction between the CD4 cells and cholangiocytes.

ORIGIN OF T CELLS MEDIATING NSDC

Although studies of T cell subset effector mechanisms supported our hypothesis of immunopathogenesis, it remained unclear whether NSDC was mediated exclusively by alloreactive donor T cells or whether the alloreaction secondarily induced an autoimmune T cell reaction. Since both mouse strains have identical MHC molecules, peptide antigens present in the antigen-binding grooves of these MHC molecules could be recognized by: (a) alloreactive T cells; (b) self-reactive T cells; or (c) a combination of the two. To investigate this possibility we isolated mononuclear inflammatory cells from both the intrahepatic portal connective tissue tree (i.e. portal tract inflammatory cells and intraepithelial lymphocytes) and parenchyma using techniques of enzymatic digestion and isopyknic centrifugation. The isolation procedure yielded proportions of total mature CD3 T cells and CD4 and CD8 T cell subsets comparable to the proportions identified in hepatic tissue sections using immunocytochemical techniques during CGVHD.

To identify the proportion of cells of B10.D2 (donor) vs BALB/c (host) origin, we performed flow cytometry using a monoclonal antibody specific for the β_2-microglobulin epitope Lym11 that is exclusively expressed by B10.D2 mice[29]. To distinguish Lym11+ T cells and non-T cells, we performed dual-label flow cytometry using anti-CD3 monoclonal antibody. Results indicated that >90% of portal cells in the BALB/c mice with CGVHD were of B10.D2 origin and ~70% of those cells were CD3+ T cells. Only 1% of portal inflammatory cells were CD3-positive BALB/c cells and approximately 3% were BALB/c non-T cells. In the parenchyma, approximately 40% of isolated mononuclear cells were of B10.D2 origin and virtually all were T cells. The remaining cells were composed of approximately 40% BALB/c CD3+ T cells and 20% BALB/c non-T cells, respectively. These data unequivocally supported the working hypothesis that NSDC in our model results from an alloimmune reaction, and does not involve induction of an autoimmune self-reactive T cell mechanism.

IMMUNOGENICITY OF CHOLANGIOCYTES

To address whether the alloreactivity mediating NSDC involved cholangiocyte-specific antigens or antigens preferentially expressed by cholangiocytes within the liver, we cloned T cells from the portal connective tree of mice with CGVHD in the presence of exogenous IL-2[30]. This method favours isolation of CD8 rather than CD4 T cells. The resulting T cell suspension was subsequently plated at low density with medium alone, B10.D2 APC, B10.D2 APC plus BALB/c liver parenchyma (containing hepatocytes and sinusoidal lining cells) and B10.D2 APC plus freshly isolated BALB/c cholangiocytes. Cholangiocytes were isolated from the portal connective tissue tree of BALB/c mice using immunomagnetic beads and a monoclonal antibody that reacts exclusively with cholangiocytes in mouse liver. Several cholangiocyte-specific CD8 T cell line/clones were obtained. In contrast, no T cell reactivity against BALB/c parenchymal cells was observed. The T cell lines and clones did not proliferate with APC alone, excluding the possibility that their proliferation was due to an autologous MLR. These data were fully compatible with the hypothesis that alloreactive TCR recognize antigens either exclusively or preferentially expressed by cholangiocytes.

We further studied the immunogenicity of BALB/c cholangiocytes by transplantation of isolated suspensions of BALB/c cholangiocytes (target of NSDC in the CGVHD model) beneath the renal capsule of B10.D2 mice[31]. Subcapsular allografts of isolated cholangiocytes were harvested on day 28 for histopathological review. During this period the cholangiocytes had formed tubular, bile duct-like structures, which were surrounded by dense periductular lymphocytic inflammatory infiltrates and focal NSDC lesions. As observed in CGVHD livers, serial sectioning demonstrated variation in the intensity of NSDC along the course of an individual bile duct-like structure. Control grafts of syngeneic B10.D2 cholangiocytes did not form bile duct-like structures or elicit an inflammatory response.

Based on this evidence of the alloreactive immunogenicity of cholangiocytes, we conducted studies to tolerize and immunize B10.D2 recipients with BALB/c cholangiocytes[32]. Tolerance was induced by injection of BALB/c cholangiocytes into the portal veins of anaesthetized B10.D2 recipients and administration of a single dose of cyclophosphamide intraperitoneally, 48 h later. Sham-tolerized mice had medium alone injected into their portal veins, followed by cyclophosphamide intraperitoneally. Immunized mice received a single subcutaneous injection of BALB/c cholangiocytes emulsified in Freund's adjuvant. After a 30-day recovery period we transplanted BALB/c cholangiocytes beneath the renal capsules of these three groups of mice. The allografts were harvested for histopathological examination 28 days later, and the spleens were removed to create grafts for induction of CGVHD in naive BALB/c recipients. Subcapsular allografts of tolerized B10.D2 mice contained few bile duct cells in clumps or occasional bile duct-like structures, and inflammation was absent. Allografts of sham-tolerized recipients contained multiple bile duct-like structures and dense lymphocytic inflammation with foci of NSDC. In contrast, allografts of immunized recipients showed dense lymphocytic inflammation and nearly total destruction of bile duct-like structures.

Sublethally irradiated BALB/c recipients of spleen cells from cholangiocyte-tolerized mice developed cutaneous scleroderma-like lesions of CGVHD; however, NSDC was absent. Conversely, spleen cell grafts of sham-tolerized mice induced both scleroderma-like lesions and NSDC. The spleen cells of B10.D2 mice immunized with BALB/c cholangiocytes caused severe portal inflammation and duct destruction, culminating in death of recipients in < 12 days. These results indicated that tolerance induced by cholangiocytes could prevent NSDC but not scleroderma-like manifestations of CGVHD. Thus, it appears likely that the cholangiocytes express antigens different from those present in skin, which argues against organ-specific injury being due to ubiquitously expressed minor histocompatibility antigenic differences in this model of CGVHD.

Our future studies will address several unresolved issues. The immunogenicity of recently immortalized mouse cholangiocyte lines will be tested *in vitro* and *in vivo*. The TCR repertoires of both CD4 and CD8 T cells responsive to cholangiocytes will be assessed. The capacity of grafts composed of sensitized T cells to mediate NSDC will also be studied. The effect of CD4 T helper 1 and 2 cytokines on cholangiocytes will be assessed, with special emphasis on the capacity of cytokines to alter the immunological phenotype of the cholangiocytes and to alter their susceptibility to apoptosis[33,34].

Acknowledgements

The author thanks the individuals who worked on the above projects (see reference citations) including William Ruderman, MD, Charles Howell, MD, Merrill Emmett, PhD, Chang-Hong Yu, MD, Ke-Qin Hu, MD, Bradley Freilich, MD, Henry Claman, MD, Dale Hammond and Mary Rosandich.

References

1. Woolf GM, Vierling JM. Disappearing intrahepatic bile ducts: the syndromes and their mechanisms. Semin Liver Dis. 1993;13:261–75.
2. Vierling JM, Hu K-Q. Immunologic mechanisms of hepatobiliary injury. In: Kaplowitz N, editor. Liver and biliary diseases, 2nd edn. Baltimore: Williams & Wilkins. 1996:55–87.
3. Desmet VJ. Vanishing bile duct disorders. In: Boyer JL, Ockner RK, editors. Progress in liver diseases, Vol. XI, Philadelphia: W.B. Saunders. 1992:89–122.
4. Freilich BF, Hu K-Q, Vierling JM. Immunopathogenesis of autoimmune hepatobiliary diseases. Curr Opin Gastroenterol. 1994;10:257–68.
5. Ben-Ezra JM, Stroup RM. Phenotype of bile ducts and infiltrating lymphocytes in graft-versus-host disease. Transplantation. 1993;56:162–5.
6. Vierling JM. Immunology of hepatic allograft rejection. In: Maddrey W, Sorrell M, editors. Transplantation of the liver. Norwalk, CT: Appleton & Lange. 1995:335–65.
7. Alpini G, Roberts S, Kuntz SM *et al.* Morphological, molecular, and functional heterogeneity of cholangiocytes from normal rat liver. Gastroenterology. 1996;110:1636–1643.
8. Charlotte F, L'Hermine A, Martin N *et al.* Immunohistochemical detection of bcl-2 protein in normal and pathological human liver. Am J Pathol. 1994;144:460–5.
9. Ayers RC, Neuberger JM, Shaw J, Joplin R, Adams DH. Intercellular adhesion molecule-1 and MHC antigens on human intrahepatic bile duct cells: effect of pro-inflammatory cytokines. Gut. 1993;34:1245–9.
10. Paradis K, Sharp HL. *In vitro* duct-like structure formation after isolation of bile ductular cells from a murine model. J Lab Clin Med. 1989;113:689–99.
11. Andus T, Bauer J, Gerok W. Effects of cytokines on the liver. Hepatology. 1991;13:364–75.
12. Tsuneyama K, Van de Water J, Leung PSC *et al.* Abnormal expression of the E2 component of the pyruvate dehydrogenase complex on the luminal surface of biliary epithelium occurs before major histocompatibility complex class II and BB1/B7 expression. Hepatology. 1995;21:1031–7.
13. Hiramatsu N, Hayashi N, Katayama K *et al.* Immunohistochemical detection of Fas antigen in liver tissue of patients with chronic hepatitis C. Hepatology. 1994;19:1354–9.
14. Kagi D, Lederman B, Burki K, Zinkernagel RM, Hengartner H. Molecular mechanisms of lymphocyte-mediated cytotoxicity and their role in immunological protection and pathogenesis in vivo. Annu Rev Immunol. 1996;14:207–32.
15. Steinhoff G, Behrend M, Schrader B *et al.* Expression patterns of leukocytes adhesion ligand molecules on human liver endothelia. Am J Pathol. 1993;142:481–8.
16. Bevilacqua M. Endothelial–leukocyte adhesion molecules. Annu Rev Immunol. 1993;11:767–804.
17. Brodsky FM, Guanguardi LE. The cell biology of antigen processing and presentation. Annu Rev Immunol. 1991;9:707–44.
18. Goodman ZD, McNally PR, Davis DR, Ishak KG. Autoimmune cholangitis: a variant of primary biliary cirrhosis. Clinicopathologic and serologic correlations in 200 cases. Dig Dis Sci. 1995;40:1232–42.
19. Sherman LA, Chattopadhy S. The molecular basis of allorecognition. Annu Rev Immunol. 1993;11:385–402.
20. Mentzer SJ, Barbosa JA, Strominger JL *et al.* Species-restricted recognition of transfected HLA-A2 and HLA-B7 by human CTL clones. J Immunol. 1986;137:408–13.
21. Lombardi R, Bal V, Rothbard JB *et al.* Co-recognition of endogenous antigens with HLA-DR1 by alloreactive human T cell clones. J Immunol. 1989;142:753–9.
22. Heath WR, Kane KP, Mescher MF, Sherman LA. Alloreactive T cells discriminate among a diverse set of endogenous peptides. Proc Natl Acad Sci USA. 1991;88:5101–5.
23. Roetzschke O, Falk K, Faath S *et al.* On the nature of peptides involved in T cell alloreactivity. J Exp Med. 1991;174:1059–71.
24. Williams FH, Thiele DL. The role of major histocompatibility complex and non-major histocompatibility complex encoded antigens in generation of bile duct lesions during hepatic graft-vs.-host responses mediated by helper or cytotoxic T cells. Hepatology. 1994;19:980–8.
25. Saitoh T, Fujiwara M, Asakura H. L3T4+ T cells induce hepatic lesions resembling primary biliary cirrhosis in mice with graft-versus-host reactions due to major histocompatibility complex class II disparity. Clin Immunol Immunopathol. 1991;59:449–61.

26. Vierling JM, Ruderman WB, Jaffee BD *et al.* Hepatic lesions in murine chronic graft-vs-host disease to minor histocompatibility antigens. Transplantation. 1989;48:717–18.
27. Hu K-Q, Yu C-H, Vierling JM. Role of T cell subsets in the pathogenesis of nonsuppurative destructive cholangitis in murine chronic graft-vs-host disease. Hepatology. 1992;16:92A (abstract).
28. Hu K-Q, Freilich BL, Yu C-H, Vierling JM. Role of infiltrating CD4 T cell in the pathogenesis of nonsuppurative destructive cholangitis (NSDC) in murine chronic graft-versus-host disease. Hepatology. 1993;18:457A (abstract).
29. Freilich BL, Hu K-Q, Yu C-H, Vierling JM. Hepatic inflammatory cell infiltrates during murine chronic graft-vs-host disease: are the cells of donor or host origin? Gastroenterology. 1994;106:A894 (abstract).
30. Freilich BL, Hu K-Q, Yu C-H, Vierling JM. Propagation of hepatic T cells that react with biliary epithelial cells (BEC) in a murine model of chronic graft-versus-host disease. Gastroenterology. 1994;106:A894 (abstract).
31. Vierling JM, Emmett M, Howell CD *et al.* Immunogenicity of isolated bile duct epithelial cells in mice exhibiting non-suppurative destructive cholangitis during chronic graft-vs-host disease. Hepatology. 1989;10:584 (abstract).
32. Vierling JM, Emmett M, Yu C-H *et al.* Tolerance to bile duct cells in mice developing non-suppurative destructive cholangitis during chronic graft-vs-host disease. Gastroenterology. 1990;98:A643 (abstract).
33. Nawaz S, Fennell RH. Apoptosis of bile duct epithelial cells in hepatic allograft rejection. Histopathology. 1994;25:137–42.
34. Koga H, Sakisaka S, Ohishi M, Sata M, Tanikawa K. Nuclear DNA fragmentation in biliary epithelial cells and in hepatocytes in primary biliary cirrhosis. Hepatology. 1995;22:121A (abstract).

16
Immunopathology of vanishing bile duct syndrome

C. GALPERIN, R. L. COPPEL, A. A. ANSARI and M. E. GERSHWIN

INTRODUCTION

Vanishing bile duct syndrome (VBDS) is a manifestation of chronic rejection and represents one of the most serious complications of liver transplantation[1]. Although the natural history of VBDS is not well understood, the involvement of immune mechanisms in its development seems to be clearly established. This is supported by the association with acute rejection histopathological alterations[2], as well as by recurrence in successive grafts[3]. Other factors reportedly associated with the development of VBDS include: HLA mismatching[4], presence of a positive lymphocytotoxic cross-match[4], and cytomegalovirus infection of the liver allograft[5,6]. While there are a few patients whose VBDS appears to reverse over time, this syndrome is generally considered to be irreversible[1,3].

In addition to chronic liver allograft rejection the characteristic histopathological features of VBDS may also be seen in primary biliary cirrhosis (PBC), and graft versus host disease (GVHD) after bone marrow transplantation[7]. A cytotoxic (CD8+) and helper/inducer (CD4+) T-lymphocyte portal tract infiltrate, that involves and damages intrahepatic bile ducts, has been shown in PBC[8], GVHD[9], and chronic liver allograft reaction[10]. VBDS has also been described as the pathological substrate in several cases of prolonged cholestasis induced by drugs[11–14]. The demonstration of a T-lymphocyte mononuclear cell portal tract infiltrate in the early biliary lesion in cases of drug-induced VBDS suggests that cell-mediated immune mechanisms may also be involved in that context. By way of illustration, chronic chlorpromazine jaundice closely resembles PBC[12]. In the typical case portal infiltration is more prominent in PBC; nonetheless, the histopathological differentiation between these two entities can be difficult, and a distinction may be possible only with the presence of serological surrogate markers of PBC[12].

Although VBDS may appear as a manifestation of distinct clinical entities, the histopathological similarity among some of them has fostered the conjecture that common immunopathological mechanisms might be involved. For instance, biliary epithelial cells, which normally express Class I antigens[15], also aberrantly express Class II HLA antigens in PBC[16,17], GVHD[18] and chronic liver rejection[19]. These findings suggest that, in these diseases, biliary antigens co-expressed with either Class I or II HLA molecules might induce an autoimmune response directed to the bile ducts. In this chapter we will discuss recent data which have provided a basis for defining the autoimmune response in PBC, and information which suggests an explanation for its selective bile duct immune damage. We believe that a better understanding of the immunological phenomenon involved in the pathogenesis of PBC will provide new insights into the effector mechanisms operating in VBDS.

PRIMARY BILIARY CIRRHOSIS: AN AUTOIMMUNE CHOLANGIOLITIS

PBC is an autoimmune destructive disease of the intrahepatic bile ducts characterized by inflammation of the portal triads of the liver followed by fibrosis and, eventually, liver failure[20,21]. A typical patient with PBC is 40–60 years of age and is female; females outnumber males by over 10 to 1 in some case series. Cases under the age of 30 are exceptional, and the incidence rises progressively with age. The onset of disease is often marked by the presence of lethargy and debilitating pruritus, with jaundice eventually occurring as the disease progresses[22]. Liver failure and portal hypertension ultimately develop in most patients with PBC, and the manifestations of these disorders are similar to those in other patients with end-stage cirrhosis. The major serological abnormality is the presence of antimitochondrial antibodies (AMA), serologically detected by immunofluorescence. AMA have long been a confirmatory marker and are found in 90–95% of patients with PBC. Recent work using recombinant autoantigens has resulted in the production of extremely reliable, sensitive and specific solid-phase tests (e.g. ELISA) for the detection of AMA[23,24].

The pathological changes in PBC are distinctively associated with the presence of widespread duct lesion, and the common scheme of histological grading of severity recognizes four stages[25]. In stage 1, a marker of early disease, small portal ductules show cellular damage and rupture, with bile leakage. There is also a dense periportal lymphoid infiltrate in which CD4+ and CD8+ T cells are found, together with monocytes, neutrophils, eosinophils and granuloma formation. In stage 2 piecemeal necrosis and/or proliferation of ductules are evident. Stage 3 is marked by the presence of septal fibrosis and/or bridging necrosis, while stage 4 is typified by overt cirrhosis. In spite of the varying rates of histological progression among individual patients, 'primary biliary cirrhosis' is clearly a misnomer for a disease that has a long precirrhotic stage. For this reason the term 'autoimmune cholangiolitis' appears to more properly characterize this disease.

EPIDEMIOLOGY AND GENETIC PREDISPOSITION

PBC, while uncommon, is present among diverse ethnic and racial populations. Nonetheless, there is great variability in the prevalence between different countries[26–30], and even between districts within the same country[31–33]. The antimitochondrial autoantibody response also varies within different ethnic groups, while the clinical manifestations of PBC appear similar among them (see Table 2)[34]. Although these data could in part reflect the different availability of diagnostic tools and a fully trained hepatologist in communities, environmental factors are also likely to be involved. Of particular interest, in one study from Sheffield, United Kingdom, the prevalence of PBC cases in relation to one water reservoir appeared to be more than ten times that of other reservoirs[33]. Although results of water analysis were inconclusive, this study was extended for a further 10 years, and the original results were confirmed.

The reported existence of familial clustering of actual cases of PBC[31], increased prevalence of various autoantibodies among relatives of PBC patients[26], and associations with Class II histocompatibility antigens[35] indicate some element, albeit low, of genetic risk for PBC. The assumption that PBC is an autoimmune disease has led to the search for genes within the major histocompatibility comlex (MHC) which may be involved in predisposition to this disease. PBC has been associated with certain Class II antigens of the MHC, including HLA-DR3, DR8, DR4 and DR2. In general, these earlier HLA correlations, based upon serological typing, were weak, and varied considerably among reporting centres and different ethnic populations. More recently, molecular studies of MHC have provided more accurate methods for defining specific HLA alleles. Therefore, to more precisely define the role of the HLA Class II genes in susceptibility of PBC, we have used the polymerase chain reaction (PCR) and sequence-specific oligonucleotide probes to type and compare the distribution of DRB1, DQA1, DQB1, and DPB1 in 51 Caucasian patients with PBC and 240 random Caucasian controls[36]. Although the allelic distribution at the DPB1 locus showed no significant variation between patients and controls, there was heterogeneity in the distribution of DR-DQ haplotypes where the frequency of the DRB1*0801-DQA1*0401/0601-DQB1*04 haplotype was significantly increased in patients, suggesting it confers susceptibility to this disease. Two other haplotypes, DRB1*1501-DQA1*0102-DQB1*0602 and DRB1*1302-DQA1*0102-DQB1*0604, were significantly reduced in patients, suggesting they confer protection. Tests for the individual loci show that resistance to this disease is more strongly associated with the DQA1*0102 allele shared by both protective haplotypes. Another attribute of HLA, linkage disequilibrium, adds an additional feature to the study of disease association with selective alleles. Instead of various alleles of each of these loci (e.g. DRB1, DQB1, etc.) being randomly assorted on human chromosomes, various combinations of them occur more often than expected, especially in a given ethnic population[37]. Because these genes lie so close to one another, the finding of a particular allelic association with a disease does not imply that it is directly playing a role in the disease. Thus, it is unclear whether multiple genes or a single locus on the susceptible DR8 haplotype are needed for PBC predisposition. Nevertheless, these data suggest that distinct HLA Class II alleles may play a role in the immunopathogenesis of this diseases, by conferring both predisposition and resistance to PBC. Recently, Morling and colleagues[38] used restriction fragment polymorphism analysis to show that susceptibility to PBC in a Danish population was associated with the extended haplotype HLA-B8, DR3, DQA1*0501, DQB1*0201. Further studies in different ethnic groups (transracial gene mapping) are expected to more precisely define the most relevant PBC predisposing gene(s).

IMMUNOLOGICAL ASPECTS

Primary biliary cirrhosis is the quintessential example of an organ-specific autoimmune disease, a group of disorders in which the antigen is broadly distributed to virtually all nucleated cells, but the immune destruction is specifically targeted to a relatively few tissues. The autoantigens recognized in PBC are predominantly components of normal mitochondria, although less commonly components of the nucleus and cytoplasm are also recognized. How a mitochondrial antigen, physically sheltered from the immune system by two membrane barriers, can elicit an immune response or, once tolerance is broken, how this 'self-reactive' immunity causes tissue damage in only some cells, is still unknown. Undeniably, though, in PBC immune damage is almost exclusively directly to the intrahepatic biliary epithelium. The present difficulties in better understanding the effector mechanisms involved in the pathogenesis of PBC stem, to a large extent, from our inability to examine the disease in its earliest stages and throughout its evolution. When patients first come to the attention of the clinician, the disease is believed to have been present for years to decades. Thus, when we come to dissect the immune response we are observing the end-stages of a process, and many of the immune responses we can detect may result from 'bystander' or secondary response to cellular components released from dying cells.

Recent advances in molecular immunology, together with other emerging technologies (such as affinity mass spectrometry), have been of cardinal importance in elucidating the identity of the autoantigens and the epitopes on the molecules targeted by T and B cell responses in PBC. While the data generated by such studies have not yet conclusively solved the critical issue of how this disease emerges, they build a compelling scenario of how the initial events in the pathogenesis of PBC may occur.

The antimitochondrial response

During the 1960s the detection of complement-fixing antibodies to tissue homogenates in the sera of a patient with PBC[39], followed by the identification by indirect immunofluorescence of a distinct antimitochondrial staining pattern produced by PBC patients' sera[40,41], established for the first time the link between this disease and autoimmunity. The mitochondrial antibody reaction was soon found in clinical studies to have a high utility for the diagnostic identification of cases of PBC, whether tested for by complement fixation or immunofluorescence[42,43]. Although the mitochondrial autoantigen was then known to be located on the inner mitochondrial membrane[44], its identity remained uncertain for nearly two decades.

In 1985 the use of immunoblotting inaugurated a new immunomolecular era for PBC, by allowing the recognition of discrete polypeptide antigens of defined molecular weight[45]. This was followed by the derivation by molecular cloning of a cDNA that encoded the major mitochondrial antigen for PBC[46], and thereafter the recognition of enzyme molecules of the 2-oxo-acid complexes as the reactants revealed by immunoblotting.

The presence of AMA is a major criterion for diagnosis of PBC. The titre of AMA does not correlate with the stages or prognosis of the disease, and whether or not these autoantibodies are involved in the pathogenesis of the disease remains unsettled. Nonetheless, antimitochondrial antibodies were the essential reagent that enabled the most critical recent development in the study of PBC: the cloning and subsequent identification of the target autoantigens in this disease[46]. The mitochondrial autoantigens of PBC have been identified as components of a functionally related enzyme family, the 2-oxo-acid dehydrogenase complexes (2-OADC), which is located on the mammalian inner mitochondrial membrane, and include the pyruvate dehydrogenase complex (PDC-E2), the branched-chain 2-oxo-acid dehydrogenase complex (BCOADC-E2), and the oxoglutarate dehydrogenase complex (OGDC-E2) (Table 1). In each case the predominant antibody reactivity to the enzyme complex is against the E2 component, which is a lipoamide acetyltransferase for PDC and BOADC and a succinyltransferase for the OGDC. In the case of PDC two additional complex components are recognized by patients' sera: protein X and E1. In PBC there is usually reactivity against two, or even all three, of the 2-oxo-acid dehydrogenase complexes, but serological cross-reactivity is found only between PDC-E2 and

Table 1 Mitochondrial autoantigens: molecular identity, earlier designation, molecular weight, function and frequency of the correspondent autoantibody in patients with PBC

Subunits of the 2-oxo-acid dehydrogenase complex				
Molecular identity	*Earlier designation**	*Molecular weight (kDa)*	*Function*	*Autoantibody frequency (%)*
PDH				
E1-α decarboxylase	M2d	41	Decarboxylates pyruvate with thiamine pyrophosphate (TPP) as a co-factor	66
E1-β decarboxylase	M2e	36	Decarboxylates pyruvate with TPP as a co-factor	1–7
E2 acetyltransferase	M2a	74	Transfers acetyl group from E1 to coenzyme A (CoA)	92
Protein X	M2c	56	Unknown	NA
BCOADC				
E2 acyltransferase	M2c	52	Transfers acyl group from E1 to CoA	54
OGDC				
E2 succinyltransferase	M2c	48	Transfers succinyl group from E1 to CoA	66

* Nomenclature a–e as cited by Berg and Klein[87]
PDH: Pyruvate dehydrogenase; BCOADC: branched-chain 2-oxo-acid-dehydrogenase; OGDC: 2-oxo-glutarate dehydrogenase

protein X. The main features of the antimitochondrial antibody response in PBC are summarized in Table 2.

The E2 subunit of PDC, of which the inner lipoyl domain is the major epitope, is the immunodominant autoantigen, being recognized by over 90% of all PBC sera by immunoblotting. Although variable, the extent of the antimitochondrial response is usually extremely high, with specific titres to PDC-E2 using dilutions of sera in the hundreds of thousands or millions. The presence of high-titre, high-affinity, and overt subclass restriction to IgG3 among anti-PDC-E2 IgG autoantibodies is clearly indicative of an influence of particular CD4+ T cells derived lymphokines, such as γ-interferon (IFNγ), during B cell maturation. Moreover, the nature of this response is certainly different from naturally occurring autoantibodies.

It has been suggested that the antibodies to mitochondrial antigens in the sera of patients with PBC arise merely as a response to hepatocyte and bile ductular injury. We have argued otherwise[47]. First, the highly directed response to the mitochondrial 74 kDa protein and the titre of antibodies are typical of what is found in other organ-specific diseases. Second, the absence of such antibodies in patients or animals with chronic biliary obstruction and/or infection with *Escherichia coli* implies that AMA are not merely a response to recurrent cholangitis. Third, the constellation of a predominance of T cells found in lesions, the presence of immune complexes, the primary involvement of biliary ductular cells and the results of *in-vitro* study of autoantibody production suggest that a target antigen is involved. Fourth, the similarities of the pathology of PBC to chronic GVHD suggest that the injury is immunologically mediated. Fifth, the reported recurrence of PBC after liver transplantation accords with the idea that PBC is indeed an organ-specific autoimmune disease.

Autoantibodies to non-mitochondrial targets, including various nuclear antigens, occasionally occur in some patients with PBC. The significance of these reactivities needs to be further addressed.

T cell response

The particular specificity of bile duct destruction, together with the portal tract lymphoid infiltration and aberrant expression of HLA-DR molecules on biliary epithelium, suggests that intrahepatic biliary ductular epithelial cells themselves are direct targets of an intense and highly focused immune response[48,49]. In early lesions, CD8+ T lymphocytes are predominant but an increased tendency towards CD4+ cells is observed in the advanced stages. Nonetheless, it is still uncertain how these cells actually cause damage to ductular cells. The evidence that T cell response participates in the pathogenesis of PBC was initially derived from staining studies of histological samples, and later by analysing lines that proliferate in the presence of putative mitochondrial autoantigens. The infiltrating T cells in PBC may be oligoclonal[50], but cloning of autoreactive T cell lines from PBC has not been extensively explored.

In initial studies we have been able to derive antigen-specific autoreactive T cell clones from liver biopsies of patients with PBC, but not from livers affected with chronic active hepatitis. The cloned T cell lines were specific for PDC-E2 and BCOADC-E2 as they produced interleukin 2 when stimulated with PDC-E2

Table 2 Characteristic features of the antimitochondrial response in PBC

	Autoantibody			
	PDC-E2	*BCOADC-E2*	*OGDC-E2*	*E1-α*
Localization of the major B cell epitope	Inner lipoyl domain[76]	Inner lipoyl domain[77]	Inner lipoyl domain[78]	TPP binding site[79]
Amino acid residues	128–221	No distinct binding sub-region	67–147	NA
Predominant Ig class and isotype	IgG3 and IgM[80–81]	NA	IgG2 and IgM[78]	NA
Inhibitory effect on the *in-vitro* enzyme catalytic activity[82–85]	+	+	+	+
Percentage of reactivity according to ethnic background[34]				
Japanese	15/23 (65%)*	16/23 (70%)	11/23 (48%)	11/23 (47%)
American Caucasian	37/39 (95%)*	17/23 (73%)	12/39 (31%)	9/23 (39%)
Murine monoclonal antibodies				
V_H gene usage[86]	Diverse array of V_H gene segments	NA	NA	NA
Human combinatorial antibodies				
V_H gene usage	Clonally related heavy chains displaying a high number of somatic mutations	NA	NA	NA

TPP: thiamine pyrophosphate
* Statistically signficant difference ($p = 0.0037$, Fisher's exact test)

and BCOADC-E2 but not with ovalbumin, tuberculin as PPD, or bovine gamma globulin (BGG)[51]. More detailed data on cloned T cell lines have now been obtained by using T cell clones specific for PDC-E2 derived from both the liver and peripheral blood of patients with PBC[52]. Interestingly, the reported T cell response differs from the B cell response in several ways. For PDC-E2 the most commonly recognized epitopic region by T cells was the outer lipoyl domain, whereas for the B cells it is the inner lipoyl domain. The frequency of patients reactive to PDC-E2 was lower for T cells, but this may reflect the limits of the assay system. As the patients studied were in advanced stages of the disease process, some of the additional epitopes may have been recognized by responses elicited secondary to tissue damage, by a process analogous to determinant spreading. Further observations involving patients at different stages of disease will help to clarify these interesting issues. Based on the concept that IL-2 and IFNγ secretion is a property of Th1-like clones, and IL-4 a property attributed to Th2-like clones, the lymphokine analysis in this study suggests that both T helper cell Th1- and Th2-like clones are present in the liver.

The T cell receptor V repertoire utilized by PDC-reactive clones infiltrating the liver was remarkable in its heterogeneity. This was especially apparent within subsets that responded to particular domains. For instance, T cell clones reactive to the inner lipoyl domain of PDC-E2 utilized multiple different V, and only a few examples of repetitive V usage were noted. Nevertheless, the relatively small number of clones used to estimate the total repertoire precludes any definite conclusions in this matter. Of all cloned lines derived there were several CD4+/CD8+ lines, but the vast majority of lines were CD4+. This is consistent with the lines being derived from patients late in the disease when CD4+ T cells in the liver are predominant. The presence of antigen-specific memory T cells in the liver was revealed by the identification of CD4RO+ phenotype among isolated clones. No satisfactory assay systems are currently available to assess the pathogenic capacity of these T-cell lines, and this remains a major unsolved issue in PBC.

LIPOIC ACID AND BACTERIAL FORMS OF PDC

Currently, one of the most intriguing areas in PBC studies is the role of lipoic acid both as an inducer and as a target of the autoimmune response. PDC-E2, BCOADC-E2 and OGDC-E2 all have one or more lipoic acid moieties bound to a lysine on the polypeptide chain. Lipoic acid has been demonstrated to have adjuvant activities in an animal model system[53], and the observation that auto-antibody epitopes are present in the lipoic acid domain is also consistent with the idea that it may have a direct role in the induction of autoimmunity. If this were the case, the presence of lipoic acid-containing enzymes in bacteria could potentially raise a cross-reactive response to mammalian enzymes.

Molecular mimicry between host autoantigens and unrelated exogenous proteins, usually bacteria or virus, is one of the hypotheses to explain how human autoantibodies to self proteins arise, break tolerance and lead to autoimmune disease[54]. Examples of amino acid sequence homology among autoantigens include: the p70 (U1)RNP[55] and topoisomerase I[56] with the p30^{gag} retroviral nucleoprotein, the 60 kDa Ro/SS-A with the nuclear capsid of vesicular stomatitis virus[57], and La/SS-B protein with the M6 protein of *Streptococcus pyogenes*[58]. On the other hand, the presence of multiple B cell epitopes, characteristic of most autoantigens studied thus far, strongly supports the notion that the autoimmune response is driven by the antigen itself. Molecular mimicry as a cause of PBC has been previously suggested, in part because of the highly conserved structure of PDC-E2, particularly its inner lipoyl domain, between bacteria, yeast and mammals. This thesis is strengthened by the fact that for PDC-E2, in contrast to most of the known autoantigens, only a single extended B cell epitope in this conserved region has been identified.

The bile ducts in PBC abnormally express Class II HLA-DR and HLA-DQ antigens[16,17]. Bourroughs *et al.* propose that the autoimmune phenomenon in PBC results from T cell epitopes of microbial proteins being mimicked by peptides derived from, and presented by, the abnormally expressed HLA-DR antigen[59]. Consistent with this hypothesis, Shimoda *et al.* have recently demonstrated the presence of molecular mimicry at the T cell clonal level between human and *E. coli* PDC-E2[60]. The reactivity of AMA with both human and bacterial mitochondria has also stimulated speculation that PBC may result from chronic bacterial infection[61]. Indeed, chronic bacteriuria[62] and colonic infection with rough-colony (R) mutants of *E. coli* have been accorded significant pathogenic significance in PBC[63]. This scenario fails to explain why there is relatively weaker reactivity of PBC sera with bacterial 2-OADC enzymes compared to mammalian enzymes[64]. However, it may be argued that late in the disease, when tolerance has been lost many years previously, the continual exposure to self-antigen induces a secondary response of higher titre and affinity to the backbone peptide sequence. Studies using sera procured early in the disease process would help resolve this issue.

BILIARY EPITHELIUM: A SELECTIVE TARGET

Several studies have suggested that autoantigens relevant to PBC may be present on the surface of hepatocytes or biliary epithelium. PBC sera react with the surface of isolated hepatocytes, and intact hepatoma cells; such reactivity is abolished by prior absorption of sera with mitochondria[65]. Sundin and Sundqvist[66] detected reactivity of PBC sera with guinea-pig hepatocytes, and with 67- and 50-kDa components of isolated rat hepatocellular plasma membranes. Using rabbit sera specific to PDC-E2, Joplin and colleagues showed in immunohistochemical studies that cultured biliary epithelial cells from patients with PBC overexpress immunologically reactive material at the cell membrane[67].

We have previously reported the development and characterization of PDC-E2-specific murine monoclonal antibodies, and human Fab monoclonal antibodies derived from a PBC lymph node Fab combinatorial library. Although most of them map to the inner lipoyl domain of PDC-E2, these antibodies exhibit distinct immunohistochemical characteristics. For instance, in immunofluorescent confocal microscope studies, two of these mAb, the murine

C355.1 and the human combinatorial SP1, demonstrate a distinct apical staining pattern on bile duct epithelium (BDE) from patients with PBC, but not other control liver diseases[68]. In contrast, all other mAb produce only a typical cytoplasmic mitochondrial staining pattern on BDE and hepatocytes from PBC and control subjects. Moreover, this unique apical staining pattern has recently been found in early or stage I PBC, before the appearance of either the co-stimulatory molecule B7 or Class II molecules, suggesting that it is the earliest detectable sign of the disease process[17]. We believe that the observation that only a selected number of anti-PDC-E2 reagents react with the apical region of BDE suggests that the elusive molecule target by these antibodies is a truncated or altered form of PDC-E2, or a cross-reactive molecule. Simultaneous examination of these sections with an anti-isotype reagent for human IgA revealed high IgA staining in the lumenal region of the BDE in patients with PBC. IgG and IgA antibodies to PDC-E2 were detected in the bile of patients with PBC but not normal controls.

To obtain insight into the nature of this elusive molecule we have recently used the PDC-E2-specific mAb C355.1 and human combinatorial SP1, described above, to screen a random phage-epitope library expressing random dodecapeptides (unpublished observations). Eight different mimotope sequences with three common amino acid motifs (W-SYP, TYVS, and VRH) were identified in 36 phage clones. Competitive inhibition of the immunohistochemical staining of PBC bile duct epithelium (BDE) was performed by incubating some of these peptides with C355.1, SP1 and control PDC-E2 specific murine and combinatorial antibodies. Interestingly, distinct peptides selectively inhibited C355.1 and SP1 unique lumenal staining of PBC BDE, suggesting that they might represent a mimotope of a cross-reactive molecule that exists primarily in the BDE of patients with PBC. Finally, using confocal microscopy, rabbit sera raised against a chosen mimotope peptide stained BDE from patients with PBC with higher intensity than controls. Comparable data were obtained with electron microscopy, which additionally identified the molecule targeted by rabbit antisera as being located on the outer side of isolated BDE cells in PBC but not in normal controls. The mimotopes generated by these studies represent powerful reagents in the pressing need to identify the target molecule responsible for the lumenal staining pattern observed when PBC BDE is stained with C355.1 and SP1.

Affinity mass spectrometry (AMS) has also been recently used by our group to evaluate the presence of tissue-specific markers in PBC (unpublished observations). Surface-enhanced laser desorption/ionization (SELDI) was used in the AMS mode with C355.1 and a control PDC-E2-specific mAb that lacks the lumenal staining pattern characteristic of C355.1. AMS was performed directly on frozen liver sections and purified bile duct epithelial cells, and the mass spectrometric signals enhanced by an *in-situ* enzyme-linked signal amplification process. Samples from patients with PBC gave strong positive signals for the antigen(s) recognized by C355.1 and no evidence of any antigen recognized by the control mAb. Conversely, in each of the negative PBC specimens evaluated, strong signals were detected for the control mAb but not for C355.1. These findings corroborate our previous studies, for they suggest the presence of an additional or altered antigenic determinant associated with PBC that is not present, or is masked, in normal liver. This technology provides a level of sensitivity in the fentomole range, that has hitherto been impossible using only tissue sections or crude cell lysates. Furthermore, by virtue of its capability to perform direct *in-situ* sequencing, AMS represents a resourceful strategy for further elucidation of the identity of the PDC-like molecule in PBC BDE.

The existence of this surface-expressed PDC-like molecule creates a compelling scenario in which the initial events in the pathogenesis of PBC would be a tissue-specific over-expression of a novel substance, with consequent presentation by Class II MHC proteins aberrantly expressed on the PBC biliary ductular surface. This would allow induction of CD4+ T cells that provide help for induction of CD8+ cytotoxic cells. It is also possible that the PDC-E2-like neo-antigen may also be surface expressed. A high level of intracellular expression of the neo-antigen would lead to an association with Class I MHC molecules; reactivity against the biliary specific neo-antigen, perhaps by CD8+ cytotoxic lymphocytes, would then lead to cell lysis and release of mitochondrial products. Presentation of released proteins to lymphocytes primed to cross-react with PDC-E2 could result in presentation of physically associated proteins such as other components of the PDC complex and synthesis of a wider range of autoantibodies. It remains to be established to what degree the biliary epithelium is able to take over the function of a 'professional presenting cell' in a way that allows provision of the essential second signal such as that provided by the co-stimulatory molecule B7.

The exclusive presence of anti-PDC-E2 IgA in the bile of patients with PBC is also of further interest; in particular the investigation on whether, during its transport, autoreactive IgA is capable of reacting with proteins in the biliary cell cytoplasm and there mediating metabolic dysfunctions that might result in cell death.

LIVER TRANSPLANTATION IN PBC

In spite of being the subject of intense examination, the issue of whether PBC recurs after liver transplantation has remained a controversial one. This stems from the fact that rejection, viral hepatitis, and drug effects may all mimic recurrent PBC biochemically and histologically. Moreover, reliable clinical criteria for PBC recurrence are largely unavailable. A number of studies have suggested disease recurrence on a histological basis, documenting the presence of granulomatous duct destruction in patients surviving more than 1 year after transplantation[69,70]. None of these patients, however, has demonstrated clinical signs of recurrence[69–71]. Recently, one group, using rabbit polyclonal affinity purified anti-PDC-E2 antibody, found that PDC-E2 was not over-expressed in post-transplant liver specimens from patients with PBC[72]. This is not in agreement with recent data obtained by our laboratory (unpublished observations). We have performed immunohistochemical and histological analyses of serial liver biopsies of 67 patients pre- and post-orthotopic liver transplantation (OLT), including 38 patients with PBC and 29 non-PBC liver disease controls. Sections were stained with mAb C355.1 or a control PDC-E2 specific mAb, and analysed as to whether there was a recurrence of the apical reactivity in the bile duct of the post-transplant biopsies. The immunohistochemical staining was correlated with the histological findings and serum biochemistries at the time of the biopsy. Our data indicated that a significant number of patients transplanted for PBC (28/38), but not controls (0/29), developed a staining pattern of liver BDE with mAb C355.1 which is indistinguishable from the pre-transplant pattern. Of the 28 patients with the apical staining pattern, eight were characterized histologically as possible recurrent PBC, two as chronic rejection, two as acute rejection, nine as non-specific changes, four as normal or near-normal, and three had other histological changes. Only 50% of the patients with apical C355.1 staining had liver enzyme levels suggestive of cholestasis.

Several interesting possibilities concerning the identity of the reactive molecule were raised by this study:

1. The absence of C355.1 characteristic staining in the control transplanted livers suggests that, whatever the reactive molecule is, it remains specific to PBC and is not induced by processes such as rejection.
2. The presence of C355.1 reactivity in the liver from genetically non-identical donors indicates that the molecule may be a tissue-specific form of a protein that is normally expressed within the biliary epithelium under certain conditions (e.g. immunological insult directed against ductal systems).
3. Alternatively, it may be that the molecule does not originate in biliary epithelial cells but may be concentrated there after transport from elsewhere in the body. It is interesting to note that a significant number of patients with PBC also have salivary gland involvement and exhibit a C355.1 ductal staining pattern similar to the liver[73]. Perhaps this tissue serves as a reservoir that maintains autosensitization of the immune system in the transplanted patient.
4. Although unlikely, the possibility of the molecule being encoded by some retrovirus, or other type of organism that became resident in biliary epithelial cells, cannot be ruled out. An infectious organism with tropism for biliary epithelial cells could remain sequestered in locations such as the salivary glands, and then regenerate the disease process by targeting newly available biliary ductal cells in the transplanted tissue host.

The implications of a PBC-specific staining pattern in the bile ducts following transplantation are unknown. Nonetheless, the recurrence of PBC following transplantation is strongly suggested by the correlation between C355.1 staining and the histological data obtained from the same tissue samples. The more important question relates to the natural history of the recurrent disease. Based on data accumulated thus far, recurrence is unlikely to be an important cause of early (i.e. < 5 years) graft loss. Over that period of time, not only is the survival rate good following transplantation, but the majority of these patients are able to return to full-time employment[74,75]. Whether recurrence of disease will have an impact on patient or graft survival over a longer period of follow-up remains to be determined. Clearly this will be influenced by a number of factors, including the immunosuppressive regimen used and the age of the patient, and will require further studies.

References

1. Manez R, Bronsther O, Kusne S, Llull R, Aguado JM, Starzl TE. Vanishing bile duct syndrome after liver transplantation: alloreactivity or viral reactivity? Transplant Proc. 1995;27:2280.
2. Freese DH, Snover DC, Sharp HL, Gross CR, Savick SK, Payne WD. Chronic rejection after liver transplantation: a study of clinical, histopathological and immunological features. Hepatology. 1991;13:882–91.
3. Ludwig J, Wiesner RH, Batts KP, Perkins JD, Krom RA. The acute vanishing bile duct syndrome (acute irreversible rejection) after orthotopic liver transplantation. Hepatology. 1987;7:476–83.
4. Batts KP, Moore SB, Perkins JD, Wiesner RH, Grambsch PM, Krom RA. Influence of positive lymphocyte crossmatch and HLA mismatching on vanishing bile duct syndrome in human liver allografts. Transplantation. 1988;45:376–9.
5. O' Grady JG, Alexander GJ, Sutherland S *et al.* Cytomegalovirus infection and donor/recipient HLA antigens: interdependent co-factors in pathogenesis of vanishing bile-duct syndrome after liver transplantation. Lancet. 1988;2:302–5.
6. Arnold JC, Portmann BC, Naoumov NV, Alexander GJ, Williams R. Cytomegalovirus infection persists in the liver graft in the vanishing bile duct syndrome [see comments]. Hepatology. 1992;16:285–92.
7. Sherlock S. The syndrome of disappearing intrahepatic bile ducts. Lancet. 1987;29:493–6.
8. Nakanuma Y, Tsuneyama K, Gershwin ME, Yasoshima M. Pathology and immunopathology of primary biliary cirrhosis with emphasis on bile duct lesions: recent progress. Semin Liver Dis. 1995;15:313–28.
9. Schulman HM, Sharma P, Amos D, Fenster LF, McDonald GB. A coded histologic study of hepatic graft-versus-host disease after human bone marrow transplantation. Hepatology. 1988;8:463–70.
10. Vierling JM, Fennell RH. Histopathology of early and late human hepatic allograft rejection: evidence of progressive destruction of interlobular bile ducts. Hepatology. 1985;5:1076–82.
11. Forbes GM, Jeffrey GP, Shilkin KB, Reed WD. Carbamazepine hepatotoxicity: another cause of the vanishing bile duct syndrome. Gastroenterology. 1992;102:1385–8.
12. Moradpour D, Altorfer J, Flury R *et al.* Chlorpromazine-induced vanishing bile duct syndrome leading to biliary cirrhosis. Hepatology. 1994;20:1437–41.
13. Dincsoy HP, Saelinger DA. Haloperidol-induced chronic cholestatic liver disease. Gastroenterology. 1982;83:694–700.
14. Turner IB, Eckstein RP, Riley JW, Lunzer MR. Prolonged hepatic cholestasis after flucloxacin therapy. Med J Aust. 1989;151:701–5.
15. Daar AS, Fuggle SV, Fabre SW, Ting A, Morris PJ. The detailed distribution of HLA A, B, Cw antigens in normal human organs. Transplantation. 1984;38:288–92.
16. Ballardini G, Bianchi FB, Doniach D, Mirakian R, Pisi E, Botazzo GF. Aberrant expression of HLA-DR antigens on bile duct epithelium in primary biliary cirrhosis: relevance to pathogenesis. Lancet. 1984;2:1009–13.
17. Tsuneyama K, Van de Water J, Leung PS *et al.* Abnormal expression of the E2 component of the pyruvate dehydrogenase complex on the luminal surface of biliary epithelium occurs before major histocompatibility complex class II and BB1/B7 expression. Hepatology. 1995;21:1031–7.
18. Miglio F, Pignatelli M, Mazzeo V *et al.* Expression of major histocompatibility complex class II antigens on bile duct epithelium in patients with hepatic graft-versus-host disease after bone marrow transplantation. J Hepatol. 1987;5:182–9.
19. Steinhoff G, Wonigeit K, Happrecht J, Johnson JP, Pichlmayr R. Expression of donor and recipient class I and class II major histocompatibility complex antigens in human liver grafts. Transplant Proc. 1987;19:3561–4.
20. Kaplan MM. Primary biliary cirrhosis. N Engl J Med. 1987;316:521–8.
21. Gershwin ME, Mackay IR. Primary biliary cirrhosis: paradigm or paradox for autoimmunity. Gastroenterology. 1991;100:822–33.
22. Kaplan MM. Primary biliary cirrhosis. Adv Intern Med. 1987;32:359–77.
23. Leung PSC, Iwayama T, Prindivelle T *et al.* Use of designer recombinant mitochondrial antigens in the diagnosis of primary biliary cirrhosis. Hepatology. 1992;15:367–72.

24. Moteki S, Leung PSC, Dickson ER, Coppel RL, Gershwin ME. Use of a designer triple expression hybrid clone for three different lypoil domains for the detection of antimitochondrial antibodies. Hepatology. 1996 (In press).
25. Dickson ER, Fleming CR, Ludwig J. Primary biliary cirrhosis. In: Popper H, Scaffner F, editors. Progress in liver disease, vol. VI. New York: Grune & Stratton. 1979:487.
26. Galbraith RM, Smith M, Mackenzie RM, Tee DED, D., Williams R. High prevalence of seroimmunologic abnormalities in relatives of patients with chronic active hepatitis and primary biliary cirrhosis. N Engl J Med. 1974;290:63.
27. Douglas JG, Finlayson ND. Are increased individual susceptibility and environmental factors both necessary for the development of primary biliary cirrhosis? Br Med J. 1979;2:419–20.
28. Salaspuro MP, Laitinen OI, Lehtola J, Makkonen H, Rasanen JA, Sipponen P. Immunological parameters, viral antibodies, and biochemical and histological findings in relatives of patients with chronic active hepatitis and primary biliary cirrhosis. Scand J Gastroenterol. 1976;11:313–20.
29. Jaup BH, Zettergren LSW. Familial occurrence of primary biliary cirrhosis associated with hypergamaglobulinemia in descendants: a family study. Gastroenterology. 1980;78:549.
30. Sasaki H, Inoue K, Higuchi K *et al.* Primary biliary cirrhosis in Japan: national survey by the subcommittee on autoimmune hepatitis. Gastroenterology. 1985;20:476.
31. Myszor M, James OFW. The epidemiology of primary biliary cirrhosis in England: an increasingly common disease? Q J Med. 1990;75:377–85.
32. Lofgren J, Jarnerot G, Danielsson D, Hemdal I. Incidence and prevalence of primary biliary cirrhosis in a defined population in Sweden. Scand J Gastroenterol. 1985;20:647–50.
33. Triger DR. Primary biliary cirrhosis: an epidemiological study. Br J Med. 1980;281:772–5.
34. Iwayama T, Leung PS, Rowley M *et al.* Comparative immunoreactive profiles of Japanese and American patients with primary biliary cirrhosis against mitochondrial autoantigens. Int Arch Allergy Immunol. 1992;99:28–33.
35. Gores GJ, Moore SB, Fischer LD, Powell FC, Dickson ER. Primary biliary cirrhosis: associations with class II major-histocompatibility complex antigens. Hepatology. 1987;7:889–92.
36. Begovich AB, Klitz W, Moonsamy PV, Van de Water J, Peltz G, Gershwin ME. Genes within the HLA class II region confer both predisposition and resistance to primary biliary cirrhosis. Tissue Antigens. 1994;43:71–7.
37. Arnett FC. HLA and autoimmunity in scleroderma (systemic sclerosis). Int Rev Immunol. 1995;12:107–28.
38. Morling N, Dalhoff K, Fugger L *et al.* DNA polymorphism of HLA class II genes in primary biliary cirrhosis. Immunogenetics. 1992;35:112–16.
39. Mackay IR. Primary biliary cirrhosis showing a high titer of autoantibody. N Engl J Med. 1958;258:185.
40. Walker JG, Doniach D, Roitt IM, Sherlock S. Serological tests in diagnosis of primary biliary cirrhosis. Lancet. 1965;1:827.
41. Berg PA, Coniach D, Roitt IM. Mitochondrial antibodies in primary biliary cirrhosis. I. Localization of the antigen to mitochondrial membranes. J Exp Med. 1967;126:227.
42. Goudie RB, Macsween RNM, Goldberg DM. Serological and histological dignosis of primary biliary cirrhosis. J Clin Pathol. 1966;19:527–31.
43. Doniach D, Roitt IM, Walker JG, Sherlock S. Tissue antibodies in primary biliary cirrhosis, active chronic (lupoid) hepatitis, cryptogenic cirrhosis and other liver diseases and their clinical implications. Clin Exp Immunol. 1966;1:237–41.
44. Berg PA, Muscatello U, Horne RW, Roitt IM, Doniach D. Mitochondrial antibodies in primary biliary cirrhosis. II. The complement fixing antigen as a component of mitochondrial inner membranes. Br J Exp Pathol. 1969;50:200–8.
45. Frazer IH, Mackay IR, Jordan TW, Whittingham S, Marzuki S. Reactivity of antimitochondrial autoantibodies in primary biliary cirrhosis: definition of two novel mitochondrial polypeptide autoantigens. J Immunol. 1985;135:1739–45.
46. Gershwin ME, Mackay IR, Sturgess A, Coppel RL. Identification and specificity of a cDNA encoding the 70 kd mitochondrial antigen recognized in primary biliary cirrhosis. J Immunol. 1987;138:3525–31.
47. Leung PSC, Van de Water J, Coppel RL, Gershwin ME. Molecular characterization of the mitochondrial autoantigens in primary biliary cirrhosis. Immunol Res. 1991;10:518–43.
48. Nakanuma Y, Ohta G. Histometric and serial observations of the intrahepatic bile ducts in primary biliary cirrhosis. Gastroenterology. 1979;76:1326–41.

49. Yamada G, Hyodo I, Tobe K *et al.* Ultrastructural immunocytochemical analysis of lymphocytes infiltrating bile duct epithelia in primary biliary cirrhosis. Hepatology. 1986;3.
50. Moebius U, Manns M, Hess G, Kober G, Meyer Zum Buschenfelde K-H. T-cell receptor gene rearrangements of lymphocytes-T infiltrating the liver in chronic hepatitis B and primary biliary cirrhosis (PBC) oligoclonality of PBC-derived T cell clones. Eur J Immunol. 1990;20:889–902.
51. Van de Water J, Ansari AA, Surh CD *et al.* Evidence for the targeting by 2-oxodehydrogenase enzymes in the T cell response of primary biliary cirrhosis. J Immunol. 1991;146:89.
52. Van de Water J, Ansari A, Prindiville T *et al.* Heterogeneity of autoreactive T cell clones specific for the E2 component of the pyruvate dehydrogenase complex in primary biliary cirrhosis. J Exp Med. 1995;181:723–33.
53. Ohmori H, Yamuchi J, Yamamoto I. Jpn J Pharmacol. 1986:42.
54. Horsfall AC. Molecular mimicry and autoantigens in connective tissue disease. Mol Biol Rep. 1992;16:139.
55. Query CC, Keene JD. A human autoimmune protein associated with U1 RNA containing a region of homology that is cross-reactive with retroviral p30gag antigen. Cell. 1987;51:211–15.
56. Maul GG, Jimenez SA, Riggs E *et al.* Determination of an epoitope of the diffuse systemic sclerosis marker antigen DNA topoisomerase I: sequence similarities with retroviral p30gag protein suggests a possible cause for autoimmunity in systemic sclerosis. Proc Natl Acad Sci USA. 1989;86:8492–6.
57. Scifield RH, Harley JB. Autoantigenicity of Ro/SSA antigen related to a nucleocapsid protein of vesicular stomatitis virus. Proc Natl Acad Sci USA. 1991;88:3343–7.
58. Horsfall AC, Rose LM. Cross-reactive maternal autoantibodies and congential heart block. J Autoimmun. 1992;5:479–93.
59. Burroughs AK, Sternberg MJE, Baum H. Molecular mimicry in liver disease. Nature. 1992;358:377–8.
60. Shimoda S, Nakamura M, Ishibashi H, Hayashida K, Niho Y. HLA DRB4 0101-restricted immunodominant T cell autoepitope of pyruvate dehydrogenase complex in primary biliary cirrhosis: evidence for molecular mimicry in human autoimmune diseases. J Exp Med. 1995;181:1835–45.
61. Stemerowicz R, Hopf U, Moller B *et al.* Are antimitochondrial antibodies in primary biliary cirrhosis induced by R(rough)-mutants of enterobacteriaceae? Lancet. 1988;2:1166–70.
62. Burroughs AK, Rosenstein IJ, Epstein O, Hamilton-Miller JM, Brumfitt W, Sherlock S. Bacteriuria in primary biliary cirrhosis. Gut. 1984;25:133–7.
63. Hopf U, Moller B, Stemerowicz R *et al.* Relation between *Escherichia coli* R(rough)-forms in gut, lipid A in liver, and primary biliary cirrhosis. Lancet. 1989;2:1419–22.
64. Teoh KL, Mackay IR, Rowley MJ, Fussey SP. Enzyme inhibitory antibodies to pyruvate dehydrogenase complex in primary biliary cirrhosis differ for mammalian, yeast and bacterial enzymes: implications for molecular mimicry. Hepatology. 1994;19:1029–33.
65. Ghadiminejad I, Baum H. Reaction pattern of mitochondrial antibodies of primary biliary cirrhosis (PBC) is species specific but not organ specific. J Bioenerg Biomembr. 1987;19:239–53.
66. Sundin U, Sundqvist KG. Plasma membrane association of primary biliary cirrhosis mitochondrial marker antigen M2. Clin Exp Immunol. 1991;83:407–12.
67. Joplin R, Wallace LL, Johnson GD *et al.* Subcellular localization of pyruvate dehydrogenase dihydrolipoamide acetyltransferase in human intrahepatic biliary epithelial cells. J Pathol. 1995;176:381–90.
68. Van de Water J, Turchany J, Leung PS *et al.* Molecular mimicry in primary biliary cirrhosis. Evidence for biliary epithelial expression of a molecule cross-reactive with pyruvate dehydrogenase complex-E2. J Clin Invest. 1993;91:2653–64.
69. Balan V, Batts KP, Porayko MK, Krom RA, Ludwig J, Wiesner RH. Histological evidence for recurrence of primary biliary cirrhosis after liver transplantation [see comments]. Hepatology. 1993;18:1392–8.
70. Hubscher SG, Elias E, Buckels JA, Mayer AD, McMaster P, Neuberger JM. Primary biliary cirrhosis. Histological evidence of disease recurrence after liver transplantation. J Hepatol. 1993;18:173–84.
71. Wong PY, Portmann B. Recurrence of primary biliary cirrhosis after liver transplantation following FK506-based immunosuppression. J Hepatol. 1993;17:284–7.
72. Neuberger J, Wallace L, Joplin R, Hubscher S. Hepatic distribution of E2 component of pyruvate dehydrogenase complex after transplantation. Hepatology. 1995;22:798–801.

73. Tsuneyama K, Van de Water J, Nakanuma Y *et al.* Human combinatorial autoantibodies and mouse monoclonal antibodies to PDC-E2 produce abnormal apical staining of salivary glands in patients with coexistent primary biliary cirrhosis and Sjögren's syndrome. Hepatology. 1994;20:893–8.
74. Scharschmidt BF. Human liver transplantation: analysis of data on 540 patients from four centers. Hepatology. 1984;4(Suppl.):95S.
75. Van Thiel DH, Tarter R, Gavaler JSEA. Liver transplantation in adults: an analysis of costs and benefits at the University of Pittsburg. Gastroenterology. 1986;90:211–37.
76. Surh CD, Coppel R, Gershwin ME. Structural requirement for autoreactivity on human pyruvate dehydrogenase-E2, the major mitochondrial autoantigen in primary biliary cirrhosis. J Immunol. 1990;144–9.
77. Leung PS, Chuang DT, Wynn RM *et al.* Autoantibodies to BCOADC-E2 in patients with primary biliary cirrhosis recognize a conformational epitope. Hepatology. 1995;22:505–13.
78. Moteki S, Leung PSC. Epitope mapping and reactivity of autoantibodies to the E2 component of 2-oxoglutarate dehydrogenase complex in primary biliary cirrhosis using recombinant 2-oxoglutarate dehydrogenase complex. Hepatology. 1996;23:436–44.
79. Iwayama T, Leung PSC, Coppel RL *et al.* Specific reactivity of recombinant human PDC-E1a in primary biliary cirrhosis. J. Autoimmun. 1991;4:769–78.
80. Surh CD, Cooper AE, Coppel RL *et al.* The predominance of IgG3 and IgM isotype anti-mitochondrial antibodies against recombinant fused mitochondrial peptide in patients with PBC. Hepatology. 1988:290–6.
81. Outschoorn I, Rowley MJ, Cook AD, Mackay IR. Subclasses of immunoglobulins and auto-antibodies in autoimmune diseases. Clin Immunol Immunopathol. 1993;66:59.
82. Van de Water J, Fregeau D, Davis P *et al.* Autoantibodies of primary biliary cirrhosis recognize dihydrolipoamide acetyltransferase and inhibit enzyme function. J Immunol. 1988;141:2321–4.
83. Fregeau DR, Davis PA, Danner DJ *et al.* Antimitochondrial antibodies of primary biliary cirrhosis recognize dihydrolipoamide acyltransferase and inhibit enzyme function of the branched chain alpha-ketoacid dehydrogenase complex. J Immunol. 1989;142:3815–20.
84. Sundin U. Antibody binding and inhibition of pyruvate dehydrogenase (PDH) in sera from patients with primary biliary cirrhosis. Clin Exp Immunol. 1990;81:238–41.
85. Uibo R, McKay IR, Rowley M, Humphries P, Armstrong MCD, McNeilage J. Inhibition of enzyme function by human autoantibodies to an autoantigen pyruvate dehydrogenase E2: different epitope for spontaneous human and induced rabbit autoantibodies. Clin Exp Immunol. 1990;80:192–6.
86. Pascual V, Cha S, Gershwin ME, Capra DJ, Leung PSC. Nucleotide sequence analysis of natural and combinatorial anti-PDC-E2 antibodies in patients with primary biliary cirrhosis. Recapitulating immune selection with molecular biology. J Immunol. 1994;152:2577–85.
87. Berg PA, Klein R. Mitochondrial antigens and autoantibodies: from anti-M1 to anti-M9 Klin Wochenschr. 1986;64:897–909.

17 Immunomodulatory properties of bile acids

Y. CALMUS, P. PODEVIN and R. POUPON

INTRODUCTION

The clinical observation that some forms of immune deficiency existed in patients with cholestatic liver disease[1–4] led us to suspect that endogenous bile acids in excess could be reponsible for this phenomenon[1–6]. On the other hand, we found that ursodeoxycholic acid (UDCA) therapy is able to correct, at least partially, some of the immunological abnormalities observed in primary biliary cirrhosis (PBC), such as abnormal hepatic HLA Class I molecule expression, high levels of circulating immunoglobulins M and antimitochondrial antibodies[7–9].

Accordingly, we designed a series of studies to evaluate the effects of cholestasis, chenodeoxycholic acid (CDCA) and UDCA on cell-mediated immunity, and to determine the mechanisms of these effects.

EFFECTS OF CHOLESTASIS AND BILE ACIDS ON CELL-MEDIATED IMMUNITY

We assessed the respective influences of cholestasis, CDCA and UDCA on mixed lymphocyte culture (MLC), a model of cellular immune response, using mouse splenic mononuclear cells[5].

Irradiated C57 BL/6 spleen mononuclear cells and fresh cells from DBA/2 mice were mixed at an optimal ratio of 1 : 4 for 5 days. Incorporation of [^{3}H] thymidine was measured at the end of the incubation period. In the first series of experiments MLC were performed with cells obtained from 3-day common bile duct-ligated mice. A significant inhibition of proliferation ($p < 0.001$) was observed in MLC when DBA responder cells were obtained from cholestatic mice and stimulator cells from normal mice (–81 ± 8%), and when both responder and stimulator cells were obtained from cholestatic mice (–87 ± 7%).

In a second series of experiments the effects of various concentrations of free bile acids (CDCA, UDCA, or a combination of both) were evaluated in MLC with splenic lymphocytes from non-cholestatic mice. In some experiments the standard culture medium was supplemented with conditioned medium. CDCA induced a dose-dependent inhibition of MLC response from non-cholestatic mice, with 50% inhibition at 25 μmol/L. In contrast, UDCA had no significant effect at concentrations ranging from 12.5 to 50 μmol/L. When incubation was performed with increasing concentrations of CDCA and a fixed concentration of UDCA (25 μmol/L), inhibition was similar to that observed with CDCA alone. Supplementation with exogenous interleukins, assessed by adding conditioned medium to the MLC, partially compensated for the inhibitory effect of 25 μmol/L CDCA.

To assess the effect of bile acids on cell viability, fresh mononuclear cells were incubated with $Na_2{}^{51}CrO_4$ for 90 min. The cells were then washed, incubated in complete medium for 60 min, then resuspended in complete medium for 24 h with various concentrations of CDCA or UDCA. At the end of the incubation period the supernatant was counted in a gamma-counter. The viability of mononuclear cells incubated for 5 days with CDCA or UDCA was not affected at concentrations up to 150 μmol/L; significant cytolysis ($p < 0.05$) was observed with 250 μmol/L CDCA and above 500 μmol/L UDCA.

EFFECTS OF BILE ACIDS ON MONONUCLEAR CELL CYTOKINE PRODUCTION

We explored whether immunosuppression could be explained by a modulating effect of bile acids on the production cytokines. Interleukin-1 (IL-1), IL-6 and tumour necrosis factor alpha (TNFα)[10], which play a critical role in the induction and regulation of the immune and inflammatory responses, and IL-2, IL-4 and IL-10 (unpublished data), produced by T lymphocytes, have been studied. IL-2 plays a critical role in the development of the cell-mediated immune response, while IL-4 and IL-10 have a negative effect on this response.

Mononuclear cell suspensions were prepared from healthy blood donors. Monocytes were isolated from total mononuclear cells by adherence and incubated for 18 h in the presence of lipopolysaccharide (LPS) or zymosan, in the presence or absence of bile acids. Purified lymphocytes were recovered from non-adherent cells and incubated with phytohaemagglutinin, in the presence or absence of bile acids. Cytokines were measured in the supernatant at the end of the incubation period. IL-1β, IL-6 and TNFα were measured using a radioimmunoassay. IL-2, IL-4 and IL-10 were measured using an enzyme-linked assay. Preliminary tests showed that CDCA and UDCA (up to 250 μmol/L) did not interfere with the assays.

IL-1β production

CDCA had a dose-dependent inhibitory effect on IL-1β secretion, with 50% inhibition at a CDCA concentration of 60 μmol/L in the culture medium. In contrast, 50% inhibition by UDCA was reached only at a concentration of 100 μmol/L.

IL-6 production

CDCA had a dose-dependent inhibitory effect, with 50% inhibition at 80 μmol/L, while 50% inhibition by UDCA was reached at concentrations above 200 μmol/L. UDCA (25μmol/L) had no significant effect on the inhibition induced by CDCA.

TNFα production

CDCA had a dose-dependent inhibitory effect on TNFα secretion by LPS-stimulated monocytes; 50% inhibition was obtained at 80 μmol/L, while 50% inhibition by UDCA was reached only at concentrations above 200 μmol/L. UDCA (25–100 μmol/L) did not reverse the inhibition induced by CDCA (100 μmol/L). CDCA also had a dose-dependent inhibitory effect on the zymosan-induced production of TNFα, with 50% inhibition at 70 μmol/L. UDCA had no significant inhibitory effect on TNFα production at 200 μmol/L.

IL-2 production

Fifty per cent inhibition was obtained at a CDCA concentration of 60 μmol/L in the culture medium; 50% inhibition by UDCA was not reached at a concentration of 200 μmol/L.

IL-4 production

CDCA had a stimulatory effect on IL-4 secretion at 50 μmol/L and 100 μmol/L (+ 190% and + 125%, respectively, of control value); an inhibition was obtained at higher concentrations; 50% inhibition by UDCA was not reached at a concentration of 200 μmol/L.

IL-10 production

Fifty per cent inhibition was obtained at a CDCA concentration of 60 μmol/L; 50% inhibition by UDCA was not reached at a concentration of 200 μmol/L.

Therefore, the immunosuppressive effect of CDCA on the cell-mediated response could be explained, at least in part, by a defective production of cytokines such as IL-2. In addition, the production of IL-4, which has a negative effect on the cell-mediated immune response, is enhanced by CDCA. These data could contribute towards explaining the immunosuppressive effects of bile acids.

MECHANISM OF THE IMMUNOSUPPRESSIVE EFFECTS OF BILE ACIDS

Monocytes/macrophages are induced by immunological stimuli to synthesize and express on their cell surface procoagulant activity (PCA), usually identified as tissue factor. Tissue factor is a membrane-bound glycoprotein that initiates the extrinsic pathway of blood coagulation, by serving as the receptor and essential cofactor for VII and VII(a). Once formed, the factor VII(a)–TF complex activates factor IX and X, leading ultimately to thrombin generation and fibrin accumulation. It is well established that T cells are involved in the production of PCA, and that PCA expression is closely correlated to cell-mediated immunity. Activation of monocytes is dependent upon transduction pathways involving both an increase in the intracellular calcium concentration and the activation of protein kinase C (PKC). Since bile acids can activate PKC activity and enhance intracellular calcium concentrations in *in-vitro* models, it is tempting to speculate that their effects on monocyte activity are mediated by a direct effect on these transducing pathways. Immunosuppressive drugs such as cyclosporine and corticosteroids have inhibitory effects on monocytes, and exert negative effects on cytokine production. Bile acids could exert their immune effects by a mechanism similar to that of immunosuppressants.

To further examine the role of bile acids we evaluated the effect of CDCA on monocyte procoagulant activity (PCA), a model of monocyte activation[11,12].

Mononuclear blood cells and monocytes were collected from medication-free volunteers. Incubations were performed in the absence or presence of LPS. Cell lysates were assayed for PCA with a one-stage clotting assay using normal human plasma as substrate. Since PCA is generated exclusively by monocytes in this system, results are expressed as PCA per 10^5 monocytes. PKC activity of monocytes was determined by measuring the incorporation of [γ-^{32}P]ATP into histone III-S. In PKC depletion studies, monocytes were depleted of PKC by 48-h treatment with phorbol myristate acetate. Then the cells were washed and stimulated by LPS in the presence of either CDCA or phorbol ester. In order to evaluate the reversibility of the inhibitory effect of CDCA, mononuclear cells preincubated with CDCA (100 μmol/L) for 4 h were washed and resuspended in complete medium for 18 h. PCA was subsequently evaluated.

CDCA inhibited PCA in a dose-dependent manner, with half-maximal and maximal inhibitions occurring at 100 and 200 μmol/L, respectively. CDCA inhibition of PCA was reversible: A 4-h treatment with 50 μmol/L CDCA followed by extensive washings did not modify mononuclear cell responsiveness to LPS, whether cells had been treated or not with CDCA; PCA after a 18-h incubation in complete medium was higher (523 ± 31 U/10^5 monocytes) than that measured in untreated cells (396 ± 29 U/10^5 monocytes). To determine whether the inhibitory effect of CDCA could result from a deleterious effect at the membrane level, sonicated membranes with high PCA obtained from LPS-stimulated cells were exposed to CDCA 25 μmol/L for 4 h. After washings, the PCA value was 727 ± 17 U/10^5 monocytes versus 688 ± 17 U/10^5 monocytes in untreated membranes sonicated. Finally, to rule out the possibility that the effect of CDCA could result from competition with LPS at the cell membrane level, we assessed the effect of CDCA on unstimulated cells. CDCA exerted a dose-dependent inhibitory effect on PCA by unstimulated mononuclear cells which was similar to that obtained with LPS-stimulated cells, the half-maximal and maximal inhibitions being obtained at CDCA concentrations of 80 and 250 μmol/L, respectively.

Two main mechanisms might explain the inhibitory effects of CDCA on effectors of the immune response. A detergent effect on the cell membrane is unlikely, as the concentrations used were far below the critical micellar concentrations, even though it has been shown that submicellar concentrations of bile acids can solubilize cholesterol[13]. The second possibility is that bile acids intercalate in cell membranes[14], modifying membrane fluidity[15] and permeability, particularly to calcium ions[16] and activating certain transduction pathways[12,17].

In an attempt to approach the signalling pathway implicated in CDCA inhibition of PCA by mononuclear cells we tested the effects of various agonists of the PKA-, PKC-, and calcium-dependent pathways for their ability to mimic the CDCA inhibitory effect on this process. Forskolin (10^{-6} mol/L and dibutyryl c-AMP (10^{-6} mol/L), two agonists of the PKA-dependent pathway, did not modify PCA by LPS-stimulated mononuclear cells. By contrast the calcium ionophore A23187 (10^{-6} mol/L) produced a marked inhibition (82 ± 9%) of PCA by mononuclear cells. Phorbol myristate acetate, a strong PKC activator, proved to be fully potent in mimicking CDCA inhibition, since the phorbol ester (160 nmol/L) produced a dramatic inhibition (87 ± 12%) of PCA, which was equivalent to that elicited by the bile acid (96 ± 10%) (200 μmol/L). Furthermore, staurosporine, a potent PKC inhibitor, could reverse, albeit partially, the inhibitory effect of CDCA (50 μmol/L) on PCA by LPS-stimulated mononuclear cells (236 ± 11 U/10^5 monocytes versus 21 ± 4 U/10^5 monocytes in untreated cells). In accordance with this finding, we observed that, after depletion of PKC activity by 48-h treatment of monocytes with 1 μg/ml PMA, CDCA inhibition of PCA was about one-half that measured in untreated monocytes. Finally, we compared the effects of CDCA and phorbol ester on endogenous substrate phosphorylation. Both these agents caused a dose-dependent increase in the phosphorylation of a 37 kDa protein, demonstrated as a PKC substrate in lymphoid tissue. PKC appears to be a major signal transduction system in macrophages and lymphoid tissue. Our results suggest the involvement of this enzyme in CDCA inhibitory effect on LPS-stimulated PCA. There are several possible mechanisms which may explain CDCA activation of PKC. The bilayer disruption by incorporation into the membrane of numerous substances, especially anionic amphiphilic compounds, is known to activate PKC. Hydrophobic bile acids such as CDCA are thought to form dimers or multimers in the outer bilayer membrane[18], and thereby to alter membrane fluidity, polarity and permeability. The altered properties of the membrane surface by hydrophobic bile acids could result in the association of PKC with membrane phospholipids promoting the liberation of diacylglycerol, the physiological endogenous activator of the enzyme. Alternatively, the ability to activate PKC may be accounted for by the ionophoretic properties of CDCA.

In addition, an intracellular effect cannot be ruled out. Indeed, in the human breast cancer cell line MCF7, submicellar bile acid concentrations (100–300 μmol/L) can influence both cell growth and oestrogen-receptor function[19].

RELEVANCE OF THE *IN VITRO* DATA TO THE IMMUNOSUPPRESSIVE EFFECT OF CHOLESTASIS

In the previous studies, bile acids were used at concentrations of 0–200 μmol/L, i.e. covering the range of bile acid concentrations commonly observed in liver tissue during chronic cholestasis[20,21]. We analysed bile acid concentrations in liver, lymph nodes and serum of 14 patients with chronic liver disease and submitted to liver transplantation. The tissue concentrations in liver and lymph nodes were 183 ± 29 and 195.5 ± 94 nmol/g of tissue, respectively, while blood concentration was 148 ± 54 μmol/L (unpublished data). Bile acid concentrations in liver and lymph nodes from patients with cholestatic disorders were 3–4-fold higher than in blood. Furthermore, because of the nature of most of the cholestatic disorders, e.g. destruction of a segment of some bile ducts, the concentration of bile acids in the portal and periportal area of the obstructed bile ducts might be higher than the average bile acid concentration in the entire liver. Finally, pharmacological effect depends on the concentration × time product rather than on concentration only. For cells which cannot easily extrude a substance, the duration of exposure becomes critical. Thus, one can imagine that 'years of cholestasis' may lead to very high concentrations of bile acids in lymphocytes which are not able to extrude them, in contrast to normal hepatocytes.

The immunosuppressive effects of endogenous bile acids could explain, at least partly, the onset of severe systemic infections during cholestasis of various origins. During PBC this immunosuppressive effect could be integrated in the pathophysiology of the disease as follows: PBC results from an activation of helper T cells, resulting in cholangitis and hepatocyte necrosis; the intrahepatic accumulation of endogenous bile acids could induce a local state of immunosuppression, explaining the slow progression of ductular destruction. This could also explain the disappointing results obtained with immunosuppressive therapies aimed at blocking T cell activation.

References

1. Roughneen PT, Gouma DJ, Kulkarni AD, Fanslow WF, Rowlands BJ. Impaired cell-mediated immunity in experimental biliary obstruction and its reversibility by internal biliary drainage. J Surg Res. 1986;41:113–25.
2. Roughneen PT, Drath DB, Kulkarni AD, Rowlands BJ. Impaired nonspecific cellular immunity in experimental cholestasis. Ann Surg. 1987;206:578–82.
3. Cainzos M, Potel J, Puente JL. Anergy in jaundiced patients. Br J Surg. 1988;75:147–9.
4. Feduccia TD, Scott-Conner CEH, Grogan JB. Profound suppression of lymphocyte function in early biliary obstruction. Am J Med Sci. 1988;296:39–44.
5. Calmus Y, Weill B, Ozier Y, Chéreau C, Houssin D, Poupon R. Immunosuppressive properties of chenodeoxycholic and ursodeoxycholic acids in the mouse. Gastroenterology. 1992;103:617–21.
6. Roughneen PT, Didlake R, Kumar SC, Kahan BD, Rowlands BJ. Enhancement of heterotopic cardiac allograft survival by experimental biliary ligation. Transplantation. 1987;43:437–8.
7. Calmus Y, Gane P, Rouger P, Poupon R. Hepatic expression of class I and class II major histocompatibility complex molecules in primary biliary cirrhosis: effect of ursodeoxycholic acid. Hepatology. 1990;11:12–15.
8. Calmus Y, Arvieux C, Gane P *et al.* Cholestasis induces major histocompatibilty complex (MHC) class I expression in hepatocytes. Gastroenterology. 1992;102:1371–7.
9. Poupon RE, Balkau B, Eschwege E, Poupon R and the UDCA–PBC study group. A multicenter double blind trial of ursodiol for the treatment of primary biliary cirrhosis. N Engl J Med. 1991;324:1548–54.
10. Calmus Y, Guéchot J, Bonnefis MT, Giboudeau J, Poupon R. Differential effects of chenodeoxycholic and ursodeoxycholic acids on IL1, IL6 and TNFα production by monocytes. Hepatology. 1992;16:719–23.

11. Calmus Y, Podevin P, Robert A, Poupon R. Differential effects of chenodeoxycholic and ursodeoxycholic acids on procoagulant activity expression by human monocytes. J Hepatol. 1994;20:466–72.
12. Podevin P, Calmus Y, Robert A *et al.* R, Chenodeoxycholic acid inhibition of procoagulant activity of human monocytes: involvement of protein kinase C activation. Hepatology. 1994;19:1164–70.
13. Vlahcevic ZR, Gurley EC, Heuman DM, Hylemon PB. Bile salts in submicellar concentrations promote bidirectional cholesterol transfer (exchange) as a function of their hydrophobicity. J Lipid Res. 1990;31:1063–71.
14. Schubert R, Schmidt KH. Structural changes in vesicles membranes and mixed micelles of various lipid composition after binding of different bile salts. Biochemistry. 1988;27:8787–94.
15. Nakashima T, Shima T, Sakamoto Y *et al.* Effects of bile acids and taurine on the lipid fluidity of hepatic microsomes in normal and bile duct-ligated rats. A spin label study. J Hepatol. 1993;18:74–9.
16. Zimniak P, Little JM, Radominska A, Oelberg DG, Anwer MS, Lester R. Taurine-conjugated bile acids act as Ca^{2+} ionophores. Biochemistry. 1991;30:8598–604.
17. Podevin P, Calmus Y, Guéchot J, Bonnefis MT, Poupon R, Cherqui G. Inhibitory effect of chenodeoxycholic acid (CDCA) on IL1β and IL6 production by human monocytes involves different signalling pathways. Hepatology. 1992;16:165A.
18. Schubert R, Schmidt. K. Structural changes in vesicule membranes and mixed micelles of various lipid composition after binding of differents bile salts. Biochemistry. 1988;27:8787.
19. Baker P, Wilton J, Jones C, Stenzel D, Watson N, Smith G. Bile acids influence the growth, oestrogen receptor and oestrogen-regulated proteins of MCF-7 human breast cancer cells. Br J Cancer. 1992;65:566–72.
20. Stiehl A. Disturbances of bile acid metabolism in cholestasis. In: Paumgartner G, editor. Clinics in gastroenterology: bile acids. London: WB Saunders; 1977:45–89.
21. Turjman N, Nair PP. Tissue-bound bile acids. In: Setchell KDR, Kritchevsky D, Nair PP, editors. The bile acids: chemistry, physiology and metabolism. New York: Plenum Press; 1988:373–8.

Section III
Clinical aspects and therapy

18
Acute and chronic liver allograft rejection

A. J. DEMETRIS, N, MURASE and T. E. STARZL

INTRODUCTION

Hepatic allograft rejection can be thought of as an iatrogenically induced autoimmune liver disease, brought about by implantation of a new liver in which there is MHC mismatching between the donor and recipient. Acute rejection is characterized by brisk portal and perivenular inflammation that damages small bile ducts and tunnels beneath the endothelium of portal and/or central veins. Inflammation is less severe in chronic rejection, the hallmark features of which are loss of small bile ducts and obliterative arteriopathy (OA). To understand pathophysiological events associated with bile duct damage during liver allograft rejection, it is important to review the functional anatomy and microenvironment of the biliary tree and surrounding portal tracts.

OVERVIEW OF MICROENVIRONMENT OF THE BILIARY TREE AND PORTAL TRACTS

This is reviewed in ref. 1. The intrahepatic biliary tract consists of a central, tree-like branching network of tubules. Starting with the trunk at the hilum, it ends after a series of *at least* 17 or 18 branches[2], in a continuous three-dimensional rete or arcade in the Hering canals[2]. Although clearly there is some functional heterogeneity of biliary epithelial cells (BEC) along the biliary tree[1], few if any studies directly address these variations from an immunological perspective. Within the liver the biliary tree is supported by a connective tissue framework recognized in tissue sections as portal tracts. These structures also normally support branches of the portal vein and hepatic artery, lymphatic capillaries that drain to hilar lymph nodes, and a few inflammatory and antigen-presenting cells.

The hepatic artery ends in three distal microcirculatory beds in or near the portal tracts[3–5]: a general plexus that supplies the portal connective tissues; a second branch that directly drains into periportal sinusoids and/or peripheral portal vein branches via arterio-portal anastomoses; and lastly, a peribiliary capillary plexus that forms an inner and outer sheath around the bile ducts up to their terminal branches[3,4]. The peribiliary microvasculature plexus provides a source of oxygenated blood to the bile ducts and facilitates exchange of substances between these two structures[6]. This arrangement is ideally suited for the important role of the peribiliary plexus in the regulation of hepatic arterial flow, in the secretion, absorption and concentration of bile, and possibly in hepatic regeneration[1,4].

Destruction of the intrahepatic artery and peribiliary plexus by intra-arterial injection of alcohol[4] or chemotherapeutic agents[7,8]; or direct immunological injury[5,9,10] can result in subsequent ischaemic damage to the biliary tree. This can manifest as atrophy and loss of small bile ducts, and/or inflammation and fibrosis of larger septal or extrahepatic bile ducts[1]. 'Ischaemic cholangitis'[11] is a term used to concisely identify this type of biliary tract injury.

Lymph vessels are found in close association with branches of the hepatic artery, portal vein and bile ducts[12]. Lymph fluid is thought to flow towards the portal tract in the space of Disse, but this is not thought to be a true lymphatic vessel. Even though direct connections between the lumen of portal lymphatics and the spaces of Disse or Mall are not observed[12], by 6 h after an intravenous carbon injection, carbon-laden macrophages migrate from the sinusoids into the interlobular connective tissue[13]. By 9–12 h they enter the lymphatic vessels of the portal tract, and by 12–24 h they end up at the corticomedullary junction of the coeliac nodes[13]. Presumably, antigens derived from the hepatic lymph follow the same route.

Professional antigen-presenting cells or dendritic cells (DC) normally lie near the small lymphatic channels in the portal tracts, where they presumably monitor the entry of potential antigens[14–21]. Mature DC express high levels of Class II MHC antigens, and a variety of adhesion and co-stimulatory molecules that enable them to efficiently prime naive T lymphocytes[14,22–26]. Acquisition of antigen by DC stimulates their emigration to regional lymph nodes, where antigen presentation to T cells occurs in the paracortex[24,26].

Although the *lymphogenous* traffic patterns of portal-based hepatic DC have not been studied in great detail, it is not unreasonable to conclude that they would behave similar to DC based at other sites. The identification of biliary antigens[27] and reactive T cells[28] in the hilar lymph nodes of patients with PBC and other inflammatory liver disorders provides indirect and circumstantial evidence for the existence of a portal-to-hilar lymph node migration route[1]. The *haematogenous* migratory routes of hepatic DC have been studied by taking advantage of alloantigens to trace the donor DC population after liver transplantation[1,18,29,30]. Within days after hepatic replacement, donor-derived DC are detected in the recipient spleen, thymus and lymph nodes[18,29]. This probably mimics the normal migratory patterns of hepatic-based DC. Although the significance of these migration patterns is unknown, it might be interesting to investigate whether traffic to the thymic medulla after antigen acquisition plays a role in oral tolerance.

The close association between the biliary tree and portal lymph vessels is illustrated by injection of dye under elevated pressures into the clamped choledochus. This results in the appearance of the dye in the hepatic lymph vessels[4].

This experiment illustrates the potential of hilar lymph nodes to serve as a processing station for antigens and other debris emigrating from immunological reactions in and around the biliary tree.

BILIARY EPITHELIAL MOLECULES OF POTENTIAL IMMUNOLOGICAL IMPORTANCE

Important to any discussion of inflammatory disorders of the biliary tree is an overview of immunologically important antigens expressed on bile epithelial cells (BEC) (Table 1; reviewed in ref. 1). Probably of greatest significance are the major histocompatibility (MHC) antigens, also known as the human leucocyte (HLA) antigens. They are highly polymorphic glycoproteins important for presentation of antigens to T cells. Class I MHC antigens are expressed to some degree on all nucleated cells including the biliary epithelium (reviewed in ref. 31). Polymorphic residues determine the specificity of a peptide-binding cleft, which is formed by two α-helices supported by an eight-strand, antiparallel β-pleated sheet[31]. This cleft binds peptides derived predominantly from cytosolic proteins, including viral antigens, which are usually eight to 11 residues in length. Expression of Class I MHC enables a cell to bind to the T cell receptor/CD8 complex on MHC identical T-lymphocytes, and initiate immune responses, such as cell-mediated lympholysis (CML)[32].

Class II MHC molecules (DR, DP and DQ) are not normally expressed on bile duct cells, but can be induced on them in an inflammatory microenvironment. Similar to Class I antigens, Class II MHC molecules can bind peptides, the usual source of which are exogenously or endogenously derived self proteins or 'ingested' foreign proteins, that are degraded in the endocytic/lysosomal compartments[31]. The bound peptides are usually derived from MHC molecules, membrane/secretory, and exogenous proteins. Cytosolic proteins are much less commonly represented. Restrictions on the length and characteristics of the peptides bound to Class II MHC molecules are less stringent than those for Class I MHC. On the cell surface the Class II/peptide complex can interact with MHC identical T cells bearing the CD4 antigen and a T cell receptor complex.

In the normal liver the BEC also express the appropriate major blood group antigens, A, B and H[33,34]; the minor antigens Lewis^{a} (Le^{a}) and Lewis^{b} (Le^{b} in secretors), sialyl Le^{x} (large ducts), sialyl Le^{a} (see also Chapter 9), Le^{y} (usually large ducts) and Pr, but are negative for I and i[33–35]. Recognition of the major blood group antigens by natural isoagglutinins is of importance in humoral liver allograft rejection. Sialyl Le^{x} antigens can serve as ligands for E- and P-selectins, which are important in neutrophil, monocyte and lymphocyte adhesion and rolling[36]. BEC also normally express the integrin molecules very late antigen (VLA)-2, 3 and 6. These are receptors for laminin and collagen, present in the surrounding basement membrane[37,38]. In addition, the integrins can also assist in binding of inflammatory cells that express surface matrix-like molecules[37].

Like the Class II MHC peptides, the adhesion molecules ICAM-1, LFA-3, and CD51 are not normally expressed on BEC. However, they can be upregulated by inflammatory cytokines (reviewed in refs 39 and 40). ICAM-1

Table 1 Summary of biliary epithelial antigens of potential importance in immunological reactions (adapted from ref. 1)

BEC molecule	*Ligand*	*BEC expression*		*Functions*
		Normal expression	*Cytokine up-regulation*	
Major blood group antigens A, B, H	React with isoagglutinins	+	+	React with isoagglutinins; of importance of humoral rejection of liver allografts
Class I MHC (A, B)	CD8 and TCR complex	+	+	Antigen presentation to CD8+ T lymphocytes for effective immunity to intracellular pathogens
Class II MHC (DR, DP, DQ)	CD4 and TCR complex	–	+	Antigen presentation to CD4+ T lymphocytes for amplification of immune responses and proliferation of reactive cells
LFA-3 (CD58)	CD2 (LFA-2)	–	+	Adhesion between activated T cells and cytotoxic targets or antigen-presenting cells; may assist in signalling for cytotoxic and helper activity of T cells
VLA-2, 3 and 6	Laminin, collagen fibronectin, invasin	+	+	Mediates adhesion to extracellular matrix and inflammatory cells that express matrix-like surface proteins; can assist the entry of bacteria into cells via invasin
ICAM-1 (CD54)	LFA-1, Mac-1	–	+	Facilitates low-frequency or low-avidity binding between Class II MHC/TCR; facilitates NK recognition of targets; ? co-mitogen for T cells; receptor for rhinovirus and *Plasmodium falciparum*
NCAM (CD56)	NCAM, heparan, sulphate, receptors on NK cells	–	+	Mediates cellular interactions in development of nervous system; may play role in NK recognition of alloantigenic targets
Sialyl Lew^{x}	E-selectin, ELAM-1, P-selectin, CD62	–	+	Mediates binding to selectins, which are a family of adhesive receptors found on leucocytes (L), platelets (P) and endothelial cells (E)
CD51	RGD sequence in ECM	–	+	Recognizes and binds to RGD sequence in the extracellular matrix proteins virtonectin, von Willebrand factor, fibrinogen and thrombospondin
BB1/B7	CD28	–	+	Co-stimulation of T cells via the CD3/T-cell receptor complex
Heat shock proteins 27, (65)*, 70, 90	Lymphocyte stimulation	+	+	May be involved in 'non-specific' pathways of BEC damage during acute and chronic rejection (see text)

* Not normally expressed but up-regulated after tissue injury (see text).

increases the efficiency of the T cell–APC binding by facilitating low-frequency or low-avidity interactions[41]. LFA-3 binding to CD2 on the surface of activated T lymphocytes assists in cell–cell adhesion, and possibly in signalling for cytotoxic and helper functional activity[39,40]. By recognizing the RGD sequence in the extracellular matrix proteins including vitronectin, von Willebrand factor, fibrinogen and thrombospondin[42], CD51 can assist in binding of BEC to matrix components.

Theoretically, expression of 27, 65, 70 and 90 kDa heat-shock protein (hsp), either normally or after BEC injury (Table 1) may also play a role in bile duct injury in liver allograft rejection, since hsp reactive lymphocytes have been isolated from rejecting cardiac allografts[43,44].

ACUTE REJECTION

Acute rejection is by far the most common manifestation of liver allograft rejection. It has recently been defined in a consensus document[45] as: ‘inflammation of the allograft, elicited by a genetic disparity between the donor and recipient, primarily affecting interlobular bile ducts and vascular endothelia, including portal and hepatic veins and occasionally the hepatic artery and its branches’[45].

Acute rejection is more frequent or can be worse in sensitized recipients, children, HLA DR mismatched recipients, and in those who receive less than adequate immunosuppression. When severe or persistent, acute rejection can predispose to chronic rejection, which is why it is covered in detail here.

Acute rejection usually first occurs between 5 and 30 days after transplantation and appears to be triggered when donor DC present in the portal tract and perivenular connective tissue directly bind and stimulate recipient T lymphocytes[16,18,46]. This results in T cell activation, proliferation and secretion of cytokines that up-regulate MHC antigens and induce adhesion molecules (reviewed in ref. 36), on the nearby microvasculature and BEC. In turn, more inflammatory cells are recruited, tissue destruction begins, and the clinical manifestations of acute liver allograft rejection appear[1]. Acute rejection occurring late (more than 30 days) after transplantation, is often associated with inadequate levels of immunosuppression[47–49].

Clinical findings are either mild or absent in early or mild acute rejection, although in late or severe cases fever, as well as enlargement, cyanosis, and tenderness of the allograft, frequently occur[45]. Bile drainage from a T tube often becomes thin and pale and the flow is decreased. Occasionally, ascites develops because of liver swelling, and increased intrahepatic pressure and production of lymphatic fluid. Liver dysfunction is usually manifest as concomitant non-selective elevations of some or all of the standard liver injury tests, including total bilirubin, alanine aminotransferase, aspartate aminotransferase, γ-glutamyl transpeptidase, and alkaline phosphatase[45]. Peripheral blood leucocytosis and eosinophilia are also frequently present. The diagnosis of acute rejection is usually suspected on the basis of clinical symptoms, and confirmed on histopathological examination of an allograft needle biopsy.

The three main histopathological features in acute rejection are: (a) predominantly mononuclear portal inflammation; (b) subendothelial inflammation of portal and/or terminal hepatic veins; and (c) bile duct inflammation and damage[1,45]. At least two of the above histopathological findings and biochemical evidence of liver damage are the minimal diagnostic criteria needed to establish the diagnosis of acute rejection.

The portal inflammation associated with acute rejection begins in the interstitium of the portal tracts where clustering between donor DC and recipient lymphocytes occurs[18]. As the reaction develops, blastic transformation of lymphocytes occurs and numerous eosinophils, macrophages and neutrophils appear. The inflammatory cells tunnel beneath the endothelium of the portal and central veins, lifting it from the underlying connective tissue[50,51]. Inflammatory cells also penetrate inside the basement membrane of bile ducts where they are associated with BEC paranuclear vacuolization, pyknosis and cytoplasmic eosinophilia. Although focal breaks in the basement membrane with subsequent lumenal disruption can occur, well-formed portal-based granulomas, like those associated with PBC, are not generally seen. The BEC can also show enlarged nuclei, an increased nuclear : cytoplasmic ratio, nucleoli and mitoses. These BEC changes presumably occur in response to the injury, or the inflammatory microenvironment. Increased proliferation of BEC using PCNA labelling has been noted in acute liver allograft rejection[52], and cytokines have been shown to enhance BEC growth, *in vitro*[53].

Several histopathological grading systems have been used to estimate the severity of acute liver allograft rejection (summarized in ref. 54). At individual centres each of the systems has been shown to have some type of predictive value and reproducibility. Recently, an international consensus has been reached for both the nomenclature[45] and the grading[55] of acute rejection. The latter is based on a combination of the severity of inflammation and the severity of damage to the bile ducts and vasculature, the latter of which manifests as ischaemic injury to the allograft. Hopefully, use of this common language and grading will allow for a better exchange of information and data regarding patient management, evaluation of new drugs and various treatment protocols.

Several methods have been used to characterize the effector mechanisms responsible for bile duct injury: immunophenotypic analysis of the inflammatory infiltrate; allograft mRNA and protein product characterization and functional analysis of graft-infiltrating lymphocytes. Immunocytochemistry studies showing a predominance of CD8+ T-lymphocytes in the portal triads and bile ducts suggest that direct CML is an important mechanism of BEC injury during acute rejection[56–58]. Although B cells comprise only a minor fraction, the presence of many macrophages and other leucocytes implicates 'non-specific' pathways of tissue injury mediated by toxic leucocyte products[56–59]. This also includes eosinophils[60] and their degranulation products, such as major basic protein.

The lymphocyte blastogenesis and eosinophilic infiltration noted on routine microscopy correlates with the up-regulation of interleukins 2 and 5 within the allografts[61–63]. Graft-infiltrating lymphocytes, expanded *in vitro* using IL-2, undergo blastogenesis and proliferate in the presence of donor MHC antigens. They can also kill cells bearing donor MHC antigens[64–66], such as BEC.

Fortunately, in most cases acute rejection is promptly reversible with augmentation of immunosuppression and the duct damage ceases. However, as mentioned above, severe or persistent acute rejection can lead to chronic rejection.

CHRONIC REJECTION

Chronic rejection has been recently defined in a consensus document as a 'usually irreversible process defined by two main histopathologic features: obliterative vasculopathy and loss of bile ducts. Although these two components usually coexist, they occasionally may occur independently.'[45] Chronic rejection has been occasionally observed as early as 2 weeks[67], but it usually does not occur before 2 months after transplantation and most frequently develops after an unresolved episode of acute rejection; multiple episodes of acute rejection; or indolently over a period of months to years, with few or no clinically apparent acute cellular rejection episodes[45].

Unresolved or indolent rejection may become apparent only because of a persistent elevation of liver injury tests. If clinical symptoms are present they usually resemble those of acute rejection, until allograft dysfunction becomes severe enough to cause jaundice. Biliary sludging or appearance of biliary strictures, hepatic infarcts, and finally loss of hepatic synthetic function (which can manifest as coagulopathy, malnutrition, and hepatosplenomegaly) are late findings presaging allograft failure[45]. Standard liver injury test abnormalities in a patient with chronic rejection usually show a progressive cholestatic pattern, with preferential elevation of γ-glutamyl transpeptidase and alkaline phosphatase. The diagnosis of chronic rejection can be supported by selective hepatic angiography that shows pruning of the intrahepatic arteries with poor peripheral filling and segmental narrowing.

Risk factors for chronic rejection indicate that severe and/or persistent immunological injury plays a major role in the development of this disorder. Poorly controlled acute rejection episodes, chronic rejection in a previous failed allograft, a positive pre-transplant lymphocytotoxic crossmatch, anti-MHC antibodies that develop after transplantation, cytomegalovirus infection, matching at the Class II MHC locus and mismatching at the MHC Class I locus, non-Caucasian recipient race, male-to-female sex mismatching, an original disease of primary biliary cirrhosis or autoimmune hepatitis, alcohol abstinence after transplantation in alcoholics, chronic viral hepatitis and treatment with α-interferon have all been cited as predisposing influences[68–84]. Thus, patients who are prone to react strongly with the allograft appear to be at greatest risk.

The minimal diagnostic criteria for establishing the diagnosis of chronic rejection in a *biopsy specimen* are the presence of foam cell obliterative arteriopathy or convincing evidence of bile duct loss (> 50% of the triads) documented by the presence of hepatic artery branches without bile ducts, or by the absence of both ducts and hepatic artery branches[45]. Unfortunately, arteries with pathognomonic foam cell obliteration are rarely present in needle biopsy specimens. Therefore, significant weight is usually placed on the loss of bile ducts, but duct loss without arteriopathy may be seen in some patients as a result of non-rejection-related complications such as bile duct strictures, drug toxicity and cytomegalovirus infection. In addition, bile duct loss can be a focal process, so appropriate caution and clinical correlation are suggested.

Histopathologically, the portal inflammation in chronic rejection is usually mild, but the biliary epithelial degenerative changes are often obvious. The infiltrate consists of an admixture of lymphocytes, plasma cells and macrophages. Degenerative BEC changes such as uneven spacing of individual epithelial cells, eosinophilic transformation of the cytoplasm, and ducts only partially lined by epithelial cells[85] occur before duct loss becomes apparent, and probably represent the earliest stages of chronic rejection[86]. However, a diagnosis of chronic rejection before there is 50% duct loss is more subject to error. Interestingly, despite the destruction of small ducts, a ductular reaction in the marginal zone is not generally seen. The reason for the lack of ductular proliferation is not known, but loss of arterialization, loss of progenitor cells or location of the injury are possible explanations.

Lobular findings in chronic rejection appear to depend on the severity of the duct loss and OA. In the early stages, before duct loss has reached 50% of the triads, lobular changes may be limited to mild spotty necrosis of hepatocytes, mild Kupffer's cell hypertrophy and, at times, mild perivenular inflammation and sclerosis. As duct destruction and loss worsens, centrilobular hepatocanalicular cholestasis, perivenular sclerosis and hepatocyte dropout usually appear. Intrasinusodial foam cell clusters are thought to represent a response to the cholestasis.

The diagnosis of chronic rejection is easier to establish in an explanted failed allograft: foam cell OA should be seen in at least some of the muscular arteries in the hilum[45]. Affected arteries show an intact but hypertrophied endothelium. Lumenal narrowing is usually attributable to subintimal deposition of lipid-laden cells that derive from macrophages and intimal and medial myocytes, but proliferation of myofibroblasts and lymphohistocytic intimal inflammation can also be seen. Occasionally there is superimposed arterial thrombosis. In the major hilar bile ducts sloughing of the epithelium, focal necrosis, intralumenal papillary hyperplasia of the epithelium, mural fibrosis and acute and chronic inflammation can be seen[45]. The same foam cells that are present in the arteries can also be seen around bile ducts and veins in the connective tissue.

Pathophysiological mechanisms that contribute to the bile duct damage and loss associated with chronic rejection include both direct immunological damage to the BEC and ischaemic injury because of OA and destruction of the peribiliary capillary plexus[5,9,10]. Thus, the bile ducts and capillary endothelium appear to be preferentially targeted for immunologically mediated damage, and these two interrelated pathways contribute to duct loss[5,9,10]. A number of immunologically active BEC molecules that might contribute to the selective damage of BEC during chronic rejection include: the expression of Class I and II MHC antigens; the up-regulation of integrin and other adhesion molecules that facilitate interactions with inflammatory cells; binding sites for receptors present on inflammatory cells[36,87]; the presence of a basement membrane and possibly the presence of as-yet-unidentified antigens on primitive epithelia.

Immunological effector mechanisms involved in chronic rejection are poorly understood. However, since chronically rejecting organs are generally devoid of donor passenger leucocytes, indirect alloantigen presentation or secondary stimulation of primed lymphocytes is the likely pathway of alloantigen recognition.

Isolation of cytotoxic T cell mediator granzyme B and pro-inflammatory cytokine mRNA, and direct contact between BEC and recipient cytotoxic lymphocytes, point towards CML effector pathways[57,68,69,88]. The presence of macrophages and B cells suggests that delayed-type hypersensitivity and allo-antibody responses may also be involved[88]. Ischaemic injury because of destruction of the arteries and peribiliary capillary plexus has been discussed above[9,10]. It has been suggested that bile ducts can participate in their own destruction by acting as antigen-presenting cells[72,78,79,89]. Actual testing of this hypothesis, *in vitro*, showed that human BEC were able to stimulate only lymphocytes that had already been primed; they were *unable* to initiate a significant proliferative response in naive or unprimed allogeneic lymphocytes[90]. Moreover, BEC were much less potent stimulators than allogeneic splenocytes or arterial endothelial cells tested in the same assay system[90].

Theoretically lymphocyte clones present in the recipient as a result of the native liver disease could contribute to the immune damage associated with both acute and chronic liver allograft rejection, because effector mechanisms may not be entirely allospecific[91–94]. An example is patients with primary biliary cirrhosis, who have a higher incidence of chronic rejection[81,95]. Perhaps the recipient immune system of such individuals is sensitized to BEC-specific or other antigens. Heat-shock proteins (hsp) are a possible candidate: normal BEC express hsp 27, 70 and 90, and hsp 65 is up-regulated during disease states, including primary biliary cirrhosis[96]. Heat-shock protein-reactive lymphocytes have also been isolated from rejecting allografts[92]. Thus, hsp-reactive clones could represent a 'non-specific' mechanism of tissue injury, called into play once the initial bile duct damage has occurred because of rejection.

Bile duct loss in chronic rejection does not appear to be an irreversible process[73,97]. Regrowth of the ducts reportedly can occur in some patients, especially if the duct loss was detected before the vasculature was destroyed[73], but this does not appear to be a common phenomenon. In such a case a ductular reaction reportedly precedes the reappearance of the ducts[73]. Treatment of patients with the earliest phases of chronic rejection has been successful if therapy is instituted before 50% duct loss and total serum bilirubin has reached 10 mg/dl[86].

FUTURE DIRECTIONS

Obliterative arteriopathy, as described above, is the hallmark feature of chronic rejection in all vascularized organ allografts. Compared to heart and kidney allografts, liver allografts are relatively resistant to this complication; there are no reliable small experimental animal models of chronic liver allograft rejection. Hepatic allografts are spontaneously accepted without immunosuppression in almost all mouse strain combinations and in many rat strains. Moreover, they induce acceptance of other organs from the same donor, and we have shown that a prior liver allograft can protect heart allografts from both severe acute[98] and chronic rejection[99].

Much of the research in chronic rejection has been devoted to studying in detail the pathophysiological mechanisms leading to arterial narrowing because of intimal myofibroblast proliferation[100]. It is thought that intimal inflammation, local release of cytokines and subsequent injury trigger intimal repair mechanisms that cause lumenal narrowing[100,101]. Little attention has been devoted to studying why the recipient immune system persistently assaults the allograft. However, if progress is to be made in studying chronic rejection, a better understanding of the underlying immunobiology is needed.

A potential breakthrough in the understanding of allograft acceptance or tolerance came with the observation that a small number of donor leucocytes (microchimaerism) could persist for decades in recipients of solid organ allografts[102,103]. It was proposed that microchimaerism represented the transfer of a miniature fragment of the donor immune system into the recipient. This fragment had the potential to redefine the immunological self of the recipient and produce allograft acceptance[103]. However, debate emerged because other investigators felt that microchimaerism was an epiphenomenon, and not causally associated with allograft acceptance[104–106]. This fuelled a series of experiments that inadvertently created an experimental animal model and provided important insights into chronic rejection[99]. In those experiments we found that a liver allograft is able to protect a subsequent cardiac allograft from chronic rejection, which was related to persistent graft inflammation and lymphatic disruption[99,107]. Protection from chronic rejection was associated with persistence of donor haematolymphoid cells in the allograft heart, donor liver and in the tissues of the recipient[107]. Although more work is needed to precisely define the immunological mechanisms responsible for graft acceptance, it appears that chronic rejection may reflect a state in which donor passenger leucocytes have been destroyed or have disappeared from the allograft and recipient. The allograft parenchyma, alone, is then unable to prevent indolent immunological injury from slowly destroying the allograft[107].

References

1. Demetris AJ. Immunopathology of the human biliary tree. In: Sirica AE, Longnecker DS, editors. New York: Marcel Dekker; 1997:127–80.
2. Landing BH, Wells TR. Considerations of some architectural properties of the biliary tree and liver in childhood. In: Abramowsky CR, Berstein J, Rosenberg HS, editors. Transplantation pathology – hepatic morphogenesis. New York: Karger; 1991;122–42.
3. Haratake J, Yamamoto O, Hisaoka M, Horie A. Scanning electron microscopic examinations of microvascular casts of the rat liver and bile duct. Sangyo Ika Daigaku Zasshi. 1990;12:19–28.
4. Rappaport AM. Physioanatomic considerations in diseases of the liver. In: Schiff ER, Schiff L, editors. Diseases of the liver, 6th edn. Philadelphia: JB Lippincott; 1987:1–46.
5. Matsumoto Y, McCaughan GW, Painter DM, Bishop GA. Evidence that portal tract microvascular destruction precedes bile duct loss in human liver allograft rejection. Transplantation. 1993;56:69–75.
6. Kono N, Nakanuma Y. Ultrastructural and immunohistochemical studies of the intrahepatic peribiliary capillary plexus in normal livers and extrahepatic biliary obstruction in human beings. Hepatology. 1992;15:411–18.
7. Doria MIJ, Shepard KV, Levin B, Riddell RH. Liver pathology following hepatic arterial infusion chemotherapy. Hepatic toxicity with FUDR. Cancer. 1986;58:855–61.
8. Ludwig J, Kim CH, Wiesner RH, Krom RAF. Floxuridine-induced sclerosing cholangitis: an ischemic cholangiopathy? Hepatology. 1989;9:215–18.

9. Oguma S, Zerbe T, Banner B, Belle S, Starzl TE, Demetris AJ. Chronic liver allograft rejection and obliterative arteriopathy: possible pathogenic mechanisms. Transplant Proc. 1989;21:2203–7.
10. Oguma S, Belle S, Starzl TE, Demetris AJ. A histometric analysis of chronically rejected human liver allografts: insights into the mechanisms of bile duct loss: direct immunologic and ischemic factors. Hepatology. 1989;9:204–9.
11. Ludwig J, Batts KP, MacCarty RL. Ischemic cholangitis in hepatic allografts [see comments]. Mayo Clin Proc. 1992;67:519–26.
12. Niiro GK, O'Morchoe CC. Pattern and distribution of intrahepatic lymph vessels in the rat. Anat Rec. 1986;215:351–60.
13. Matsuno K, Miyakawa K, Ezaki T, Kotani M. The liver lymphatics as a migratory pathway of macrophages from the sinusoids to the celiac lymph nodes in the rat. Arch Histol Cyto. 1990;53:179–87.
14. Steinman RM. The dendritic cell system and its role in immunogenicity. Annu Rev Immunol. 1991;9:271–96.
15. Hart DN, Fabre JW. Demonstration and characterization of Ia-positive dendritic cells in the interstitial connective tissues of rat heart and other tissues, but not brain. J Exp Med. 1981;154:347–61.
16. Prickett TCR, McKenzie JL, Hart DNJ. Characterization of interstitial dendritic cells in human liver. Transplantation. 1988;46:754–61.
17. Hart DNJ, McKenzie JL. Interstitial dendritic cells. Int Rev Immunol. 1990;6:128–49.
18. Demetris AJ, Qian S, Sun H *et al.* Early events in liver allograft rejection: delineation of sites of simultaneous intragraft and recipient lymphoid tissue sensitization. Am J Pathol. 1991;138:609–18.
19. van den Oord JJ, Volpes R, Desmet VJ. Dendritic cells and the liver. [Review]. APMIS. Suppl. 1991;23:68–76.
20. Rao AS, Roake JA, Larsen CP, Hankins DF, Morris PJ, Austyn JM. Isolation of dendritic leukocytes from non-lymphoid organs. [Review]. Adv Exp Med Biol. 1993;329:507–12.
21. Lu L, Woo J, Rao AS *et al.* Propagation of dendritic cell progenitors from normal mouse liver using granulocyte/macrophage colony-stimulating factor and their maturational development in the presence of type-1 collagen. J Exp Med. 1994;179:1823–34.
22. Jenkins MK, DeSilva DR, Johnson JG, Norton SD. Costimulating factors and signals relevant for antigen presenting cell function. In: Kamperdijk EWA, Nieuwenhuis P, Hoefsmit ECM, editors. Advances in experimental medicine and biology: dendritic cells in fundamental and clinical immunology. New York: Plenum Press; 1993:87–92.
23. June CH, Ledbetter JA, Linsley PS, Thompson CB. Role of the CD28 receptor in T-cell activation. [Review]. Immunol Today. 1990;11:211–16.
24. Knight SC, Stagg AJ. Antigen-presenting cell types. [Review]. Curr Opin Immunol. 1993;5:374–82.
25. Linsley PS, Ledbetter JA. The role of the CD28 receptor during T cell responses to antigen. [Review]. Annu Rev Immunol. 1993;11:191–212.
26. MacPherson GG, Liu L. Dendritic cells 'in vivo': Migration and antigen handling. In: Kamperdijk EWA, Nieuwenhuis P, Hoefsmit ECM, editors. Advances in experimental medicine and biology: dendritic cells in fundamental and clinical immunology. New York: Plenum Press; 1993:327–32.
27. Joplin R, Lindsay JG, Hubscher SG *et al.* Distribution of dihydrolipoamide acetyltransferase (E2) in the liver and portal lymph nodes of patients with primary biliary cirrhosis: an immunohistochemical study. Hepatology. 1991;14:442–7.
28. Saidman SL, Demetris AJ, Zeevi A, Duquesnoy RJ. Propagation and characterization of lymphocytes infiltrating livers of patients with primary biliary cirrhosis and autoimmune hepatitis. Hum Immunol. 1990;28:237–44.
29. Demetris AJ, Murase N, Fujisaki S, Fung JJ, Rao AS, Starzl TE. Hematolymphoid cell trafficking, microchimerism, and GVH reactions after liver, bone marrow, and heart transplantation. Transplant Proc. 1993;25:3337–44.
30. Qian S, Demetris AJ, Murase N, Rao AS, Fung JJ, Starzl TE. Murine liver allograft transplantation: tolerance and donor cell chimerism. Hepatology. 1994;19:916–24.
31. Urban RG, Chicz RM, Vignali DAA, Strominger JL. The dichotomy of peptide presentation by Class I and Class II MHC proteins. In: Sette A, editor. Naturally processed peptides. Basel: Karger; 1993:197–234.

32. Johnson AH, Hurley CK, Hartzman RJ, Alper CA, Yunis EJ. HLA. The major histocompatibility complex of man. In: Henry JB, editor. Clinical diagnosis and management by laboratory methods, 18th edn. Philadelphia: WB. Saunders; 1991:761–94.
33. Rouger P, Poupon R, Gane P, Mallissen B, Darnis F, Salmon C. Expression of blood group antigens including HLA markers in human adult liver. Tissue Antigens. 1986;27:78–86.
34. Nakanuma Y, Saski M. Expression of blood group-related antigens in the intrahepatic biliary tree and hepatocytes in normal livers and various hepatobiliary diseases. Hepatology. 1989;10:174–8.
35. Terada T, Nakanuma Y. Profiles of expression of carbohydrate structures during human intrahepatic bile duct development and maturation: a lectin-histochemical and immunohistochemical study. Hepatology. 1994;20:388–97.
36. Steinhoff G, Behrend M, Schrader B, Pichlmayr R. Intercellular immune adhesion molecules in human liver transplants: overview on expression patterns of leukocyte receptor and ligand molecules. Hepatology. 1993;18:440–53.
37. Shimizu Y, Shaw S. Lymphocyte adhesion mediated by VLA(beta 1) integrins. In: Hogg N, editor. Integrins and ICAM-1 in immune responses. Basel: Karger; 1991:34–54.
38. Steinhoff G, Behrend M, Schrader B, Duijvestijn AM, Wonigeit K. Expression patterns of leukocyte adhesion ligand molecules on human liver endothelia. Lack of ELAM-1 and CD62 inducibility on sinusoidal endothelia and distinct distribution of VCAM-1, ICAM-1, ICAM-2, and LFA-3. Am J Pathol. 1993;142:481–8.
39. Imhof BA, Dunon D. Leukocyte migration and adhesion. In: Dixon FJ, editor. Advances in immunology. San Diego: Academic Press;1995:345–416.
40. Dustin ML, Springer TA. Role of lymphocyte adhesion receptors in transient interactions and cell locomotion. In: Paul WE, Fathman CG, Metzger H, editors. Annual review of immunology Palo Alto: Annual Reviews; 1991:27–66.
41. Hogg N, Bates PA, Harvey J. Structure and function of intercellular adhesion molecule-1. In: Hogg N, editor. Integrins and ICAM-1 in immune responses. Basel: Karger; 1991:98–115.
42. Barclay AN, Birkeland ML, Brown MH *et al.* The leucocyte antigens. In: The leucocyte antigen factsbook. San Diego: Academic Press; 1993:101–412.
43. Moliterno R, Woan M, Bentlejewski C *et al.* Heat shock protein-induced T-lymphocyte propagation from endomyocardial biopsies in heart transplantation. J Heart Lung Transplant. 1995;14:329–37.
44. Duquesnoy RJ, Moliterno R, Qian J, Donovan-Peluso M, Pan F, Valdivia L. Role of heat shock protein immunity in allograft rejection. [Review]. Transplant Proc. 1995;27:468–70.
45. Panel IW. Terminology for hepatic allograft rejection. Hepatology. 1995;22:648–54.
46. Hytiroglou P, Lee R, Sharma K *et al.* FK506 versus cyclosporine as primary immunosuppressive agent for orthotopic liver allograft recipients. Histologic and immunopathologic observations. Transplantation. 1993;56:1389–94.
47. Pappo O, Ramos H, Starzl TE, Fung JJ, Demetris AJ. Structural integrity and identification of causes of liver allograft dysfunction occurring more than 5 years after transplantation. Am J Surg Pathol. 1995;19:192–206.
48. Anand AC, Hubscher SG, Gunson BK, McMaster P, Neuberger JM. Timing, significance, and prognosis of late acute liver allograft rejection. Transplantation. 1995;60:1098–103.
49. Soin AS, Rasmussen A, Jamieson NV *et al.* CsA levels in the early posttransplant period – predictive of chronic rejection in liver transplantation? Transplantation. 1995;59:1119–23.
50. Snover DC, Sibley RK, Freese DK. Orthotopic liver transplantation: a pathologic study of 63 serial liver biopsies from 17 patients with specific reference to the diagnostic features and natural history of rejection. Hepatology. 1984;4:1212–22.
51. Snover DC, Freese DK, Sharp HL, Bloomer JR, Najarian JS, Ascher NL. Liver allograft rejection. An analysis of the use of biopsy in determining outcome of rejection. Am J Surg Pathol. 1987;11:1–10.
52. Ray M, Schroeder TJ, Michaels SE, Park S, Hanto DW. Increased expression of proliferating nuclear antigen (PCNA) in liver allograft rejection. Lab Invest. 1993;68:114A.
53. Matsumoto K, Fujii H, Michalopoulos G, Fung JJ, Demetris AJ. Human biliary epithelial cells secrete and respond to cytokines and hepatocyte growth factors *in vitro*: interleukin-6, hepatocyte growth factor and epidermal growth factor promote DNA synthesis *in vitro*. Hepatology. 1994;20:376–82.

54. Demetris AJ, Tsamandas AC, Delaney CP, Abu-Elmagd K, Fung JJ, Starzl TE. Pathology of liver transplantation. In: Klintmalm GB, Bussitill R, editors. Transplantation of the liver. Philadelphia: WB Saunders; 1996:681–723.
55. Panel. The Banff Schema for grading acute liver allograft rejection. Hepatology. 1997 (In press).
56. Demetris AJ, Lasky S, Thiel DHV, Starzl TE, Whiteside T. Induction of DR/IA antigens in human liver allografts: an immunocytochemical and clinicopathologic analysis of twenty failed grafts. Transplantation. 1985;40:504–9.
57. McCaughan GW, Davies JS, Waugh JA *et al.* A quantitative analysis of T lymphocyte populations in human liver allografts undergoing rejection: the use of monoclonal antibodies and double immunolabeling. Hepatology. 1990;12:1305–13.
58. Ibrahim S, Dawson DV, Killenberg PG, Sanfilippo F. The pattern and phenotype of T-cell infiltration associated with human liver allograft rejection. Human Pathol. 1993;24:1365–70.
59. Steinhoff G, Wonigeit K, Sorg C *et al.* Patterns of macrophage immigration and differentiation in human liver grafts. Transplant Proc. 1989;21:398–400.
60. de Groen PC, Kephart GM, Gleich GJ, Ludwig J. The eosinophil as an effector cell of the immune response during hepatic allograft rejection. Hepatology. 1994;20:654–62.
61. Martinez OM, Villanueva JC, Lake J, Roberts JP, Ascher NL, Krams SM. IL-2 and IL-5 gene expression in response to alloantigen in liver allograft recipients and in vitro. Transplantation. 1993;55:1159–66.
62. Martinez OM, Krams SM, Sterneck M *et al.* Intragraft cytokine profile during human liver allograft rejection. Transplantation. 1992;53:449–56.
63. Martinez OM, Ascher NL, Ferrell L *et al.* Evidence for a nonclassical pathway of graft rejection involving interleukin 5 and eosinophils. Transplantation. 1993;55:909–18.
64. Saidman SL, Demetris AJ, Zeevi A, Duquesnoy RJ. Propagation of lymphocytes infiltrating human liver allografts. Correlation with histologic diagnosis of rejection. Transplantation. 1990;49:107–12.
65. Markus BH, Fung JJ, Zeevi A, Starzl TE, Demetris AJ, Duquesnoy RJ. Analysis of T lymphocytes infiltrating human hepatic allografts. Transplant Proc. 1987;19:2470–3.
66. Kolbeck PC, Wood RP, Markin RS. The immunopathology and clinical relevance of lymphocyte cultures in liver transplantation. Mod Pathol. 1993;6:307–12.
67. Ludwig J, Wiesner RH, Batts KP, Perkins JD, Krom RA. The acute vanishing bile duct syndrome (acute irreversible rejection) after orthotopic liver transplantation. Hepatology. 1987;7:476–83.
68. Fennell RH. Ductular damage in liver transplant rejection: its similarity to that of primary biliary cirrhosis and graft-versus-host disease. Pathol Annu. 1981;16:289–294.
69. Vierling JM, RH. Fennell J. Histopathology of early and late human hepatic allograft rejection. Evidence of progressive destruction of interlobular bile ducts. Hepatology. 1985;4:1076–82.
70. Grond J, Gouw AS, Poppema S, Sloof MJH, Gips CH. Chronic rejection in liver transplants: a histopathologic analysis of failed grafts and antecedent serial biopsies. Transplant Proc. 1986;18:128–35.
71. Demetris AJ, Markus BH, Burnham J *et al.* Antibody deposition in liver allografts with chronic rejection. Transplant Proc. 1987;19:121–5.
72. O'Grady JG, S. Sutherland, Harvey F *et al.* Cytomegalovirus infection and donor/recipient HLA antigens. Interdependent co-factors in pathogenesis of vanishing bile duct syndrome after liver transplantation. Lancet. 1988;1:302–5.
73. Freese DK, Snover DC, Sharp HL, Gross CR, Savick SK, Payne WD. Chronic rejection after liver transplantation: a study of clinical, histological and immunological features. Hepatology. 1991;13:882–91.
74. Hoek BV, Wiesner R, Krom R, Ludwig J, Moore S. Severe ductopenic rejection following liver transplantation: incidence, time of onset, risk factors, treatment and outcome. Semin Liver Dis. 1992;12:41–50.
75. Arnold JC, Portmann BC, O'Grady JG, Naoumov NV, Alexander GJM, Williams R. Cytomegalovirus infection persists in the liver graft in the vanishing bile duct syndrome. Hepatology. 1992;16:285–92.
76. Devlin J, O'Grady J, Tan K, Calne R, Williams R. Ethnic variations in patient and graft survival after liver transplantation. Identification of a new risk factor for chronic allograft rejection. Transplantation. 1993;56:1381–4.

77. Lowes J, Hubscher S, Neuberger J. Chronic rejection of the liver allograft. Gastroenterol Clin N Am. 1993;22:401–20.
78. Manez R, White LT, Linden P *et al.* The influence of HLA matching on cytomegalovirus hepatitis and chronic rejection after liver transplantation. Transplantation. 1993;55:1067–71.
79. Manez R, White LT, Kusne S *et al.* Association between donor-recipient HLA-DR compatibility and cytomegalovirus hepatitis and chronic rejection in liver transplantation. Transplant Proc. 1993;25:908–9.
80. Dousset B, Conti F, Houssin D, Calmus Y. Acute vanishing bile duct syndrome after interferon therapy for recurrent HCV infection in liver transplant recipients. N Engl J Med. 1994;330:1160–1.
81. Candinas D, Gunson BK, Nightingale P, Hubscher S, McMaster P, Neuberger JM. Sex mismatch as a risk factor for chronic rejection of liver allografts. Lancet. 1995;346:1117–21.
82. Feray C, Samuel D, Gigou M *et al.* An open trial of interferon alfa recombinant for hepatitis C after liver transplantation: antiviral effects and risk of rejection. Hepatology 1995;22:1084–9.
83. Lautenschlager I, Nashan B, Schlitt HJ, Ringe B, Wonigeit K, Pichlmayr R. Early intragraft inflammatory events of liver allografts leading to chronic rejection. Transplant Int. 1995;8:446–51.
84. Van Thiel DH, Bonet H, Gavaler J, Wright HI. Effect of alcohol use on allograft rejection rates after liver transplantation for alcoholic liver disease. Alcohol Clin Exp Res. 1995;19:1151–5.
85. Demetris AJ, Lee RG, Randhawa P *et al.* Liver allograft rejection. In: Wiesner RH, Lake J, Ascher N, editors. Liver Transplantation, Second Edition. New York: Wiley-Liss; 1997: (in press).
86. Demetris AJ, Fung JJ, Todo S *et al.* Conversion of liver allograft recipients from cyclosporine to FK506 immunosuppressive therapy – a clinicopathologic study of 96 patients. Transplantation. 1992;53:1056–62.
87. Sousa MD, Tilney NL, Kupiec-Weglinski JW. Recognition of self within self: specific lymphocyte positioning and the extracellular matrix. Immunol Today. 1991;12:262–6.
88. Hayashi M, Martinez OM, Garcia-Kennedy R, So S, Esquivel CO, Krams SM. Expression of cytokines and immune mediators during chronic liver allograft rejection. Transplantation. 1995;60:1533–8.
89. Donaldson PT, Alexander GJ, O'Grady J *et al.* Evidence for an immune response to HLA class I antigens in the vanishing-bile duct syndrome after liver transplantation. Lancet. 1987;1:945–51.
90. Saidman SL, Duquesnoy RJ, Zeevi A, Fung JJ, Starzl TE, Demetris AJ. Recognition of major histocompatibility complex antigens on cultured human biliary epithelial cells by alloreactive lymphocytes. Hepatology. 1991;13:239–46.
91. Duquesnoy RJ, Saidman S, Markus BH, Demetris AJ, Zeevi A. Role of HLA in intragraft cellular immunity in human liver transplantation. [Review]. Transplant Proc. 1988;20:724–7.
92. Duquesnoy RJ, Murase N, Suzow J *et al.* Evidence for heat shock protein immunity in a rat cardiac allograft model of chronic rejection. J Heart Lung Transplant. 1996;15:S63.
93. Markus BH, Duquesnoy RJ, Gordon RD *et al.* Histocompatibility and liver transplant outcome. Does HLA exert a dualistic effect? Transplantation. 1988;46:372–7.
94. Delaney CP, Murase N, Chen-Woan M *et al.* Allogeneic hematolymphoid microchimerism and prevention of autoimmune disease in the rat: a relationship between allo- and autoimmunity. J Clin Invest. 1996;97:217–25.
95. Demetris AJ, Markus BH, Esquivel C *et al.* Pathologic analysis of liver transplantation for primary biliary cirrhosis. Hepatology. 1988;8:939–47.
96. Broome U, Scheynius A, Hultcrantz R. Induced expression of heat-shock protein on biliary epithelium in patients with primary sclerosing cholangitis and primary biliary cirrhosis. Hepatology. 1993;18:298–303.
97. Hubscher SG, Buckels JA, Elias E, McMaster P, Neuberger J. Vanishing bile-duct syndrome following liver transplantation – is it reversible? Transplantation. 1991;51:1004–10.
98. Kamada N. The immunology of experimental liver transplantation in the rat. Immunology. 1985;55:369–89.
99. Murase N, Starzl TE, Tanabe M *et al.* Variable chimerism, graft versus host disease, and tolerance after different kinds of cell and whole organ transplantation from Lewis to Brown-Norway rats. Transplantation. 1995;60:158–71.

100. Hayry P, Isoniemi H, Yilmaz S *et al.* Chronic allograft rejection. Immunol Rev. 1993;134:33–81.
101. Oguma S, Banner B, Zerbe T, Starzl T, Demetris AJ. Participation of dendritic cells in vascular lesions of chronic rejection of human allografts. Lancet. 1988;2:933–6.
102. Starzl TE, Demetris AJ. Transplantation milestones: viewed with one- and two-way paradigms of tolerance. J Am Med Assoc. 1995;273:876–9.
103. Demetris AJ, Noriko M, Rao AS, Starzl TE. The role of passenger leukocytes in rejection and 'tolerance' after solid organ transplantation: a potential explanation of a paradox. In: Touraine JL *et al.* editors. Rejection and tolerance. Dordrecht: Kluwer; 1994:325–92.
104. Schlitt HJ, Hundrieser J, Ringe B, Pichlmayr R. Donor-type microchimerism associated with graft rejection eight years after liver transplantation [Letter]. N Engl J Med. 1994;330:646–7.
105. Schlitt HJ, Hundrieser J, Hisanaga M *et al.* Patterns of donor-type microchimerism after heart transplantation. Lancet. 1994;343:1469–71.
106. Bushell A, Pearson TC, Morris PJ, Wood KJ. Donor–recipient microchimerism is not required for tolerance induction following recipient pretreatment with donor-specific transfusion and anti-CD4 antibody. Evidence of a clear role for short-term antigen persistence. Transplantation. 1995;59:1367–71.
107. Demetris AJ, Murase N, Ye Q *et al.* Obliterative arteriopathy and quilty lesions: leukocyte trafficking, microchimerism and the immunolymphatic theory of chronic rejection. Am J Pathol. 1996 (Submitted).

19
Transplantation for vanishing bile duct syndromes

J. NEUBERGER

INTRODUCTION

The continuing use of liver transplantation for patients with chronic cholestatic disease is a clear indication of the relative lack of success of therapeutic interventions to prevent progression of the disease and to obviate the effects of liver fibrosis and cirrhosis. Although the number of patients transplanted in Europe for chronic cholestatic disease has remained roughly constant, these patients represent a falling proportion of the numbers transplanted, as viral hepatitis and alcoholic liver disease are becoming increasingly common indications. Nonetheless, transplantation for primary biliary cirrhosis (PBC) and primary sclerosing cholangitis (PSC) remains a continuing problem. Thus, in data from the European Liver Transplant Registry[1], cholestatic disease was the indication for transplantation in 2025 cases between 1988 and 1995, accounting for 12% of the indications. Of those grafted for cirrhosis, PBC accounted for 19%, compared with 25% with alcoholic cirrhosis and 41% with post-hepatitic cirrhosis. In 1989 PBC was the primary indication in 40% of those grafted for cirrhosis; in 1995 it accounted for less than 20%. Although it might appear that the excellent 1- and 5-year survival, at 81% and 76%, represent a cause for congratulation, there is still room for improvement. The long-term consequences of immunosuppressive therapy only emphasize the need for increasing efforts to find safe and effective remedies for the underlying condition, so that liver replacement for chronic cholestatic diseases is no longer required.

INDICATIONS FOR LIVER TRANSPLANTATION

In general, indications for liver transplantation are two-fold:

1. liver disease which makes the quality of life unacceptable to the patient,
2. anticipated length of life (due to liver disease) of 1 year or less.

These principles are relatively easy to define but are often more difficult to extrapolate to the individual patient.

Transplantation for symptomatic disease in patients with chronic cholestasis

The main symptomatic indications for transplantation are lethargy and intractable pruritus. The lethargy of chronic cholestasis is of unknown aetiology. Recent work by Swain and Maric[2] has suggested this may be due to defective corticotropin-releasing hormone responses associated with cholestasis, but there is little conclusive work in humans, and extrapolation into the clinical therapeutic area remains for the future. Nonetheless, lethargy can result in major debilitation, significantly affecting the quality of a patient's life. It must, however, be remembered that there are many other, potentially treatable, causes of lethargy in patients with chronic cholestasis, and these are shown in Table 1. It is important that these are excluded before the patient is considered for transplantation in this situation. Perhaps the most difficult diagnosis to exclude is that of depression. It is not surprising that many patients, given the diagnosis of a chronic progressive disease not of their own making, will become depressed. It is often worth instituting a trial of antidepressant therapy in such patients. Other conditions such as thyroid disease or Addison's disease can be readily excluded using the appropriate serological tests. The medication should be reviewed; in particular antihistamines given for the treatment of pruritus usually have little effect on the pruritus, but do cause lethargy and drowsiness.

The pathogenesis of pruritus in patients with chronic cholestasis remains uncertain. It used to be believed that this was due to elevated levels of bile acids, but this has never really been conclusively shown. Work by Bergasa and Jones[3] has implicated the opioid system in the pathogenesis of pruritus. Whether this represents the entire mechanism behind the pruritus of chronic cholestasis remains to be seen. The concept has led to new therapeutic interventions with opioid receptor antagonists such as nelmefene and naltroxone. Intractable pruritus can cause immense distress to the patient and can even lead to suicide. Transplantation is a highly effective therapy for pruritus, but it is important that other therapies (Table 2) should be considered before transplantation is undertaken for this indication.

In both indications the lethargy and the pruritus improve dramatically within days after surgery. In chronic cholestatic liver disease, end-stage disease may develop before the establishment of a true cirrhosis; therefore the decision to consider transplantation must depend on factors other than histological stage. The clinical and serological features suggesting end-stage liver disease are listed in Table 3.

Table 1 Potential causes of lethargy in patients with chronic cholestatic liver disease

The liver disease itself
Myxoedema/thyrotoxicosis
Addison's disease
Coeliac disease
Depression
Medication (especially sleeping tablets and antihistamines)

Table 2 Therapies for pruritus

Medication
Cholestyramine
Colestipol
Antihistamines*
Vitamin D*
Oil of evening primrose*
Ursodeoxycholic acid
Opioid receptor antagonists: naloxone, naltrexone
Propofol
Rifampicin
Phenobarbitone
Androgenic steroids: stanozolol
Mechanical
External biliary diversion
Other
Ultraviolet therapy*

* Of uncertain effectiveness

The time for consideration of transplantation must in part depend on the length of time on the waiting list and the method of organ allocation. Both factors vary in different countries. However, nearly all countries report a major increase in the number of transplant recipients without a comparable rise in donor organs. It seems to be an unfortunate consequence of the success of liver transplantation in general that waiting times are increasing throughout the world, and that many systems of organ allocation almost require that the patient is in the intensive care unit before he/she stands a good chance of being allocated a liver graft. As the length of time on the waiting list increases, patients' conditions will deteriorate, and this will reduce the success of transplantation[4]. It is unlikely that new advances in the field of xenografting will have a significant clinical impact, at least in the near future.

Chronic cholestatic diseases tend to regress in a relatively slow and predictable fashion, and it has been possible to develop prognostic models to predict patient survival[5]. Nonetheless, it must be remembered that there may be

Table 3 General indications for transplantation for chronic cholestatic disease

Serum bilirubin >180 μmol/L for > 6 months
Ascites resistant to treatment
Spontaneous bacterial peritonitis
Hepatic encephalopathy
Progressive muscle wasting*
Recurrent variceal bleeding
Development of primary liver cell cancer
Intractable pruritus/lethargy
Progressive osteopenia*
Hepatopulmonary syndrome*

* These may also, paradoxically, be contraindications to liver replacement

unpredictable deterioration in the patient's condition, which may prove fatal, such as the development of liver cell cancer, severe infection or variceal haemorrhage.

Both for PBC[6–12] and PSC[13–15] prognostic models have been developed. These models, when compared with each other, compare well[16]. With the exception of the time-dependent model of Christensen *et al.*[17], all these models are static; that is to say, they can technically be applied only once, at the time of presentation, and it is not strictly valid to apply models repeatedly during the course of the illness. Furthermore, models are most accurate when the patients tested are similar to those in the median range of the population from which the model is derived. In most cases models are derived from patients presenting for treatment to various centres, and who are thus relatively well; inevitably those in whom the model will be applied will be at one extreme. The prognostic models give either the survival probability of the patient surviving for, say, 1 year or else the median survival time; in both instances there will be a confidence interval which may be so wide as to be clinically unhelpful. In addition, models are determined from retrospective studies; prospective application of such models may not be valid in the light of therapeutic advances. This problem is well illustrated by the introduction into clinical practice of ursodeoxycholic acid (UDCA). Many studies have clearly demonstrated that UDCA has a significant beneficial effect on improving liver tests[18], although whether there is a benefit in survival remains uncertain. Whether treatment with UDCA alters prognostic markers is also uncertain, since Poupon *et al.*[19] found (using multivariate analysis) that in patients with PBC treated with UDCA, serum bilirubin was no longer a major prognostic marker and, after adjustment for age, hyaluronic acid was most associated with treatment failure. In contrast, in the meta-analysis by Heathcote *et al.*[20], which included data from the Poupon trial, serum bilirubin was a valid marker. In addition, alteration of prognostic markers does not necessarily imply a change in outcome: for example, the peripheral CD4 lymphocyte count is a valid prognostic marker in people infected with HIV; therapy with zidovudine has a beneficial effect on the CD4 count, but no demonstrable effect on survival[21]. Other advances, such as the use of variceal banding or placement of transjugular intrahepatic portal systemic stent shunts, may alter prognosis. Finally, of course, it must be remembered that those risk factors for survival in the absence of transplantation do not necessarily mirror those risk factors for survival after transplantation[22]. Although one such model[22] has been developed, this has not been confirmed in other studies.

PROGNOSTIC MODELS OF PBC

Since the work by Shapiro and colleagues[23], emphasizing the importance of serum bilirubin as a prognostic marker for PBC, others have developed prognostic markers, and there are now several models that have been described (Table 4). As can be seen, serum bilirubin remains the major prognostic factor, and the presence of cirrhosis, age and serum albumin are also prognostic important factors. It is possible to give a numeric value to these individual parameters and these values can be translated into a figure which can give an estimate of

Table 4 Prognostic factors in different models for prognosis in PBC

	Age	*Variceal bleeding*	*Ascites*	*Bilirubin*	*Prothrombin time*	*Hepatomegaly*	*Fibrosis /cirrhosis*	*Cholestasis*	*Mallory's hyaline*	*Albumin*
European	+			+			+	+		+
Mayo	+		(+)	+	+					+
Yale	+			+		+	+			
Australia	+			+						+
Glasgow	+	+	+	+			+	+	+	
Oslo		+		+						
Royal Free	+		+	+						+

(+) = oedema

1-, 2- or 3-year survival, or a median survival probability. It must be remembered that the confidence interval on prognostic time is often wide and, therefore, as indicated above, application to the individual may be of less benefit. Nonetheless, these prognostic models are of great value not only in allowing survival with and without transplantation to be compared, but also in identifying those major prognostic factors. In practice, in my experience, very few of these models are actually applied to the individual patient.

Other prognostic variables have been described: these include serum hyaluronic acid[24], procollagen peptide type III[25] and dynamic liver function tests such as the lignocaine metabolism (MEGX test), indocyanine green clearance, caffeine clearance and galactose elimination capacity[26,27]. Although many of these markers and tests have been shown to correlate well with survival, none has yet achieved widespread use in clinical practice.

PROGNOSTIC MODELS FOR PSC

Fewer models for PSC have been described, and prognostic variables are defined in Table 5. In contrast to PBC the clinical pattern of PSC is more varied. The disease appears to run a more fluctuating course, which may in part depend on the presence of coincidental cholangitis.

SPECIFIC PROBLEMS OF PSC

Compared with PBC, selection and timing of transplantation in patients with PSC is associated with two additional problems: the presence of inflammatory bowel disease and the probability of cholangiocarcinoma.

Table 5 Prognostic factors in different models for prognosis in PSC

	Age	*Bilirubin*	*Inflammatory bowel disease*	*Hepatomegaly*	*Splenomegaly*	*Alkaline phosphatase*	*Histological stage*	*Haemoglobin*
Mayo	+	+	+				+	+
King's	+			+	+	+	+	
Multicentre	+	+			+		+	

In many patients with PSC there is coexisting inflammatory bowel disease, usually ulcerative colitis. In many patients the ulcerative colitis is often mild and may indeed be subclinical. There remains controversy in the literature as to whether patients with PSC who have ulcerative colitis do have increased risk of colonic neoplasia[28,29]. It is likely that further studies are required to answer this point. Nonetheless, it would appear sensible to perform colonoscopy in all patients who are potential transplant candidates, in order not only to exclude the possibility of an undiagnosed colonic neoplasm, but also to look for evidence of colitis. It is usually considered inappropriate to transplant patients with active colitis, although once this is under control there is no reason why transplantation should be withheld. There is no evidence that surgery for colitis significantly adversely affects the outcome. Although the Mayo Clinic have suggested that patients with PSC and ulcerative colitis have a worse prognosis than those without clinical colitis[30], our own data do not support this (unpublished data, see below).

In general, non-transplant surgical intervention in patients with PSC is unhelpful, and may indeed increase the morbidity of transplantation[31,32], although in the rare cases of a single dominant extrahepatic stricture in the patient without advanced cirrhosis, stenting, dilatation or biliary resection may be useful.

CHOLANGIOCARCINOMA

The major diagnostic problem in patients with sclerosing cholangitis is due to the increased risk in these patients of cholangiocarcinoma. Many studies have shown convincingly that the presence of cholangiocarcinoma has a significant adverse effect on survival after transplantation[33,34]. In most cases the cholangiocarcinoma developed insidiously, and it is often very difficult to diagnose this condition pre-transplant. Serum markers for cholangiocarcinoma, such as CEA and CA 19–9, lack the necessary sensitivity and specificity required for a certain diagnosis of cholangiocarcinoma[35,36]. These tumours are often difficult to visualize on imaging, whether by ERCP, PTC, ultrasound, CT scanning or MRI scanning[37,38]. We have found (Mirza, unpublished data) that biopsy of any possible stricture is highly specific but not very sensitive. Although brushings or bile cytology may be of value in this instance, it is often difficult to obtain satisfactory brushings of hilar lesions in those with extensive extrahepatic sclerosing cholangitis[39,40]. Furthermore, there is a significant risk of inducing biliary sepsis, which may be impossible to control and may be fatal. In some cases laparoscopic biopsy may be of help in diagnosis. A high clinical suspicion and, where appropriate, frozen section histology during the laparotomy preceding hepatectomy, will reduce the number of liver replacements in this condition.

CONTRAINDICATIONS TO TRANSPLANTATION

Contraindications to liver transplantation with chronic cholestatic disease are similar to those in any other condition. In general these can be divided into those conditions which preclude good survival after surgery and those conditions

Table 6 Contraindications for liver transplantation (although these will vary to some extent between centres)

Advanced age
Extensive portal and mesenteric vein thrombosis
Active bacterial/fungal sepsis
HIV infection
Extrahepatic primary malignancy
Primary liver cell cancer extending outside the liver
Cholangiocarcinoma
Severe extrahepatic disease (cardiac, respiratory, neurological) preventing successful transplantation or rehabilitation

which make it unlikely the patient will survive surgery. A summary is given in Table 6.

SURVIVAL AFTER TRANSPLANTATION

In discussing survival after transplantation I will use data from our own registry, primarily because of ease of access! Comparison of outcome between centres is usually difficult because of differences in case-mix. Indeed, a centre with a 5-year survival of 85% may actually be doing worse than another with a 5-year survival of only 70% if the former are operating on less sick and lower-risk patients.

Survival after transplantation for PBC

Between 1982 and 1995, in the Birmingham Liver Transplant Unit, 312 patients were grafted for PBC. The overall 1-, 2- and 5-year survival values are 82.5%, 81.7% and 76%, respectively. As may be hoped for, results have improved during the lifetime of the unit with 1-, 2- and 5-year survival of 72.5%, 70.5% and 69.6% in patients grafted during the 1980s, compared with the respective figures in patients grafted in the 1990s of 87.4%, 86.8% and 77.2%. This apparent gratifying improvement in outcome may reflect a number of factors, including better selection, as well as improved immunosuppression and better surgical, anaesthetic and microbiological techniques.

The majority of postoperative deaths occur in the first months after transplantation; common causes of death include bleeding, sepsis and multi-organ failure. After 6 months the causes of death include tumour and technical problems. The relatively low level of *de-novo* tumours in this group of patients may reflect the relatively low degree of immunosuppression used in this centre: of the last 500 adult liver allograft recipients none has received antilymphocyte immunoglobulin, and corticosteroids are usually stopped within 3 months; it is possible that the price for this relatively low immunosuppressive regime is an increased graft loss from rejection (although we are unaware of any evidence that this is so).

Survival after transplantation for PSC

The number of patients transplanted for PSC is lower than for PBC, with 101 grafted between 1986 and 1995 in our unit. The overall 1-, 2- and 5-year survival is currently 79%, 75% and 68%; as with patients with PBC, there has been an improvement in survival in patients grafted during the 1980s and the 1990s – with 1-, 2- and 5-year survival of 60%, 55% and 50% before 1990 compared with 84%, 80% and 73%. Seven patients had a cholangiocarcinoma, and in these patients 1-year survival was 29%. Of the 101 patients with PSC, 65% had ulcerative colitis. The 1-, 2- and 5-year survival in these patients is, if anything, higher in these patients than in those without colitis, at 83%, 79% and 69%. Our own experience shows that there appears to be a higher rate of post-transplantation malignancy, with 32 of the 101 patients developing *de-novo* tumours (compared with only eight of the 312 patients grafted for PBC); reasons for this discrepancy are uncertain and are currently being investigated.

QUALITY OF LIFE AFTER TRANSPLANTATION

Now that many of the technical problems of transplantation have been overcome, clinicians are starting to assess the quality of life after transplantation. While this can never be stated to be normal, it is better than no life at all[41,42]. Several studies have confirmed that the actual, observed survival after transplantation is superior to the length of life predicted from prognostic models[43–46].

RECURRENT DISEASE

Recurrence of both PBC and PSC after transplantation has been suggested, but remains controversial. For both conditions the diagnosis of recurrent disease is difficult, and the criteria used to define disease in the native liver may be different from those in the allograft. It must be remembered that the effect of a different HLA phenotype in the graft, the effect of immunosuppressive therapy and the possibility of other factors affecting the graft must be excluded. The latter conditions include acute and chronic rejection, infection, drug toxicity, ischaemia and sepsis. It has variously been suggested that patients grafted for either PBC or PSC may be at greater risk of developing acute or ductopenic rejection, but results are conflicting and, as yet, few firm conclusions can be drawn.

RECURRENT PBC

It is clear that many of the serological abnormalities and associated extrahepatic manifestations in PBC persist or recur after transplantation. These include the presence of elevated serum IgM and antimitochondrial antibodies (AMA) and development of extrahepatic manifestations of PBC such as sicca syndrome or thyroid disorders. Of course, these do not prove recurrent disease. AMA have not been shown to be pathogenic of the disease, although they are diagnostic of PBC in patients with a native liver.

The major, if not the only, way confidently to diagnose recurrent disease must be liver histology. Differential diagnosis of PBC and chronic rejection is not difficult, since the features of PBC which are not present in rejection include granulomas, lymphoid follicles, bile duct proliferation, fibrosis, and the development of copper-associated protein in the absence of extrahepatic biliary obstruction.

The initial report that PBC may recur in the graft was based on three patients who had survived more than 3 years after transplantation and had histological features consistent with PBC in the allograft[47]. The diagnosis was based on clinical, immunological and histological features. In the subsequent paper[48] three more patients were described, all of whom had disease recurrence. In two patients the disease had progressed to histological stage 3. Biliary obstruction had been excluded radiologically. One patient died of a myocardial infarct 5 years later, and another ran a progressive course; she died with sepsis which was associated with cholangitis due to a gallbladder conduit and renal failure nearly 10 years after transplantation. Examination of the graft[49] showed features of chronic ductopenic rejection, cholestasis and nodular regenerative hyperplasia. Although no evidence of recurrent PBC was noted in the hepatectomy specimen, it is believed that the features of PBC were not apparent because of the portal tract damage and fibrosis. Four other long-term survivors in the Addenbrookes/King' College Hospital series had features of recurrent PBC.

In our own unit in Birmingham, patients have undergone annual biopsy post-liver transplant on a prospective basis[50]. Of 188 patients followed up to 8 years 83 were grafted for PBC. Patients were maintained on triple therapy initially with cyclosporine, corticosteroids and azathioprine, but corticosteroids were reduced, and were stopped after 3 months. Of the 83 patients who underwent transplantation for PBC, histological evidence of disease recurrence was found in 13. The features suggesting recurrence included mononuclear cell portal infiltrate, lymphoid aggregates in the portal tract, bile duct damage and portal epithelioid granulomas. None of the patients grafted for conditions other than PBC had comparable features. One of the 12 patients for recurrent PBC was already at the cirrhotic stage, whereas the others were end-stage 1 and 2. These results are supported by other studies such as that by Balan and colleagues, who found features suggestive of recurrent disease in five of 72 patients transplanted for PBC[51].

However, it must be recognized that not all studies have confirmed these results. In the early years of transplantation Fennell *et al.*[52] and Esquivel *et al.*[53] failed to find evidence of recurrent PBC in failed allografts. More recently Gouw and colleagues, in the Netherlands[54], reported a prospective study of 19 patients transplanted for PBC who underwent annual biopsies. With a follow-up period of up to 11 years there was no evidence of recurrent disease.

Although portal tract granulomas are suggestive of PBC (at least in the native liver), it should be recognized that granulomas are not specific to recurrent PBC. Ferrell and colleagues[55] assessed the significance of hepatic granulomas in the allograft in over 3600 liver biopsies from 563 patients. Forty-two patients were found to have hepatic granulomas, and causes other than recurrent PBC included acute rejection, tuberculosis and a foreign body reaction. However, 12% of patients with hepatic granulomas were shown have additional histological features suggesting the diagnosis of recurrent PBC.

It is difficult to reconcile these conflicting data. One factor might relate to immunosuppression. Wong *et al.*[56] initially reported recurrent PBC in two patients maintained on immunosuppression with tacrolimus. Subsequent studies reported by ourselves[57] showed that patients participating in a prospective controlled trial comparing cyclosporine with FK-based immunosuppression were more likely to have evidence of recurrent PBC if they were receiving immunosuppression with tacrolimus. Furthermore, evidence of recurrent PBC was likely to occur at an earlier stage. These results suggest that increased immunosuppression may lead to a more aggressive form of recurrent disease; an apparent paradox for an autoimmune disease and more in keeping with an infective aetiology for PBC.

Another factor for this apparent paradox may relate to the number of patients studied. Our initial experience in Birmingham led us to believe there was no evidence of recurrence of PBC in the allograft[58]. However, more patients were studied over a longer time period, and we found evidence of PBC recurrence in a proportion of patients[50].

Thus it seems at present that PBC probably does recur after transplantation in the allograft, and this may be related to the degree of immunosuppression. Further studies are required to confirm these observations, and it may be that intervention strategies may be helpful in preventing further progression.

RECURRENCE OF PRIMARY SCLEROSING CHOLANGITIS

The diagnosis of PSC depends on clinical, serological and histological observations, although imaging of the biliary tree is most useful. Histological features which may show the characteristic fibro-obliterative lesions are not specific. Radiological imaging of the biliary tree, either by endoscopic or percutaneous techniques, will show the presence of sclerosing cholangitis but cannot reliably differentiate primary from secondary disease. Most patients transplanted for PSC have a roux loop fashioned as the extrahepatic biliary tree is resected in order to reduce the risk of cholangiocarcinoma. The presence of roux loop is often associated with biliary sludge and recurrent cholangitis and it is therefore difficult to differentiate primary and secondary cholangitis. A study by Sebagh and colleagues[59] of 24 patients with non-anastomotic biliary strictures showed that sclerosing cholangitis in the graft was associated with a number of factors including ABO blood group incompatibility, hypoxia associated with hepatic artery thrombosis, focal arterial fibrointimal hyperplasia, chronic ductopenic arteriopathic rejection and preservation-related ischaemia.

We have compared histological features of PSC in patients grafted for PSC and those with roux loops fashioned for other reasons[60]. It is accepted that the latter group is a comparison rather than a control group. There were 22 patients in each group. Histological evidence of periductular fibrosis and fibro-obliterative disease were significantly more common in those transplanted for PSC than in those transplanted for other conditions. Our own experience has suggested that the antineutrophil cytoplasmic antibody (ANCA), which has been suggested to be a marker of PSC in the non-transplant situation, is unhelpful in distinguishing PSC recurrence from other conditions.

CONCLUSIONS

Chronic cholestatic disease remains a common indication for liver transplantation. The development of prognostic models for both PBC and for PSC has been of considerable benefit in helping define the time of transplantation. Nonetheless, care must be taken in extrapolating results from prognostic models to the individual patients. Transplantation offers a considerable improvement in survival and a relief of symptoms. Five-year survival is at present acceptable, but there is a not inconsiderable mortality and morbidity as a consequence of immunosuppression. The presence of recurrent disease after transplantation appears well documented but occurs in a minority of patients.

References

1. Registry of the European Liver Transplant Registry. Hôpital Paul Brousse, 1996.
2. Swain M, Maric M. Defective corticotropin-releasing hormone mediated neuroendocrine and behavioural responses in cholestatic rats. Hepatology. 1995;22:1560–4.
3. Jones EA, Bergasa N. The pruritus of cholestasis: from bile acids to opiate agonists. Hepatology. 1990;11:884–7.
4. Wiesner R, Porayko M, Dickson ER *et al.* Selection and timing of liver transplantation in primary biliary cirrhosis and primary sclerosing cholangitis. Hepatology. 1992;16:1296–9.
5. Christensen E. Multivariate survival analysis using Cox's regression model. Hepatology. 1987;7:1346–50.
6. Roll J, Boyer JL, Barry D, Klatskin G. The prognostic importance of clinical and histologic features in asymptomatic and symptomatic primary biliary cirrhosis. N Engl J Med. 1983;308:1–8.
7. Christensen E, Neuberger J, Crowe J *et al.* Beneficial effect of azathioprine and prediction of prognosis in primary biliary cirrhosis: final result of an international trial. Gastroenterology. 1985;89:1084–91.
8. Dickson E, Grambsch P, Fleming T, Fisher L, Langworthy A. Prognosis in primary biliary cirrhosis: model for decision making. Hepatology. 1989;10:1–7.
9. Rydning A, Schrumpf E, Abdel-noor M, Elgio K, Jenssen E. Factors of prognostic importance in primary biliary cirrhosis. Scand J Gastroenterol. 1990;25:119–26.
10. Goudie B, Burt AD, Macfarlane G *et al.* Risk factors and prognosis in primary biliary cirrhosis. Am J Gastroenterol. 1989;84:713–16.
11. Jeffrey G, Reed W, Shilkin K. Natural history and prognostic variables in primary biliary cirrhosis. Hepatology. 1990;12:955.
12. Hughes M, Raskino C, Pocock S, Biagini M, Burroughs A. Prediction of short-term survival with an application in primary biliary cirrhosis. Stat Med. 1992;11:1731–45.
13. Wiesner R, Grambsch P, Dickson ER *et al.* Primary sclerosing cholangitis: natural history, prognostic factors and survival analysis. Hepatology. 1989;10:430–6.
14. Farrant M, Hayllar K, Wilkinson M *et al.* Natural history and prognostic variables in primary sclerosing cholangitis. Gastroenterology. 1991;100:1710–17.
15. Dickson ER, Murtaugh P, Wiesner R *et al.* Primary sclerosing cholangitis: refinement and validation of survival models. Gastroenterology 1992;103:1893–901.
16. Klion F, Fabry T, Palmer M, Schaffner F. Prediction of survival of patients with primary biliary cirrhosis: examination of the Mayo Clinic model on a group of patients with known end-point. Gastroenterology. 1992;102:310–13.
17. Christensen E, Altman D, Neuberger J, de Stavola B, Tygstrup N, Williams R. Updating prognosis in primary biliary cirrhosis using a time-dependent Cox regression model. Gastroenterology. 1993;105:1865–76.
18. Lim A, Jazawri R, Northfield T. The ursodeoxycholic acid story in primary biliary cirrhosis. Gut. 1995;37:301–4.
19. Poupon R, Balkau B, Guechot J, Heintzman F. Predictive factors in ursodeoxycholic acid-treated patients with primary biliary cirrhosis. Hepatology. 1994;19:635–40.

20. Heathcote EJ, Lindor K, Poupon R *et al.* Combined analysis of French, American and Canadian randomised controlled trials of ursodeoxycholic acid therapy in primary biliary cirrhosis. Gastroenterology. 1995;108:A1082.
21. Concorde Co-ordinating Committee. Concorde MRC/ANRS randomised double-blind, controlled trial of immediate and deferred zidovudine in symptom-free HIV infection. Lancet. 1994;343:871–81.
22. Neuberger J, Altman D, Polson R *et al.* Prognosis after liver transplantation for primary biliary cirrhosis. Transplantation. 1989;48:444–7.
23. Shapiro J, Smith H, Schaffner F. Serum bilirubin: a prognostic factor in primary biliary cirrhosis. Gut. 1979;20:137–40.
24. Nyberg A, Engstrom-Laurent A, Loof L. Serum hyaluronate in primary biliary cirrhosis: a biochemical marker for progressive liver damage. Hepatology. 1988;8:142–6.
25. Eriksson E, Zettervall O. The N-terminal propeptide of collagen type III in serum as a prognostic indicator in primary biliary cirrhosis. J Hepatol. 1982;2:370–8.
26. Clements D, Elias E, McMaster P. Preliminary study of indocyanine green clearance in primary biliary cirrhosis. Scand J Gastroenterol. 1991;26:119–23.
27. Reichen J, Widmer T, Cutting J. Accurate prediction of death by serial determination of galactose elimination capacity in primary biliary cirrhosis: a comparison with the Mayo model. Hepatology. 1991;14:504–10.
28. Brentali T, Haggitt R, Rabonivitch P *et al.* Risk and natural history of colonic neoplasia in patients with primary sclerosing cholangitis and ulcerative colitis. Gastroenterology. 1996;110:331–8.
29. Loftus E, Sandborn W, Tremaine W *et al.* Risk of colorectal neoplasia in patients with primary sclerosing cholangitis. Gastroenterology. 1996;110:432–44.
30. Shaked A, Colonna J, Goldstein L, Busuttil R. The interrelationship between sclerosing cholangitis and ulcerative colitis in patients undergoing liver transplantation. Ann Surg. 1992;215:598–605.
31. Ismail T, Angrisani L, Powell J *et al.* Primary sclerosing cholangitis: surgical options, prognostic variables and outcome. Br J Surg. 1991;78:564–7.
32. Thompson J, Wood P, Burnett D, Shae B, Rikkers L. The role of non-transplant procedures for sclerosing cholangitis. Am J Surg. 1988;156:506–8.
33. Wiesner R, Grambsch P, Dickson E *et al.* Primary sclerosing cholangitis: natural history, prognostic factors and survival analysis. Hepatology. 1989;10:430–36.
34. Rosen C, Nagorney D, Wiesner R, Coffey R, LaRusso N. Cholangiocarcinoma complicating primary sclerosing cholangitis. Ann Surg. 1991;213:21–5.
35. Fisher A, Thiese N, Min A *et al.* CA19-9 does not predict cholangiocarcinoma in patients with primary sclerosing cholangitis undergoing liver transplantation. Liver Transplant Surg. 1995;1:94–8.
36. Ramage J, Farrant JM, lorns R, Williams R. Serum tumour markers for diagnosis of cholangiocarcinoma in patients with primary sclerosing cholangitis. Gut. 1992;33:S1.
37. Takayasu K, lkeya S, Mukai K, Muramatsu Y, Makuuchi M, Hasegawa H. CT of hilar cholangiocarcinoma: late contrast enhancement in six patients. Am J Roentgenol. 1990;154:1203–6.
38. Shulte S, Baron R, Teefey S *et al.* CT of the extrahepatic bile ducts: wall thickness and contrast enhancement in normal and abnormal ducts. Am J Roentgenol. 1990;154:79–85.
39. Cobb C, Floyd W. Usefulness of bile cytology in the diagnostic management of patients with biliary tract obstruction. Acta Cytol. 1985;29:93–100.
40. Davidson B, Varsamidakis N, Dooley J *et al.* Value of exfoliative cytology for investigating bile duct strictures. Gut. 1992;33:1408–11.
41. Hunt C, Tart J, Dowdy E, Bute B, Williams D, Clasen P. Effect of orthotopic liver transplantation on employment and health status. Liver Transplant Surg. 1996;2:148–53.
42. Adams PC, Ghent C, Grant D, Wall W. Employment after liver transplantation. Hepatology. 1995;21:140–4.
43. Keiding S, Ericzon B, Eriksson B *et al.* Survival after liver transplantation of patients with PBC in the Nordic countries. Scand J Gastroenterol. 1990;25:11–18.
44. Markus B, Dickson ER, Grambsch P *et al.* Efficacy of liver transplantation in patients with primary biliary cirrhosis. N Engl J Med. 1989;320:1709–13.
45. Bonsel G, Klompmaker I, van de Veer F, Habbema J, Slooff M. Use of prognostic models for assessment of value of liver transplantation in primary biliary cirrhosis. Lancet. 1990;335:493–7.

46. Neuberger J, Gunson B, Buckels J, Elias E, McMaster P. Referral of patients with primary biliary cirrhosis for liver transplantation. Gut. 1990;31:1069–72.
47. Neuberger J, Portmann B, MacDougall B *et al.* Recurrence of primary biliary cirrhosis after liver transplantation. N Engl J Med. 1982;306:1–4.
48. Polson R, Portmann B, Neuberger J *et al.* Evidence for disease recurrence after liver transplantation for primary biliary cirrhosis. Gastroenterology. 1989;97:715–25.
49. Lerut J, Zimmerman A, Geretsch P, Preisig R, Blumgart L. Chronic rejection and extra-hepatic biliary obstruction 8 years after orthotopic liver transplantation with gall bladder conduit. HPB Biliary Surg. 1991;5:17–22.
50. Hubscher S, Elias E, Buckels J, Neuberger J. Primary biliary cirrhosis: histological evidence of disease recurrence after liver transplantation. J Hepatol. 1993;18:173–84.
51. Balan V, Batts K, Porayko M *et al.* Histological evidence for recurrence of primary biliary cirrhosis after liver transplantation. Hepatology. 1993;18:1392–8.
52. Fennell R, Shikes G, Vierling J. Relationship of pre-transplant hepatobiliary disease to bile duct damage occurring in the liver allograft. Hepatology. 1983;3:84–9.
53. Esquivel C, Van Thiel D, Demetris A *et al.* Transplantation for primary biliary cirrhosis. Gastroenterology. 1988;94:1207–16.
54. Gouw A, Haagsma E, Manns M *et al.* Is there recurrence of primary biliary cirrhosis after liver transplantation? J Hepatol. 1994;20:500–7.
55. Ferrell L, Lee R, Brixko C *et al.* Hepatic granulomas following liver transplantation. Hepatology. 1995;60:926–30.
56. Wong P, Portmann B, O'Grady J, Williams R. Recurrence of primary biliary cirrhosis after liver transplantation following FK506 based immunosuppression. J Hepatol. 1993;17:284–7.
57. Dmetrewski J, Mayer AD, Hubscher S, Neuberger JM. Histopathological recurrence of primary biliary cirrhosis after liver transplantation: effect of immunosuppression. J Hepatol. 1996;24:253–7.
58. Buist L, Hubscher S, Vickers C, Neuberger J, McMaster P. Does liver transplantation cure primary biliary cirrhosis? Transplant Proc. 1989;21:2402.
59. Sebagh M, Farges O, Khalil A *et al.* Sclerosing cholangitis following human orthotopic liver transplantation. Am J Pathol. 1995;19:81–90.
60. Harrison R, Davies M, Neuberger J, Hubscher S. Sclerosing cholangitis in the liver allograft: histological evidence of disease recurrence. Hepatology. 1994;20:356–61.

20
Medical treatment of vanishing bile duct syndrome

U. LEUSCHNER

INTRODUCTION

Liver disorders associated with ductopenia (vanishing bile duct syndrome) are found in neonates, children and adults[1] (Table 1). Since there is only little experience with the treatment of vanishing bile duct syndrome in Alagille's syndrome, in the rare defects of bile salt metabolism, the acquired immune deficiency syndrome (AIDS), and since surgical aspects and the treatment with ursodeoxycholic acid (UDCA) have been discussed by others in this book, I will concentrate on non-bile-salt therapy of primary biliary cirrhosis (PBC) and primary sclerosing cholangitis (PSC).

Table 1 Liver disorders associated with ductopenia (vanishing bile duct syndrome)

Neonates and children	
Extrahepatic biliary atresia	
Paucity of interlobular bile ducts	
Syndromic: Alagille's syndrome	
Non-syndromic:	α_1 antitrypsin defect
	bile salt defects
	idiopathic
Adults	
Primary biliary cirrhosis (autoimmune cholangitis)	
Sarcoidosis	
Primary sclerosing cholangitis	
Primary/secondary immunodeficiency (AIDS)	
Ischaemic:	liver allograft
	intra-arterial infusions of cytotoxic drugs
Idiopathic	
Hepatic allograft rejection	
Graft-versus-host disease	

Data from ref. 1

GENERAL ASPECTS

PBC, which is believed to be a model autoimmune disease, is characterized by two major factors which may be important for therapy: inflammation and cholestasis. Autoimmune chronic active hepatitis is usually not accompanied by cholestasis, and can be treated with immunosuppressives, e.g. glucocorticoids and azathioprine, but not with bile acids. PBC, in which cholestasis is a major feature, reacts to bile acids, but not to immunosuppressives. This raises the questions of whether bile prevents the beneficial effect of immunosuppressives and whether the pretreatment of cholestasis with bile acids renders the inflammatory process more susceptible to immunosuppressives.

That a combination therapy with UDCA plus glucocorticoids may be superior to monotherapy with UDCA has been shown recently[2]. The drawback with using glucocorticoids is the induction of bone loss. A currently ongoing controlled study with budenoside, which will be terminated in early 1997, will show whether budenoside has comparable effects with fewer side-effects.

The question of whether a triple therapy with choleretic UDCA (the mode of action of UDCA is still unknown), immunosuppressive and antifibrotic substances will be superior to monotherapy with bile salts, or the above-mentioned combination therapy with UDCA and immunosuppressives, remains open. In the past many compounds have been used in the treatment of primary biliary liver diseases, all of which had some positive but also negative effects. Therefore the question arises as to which of the hitherto-used compounds would be most suitable for monotherapy or combination therapy.

MEDICAL THERAPY OF PBC

Rationale for medicamentous therapy

The rationale for using glucocorticoids, azathioprine, chlorambucil, methotrexate, cyclosporine, D-penicillamine, colchicine or thalidomide is based on the immunosuppressive and anti-inflammatory properties of these substances (Table 2). Two drugs are said to have additional antifibrotic properties. D-penicillamine impairs hepatic collagen maturation[3] while copper chelation, useful in Wilson's disease, is of no importance in primary biliary liver diseases[4]. Colchicine is an

Table 2 Rationale for medicamentous therapy in primary biliary liver diseases

Glucocorticoids	Immunosuppressive, anti-inflammatory
Cyclosporine	Inhibits T-cell function, immunosuppressive, decreases sex hormone binding globulin and oestradiol
Azathioprine	Immunosuppressive
D-penicillamine	Immunosuppressive, inhibits collagen metabolism (chelation of copper)
Methotrexate	Inhibits IL-1 (immunomodulatory), anti-inflammatory, folic acid antagonist
Chlorambucil	Immunosuppressive
Colchicine	Antifibrotic, anti-inflammatory, increases collagenases, decreases collagen synthesis
Thalidomide	Successful in graft-versus-host disease and other immunological diseases

anti-inflammatory drug, but additionally it increases collagenase activity and decreases collagen synthesis[5,6].

Cyclosporine inhibits T-cell function, but has also been shown to decrease sex hormone-binding serum globulins and total and free oestradiol concentrations[7], which is of interest since PBC is a disease occurring predominantly in middle-aged women.

The rationale for using thalidomide[8] is not clear, but it has been useful in the treatment of graft-versus-host disease[9], erythema nodosum leprosum, AIDS-related aphthous ulcerations[10] and chronic actinic prurigo, which are presumed to be immunologically mediated diseases.

Clinical trials

Studies with monotherapy

Azathioprine. There are two studies using azathioprine in a total of 293 patients. In one study symptoms, laboratory data and liver histology did not improve[11]; in the second one these data were not given[12]. Side-effects in both trials were mild. In the second study the actual Kaplan–Meier survival curves showed no difference after 120 months, but when adjusted because of the more severe cases in the azathioprine group, survival became significantly longer (p=0.01) in the azathioprine group[12]. Azathioprine reduced the risk of dying to 59% of that observed with placebo (Table 3). The patient number in the study from the Royal Free Hospital[11] was 45; therapy dose was 1.2 mg/kg per day for 36 months. In the multinational study from Copenhagen[12] 248 patients were included; the treatment dose was 2 mg/kg per day for 48 months. This means that although the influence on symptoms, laboratory data and histology is marginal or totally absent, azathioprine has only minor side-effects and seems to improve life expectancy.

Colchicine. There are four controlled trials with colchicine[13–16], comprising a total of 271 patients. Treatment dose was 1–1.2 mg/day (Table 3). Symptoms and some laboratory data in three studies, histology only in one study improved by trend. In one study[17] cumulative mortality in the colchicine group was 21% and in the placebo group 47% ($p < 0.05$) after 4 years of therapy.

Interesting data were obtained by Vuoristo *et al.*[16]. In their study colchicine at a dose of 1 mg/day, like UDCA in a dosage of 12–15 mg/kg per day, was unable to reduce the increased S-PIIINP-levels (serum concentrations of the amino-terminal propeptide of type III procollagen). Since PIIIP reflects the production and degradation of type III procollagen, in this study colchicine showed no antifibrotic properties (colchicine reduced S-PIIIP by 1%, UDCA by 16%, decrease for both substances being statistically not significant). Colchicine also had no influence on S-PICP (serum concentrations of the carboxyterminal propeptide of type I procollagen). Because S-PICP levels are associated with the turnover of type I collagen in bone tissue, this study shows that colchicine is also unable to prevent osteoporosis. On the other hand UDCA did prevent it ($p < 0.05$ after 12 months therapy).

Table 3 Medical therapy of primary biliary cirrhosis: controlled trials

Drugs	*Studies*	*Patients*	*Dosage*	*Symptoms*	*Laboratory*	*Histology*	*Toxicity*	*Survival*
D-penicillamine[19–26]	8	767	0.6–1.2 g	5–	5–/3+	6–/1+	6+	6–
Colchicine[13–16]	4	271	1–1.2 mg	1–/3(+)	3+	(+)/2–	(+)	+/(+)
Azathioprine[11,12]	2	293	1.2–2 mg/kg	–/+	–	–	–/(+)	–/+
Cyclosporine[29–31]	3	41	2.5–4.0 mg/kg	–/+	–/+	–/+	2+	
Prednisolone[18]	1	36	30 → 10 mg/kg	+	(+)	+	(+)	
Chlorambucil[28]	1	24	0.5–4 mg		+	(+)	+	
Thalidomide[8]	1	18	50 → 100 mg	–	–	–	+	

+, Improved or present; –, deteriorated or absent; (+): trend

Prednisolone. There is only one controlled study in 36 patients with the classical immunosuppressive glucocorticoid prednisolone[18]. The starting dose was 30 mg/day, the maintenance dose was 10 mg/day, the total treatment time was 3 years. In the prednisolone group symptoms improved, laboratory data improved slightly and liver histology deteriorated in one patient, but improved in four of nine patients who had consented to a second biopsy. Of the seven patients who had consented in the placebo group, none had improved and four had deteriorated.

Unfortunately in some patients prednisolone treatment was accompanied by an increase in osteoporosis, although the rate of fall in densitometry values in the treated group for either the femur or the forearm could not be demonstrated to be significantly different from the placebo group. Spinal measurements, available only in a few patients, also failed to show any difference compared with untreated PBC patients not included in this study after a mean of 4 years. However since there were some individuals who demonstrated more bone loss than expected, a larger study group might have confirmed this impression.

Since Vuoristo's study[16] has shown that UDCA therapy seems to be able to prevent bone loss by lowering S-PICP metabolism, this could be the explanation for the observation that combination therapy with UDCA plus prednisolone (10 mg/day) did not increase osteoporosis as shown with EDXA[2] during a treatment period of 9 months. Therefore, when we compare the benefit of azathioprine, colchicine and prednisolone for combination therapy with UDCA, we favour the glucocorticoids.

D-penicillamine, thalidomide, methotrexate, chlorambucil and cyclosporine need to be discussed only briefly, because of their ineffectiveness and severe side-effects.

D-*penicillamine, thalidomide.* There are eight controlled studies with penicillamine (600–1200 mg/day) comprising the data of 767 patients, a sufficiently large number to eliminate a type 2 error[19–26]. Only in three studies had some laboratory data improved, but six studies reported on side-effects in about 30% of the treated patients, and several deaths (Tables 3 and 4). Although a preliminary report suggests that penicillamine might improve survival, this has not been corroborated by six controlled trials. D-penicillamine has no place in the treatment of vanishing bile duct syndrome.

Thalidomide has been used in only one placebo-controlled study, with 18 patients[8] and with a starting dose of 50 mg at night and a maintenance dose of 100 mg daily. The only effects seen were fatigue and sedation. The positive effects seen in the treatment of steroid-resistant graft-versus-host disease was with a dose of 800 mg/day.

Methotrexate (MTX). No controlled trials have been published with methotrexate. M. Kaplan has shown that laboratory data and liver histology of five patients treated with low-dose pulse MTX (15 mg/week for 12–34 months) improved markedly compared to the data of a historical group of 28 patients treated with colchicine[17,27]. When treatment was interrupted, all data deteriorated dramatically, but attempts to reinstitute MTX were not successful because the platelet count was maintained below 100 000. At a lower dosage of

Table 4 Side-effects of drugs used in the treatment of primary biliary liver diseases

Glucocorticoids	Bone loss, hypertension, peripheral oedema
D-penicillamine	30%: proteinuria, thrombopenia, autoimmune reactions
Azathioprine	*Few*: bone marrow suppression, gastrointestinal discomfort
Colchicine	*Minimal*: granulocytopenia
Chlorambucil	Bone marrow suppression (30%), acute non-lymphocytic leukaemia
Cyclosporine	Renal insufficiency, hypertension (50%), paraesthesias, hirsutism
Methotrexate	Bone marrow suppression, interstitial pneumonitis, hepatotoxicity

7.5 mg/week, or a full dose followed by folinic acid therapy, liver function tests have not improved. Since MTX may be accompanied by bone marrow suppression, hepatotoxic reactions (initial increases of transaminases) or an unpredictable life-threatening interstitial pneumonitis even at low doses (Table 4), MTX should be used only in experienced centres.

Chlorambucil, cyclosporine. Chlorambucil has been used in a controlled study with 24 patients[28] over a period of 4.1 years. Treatment dose was 10 mg/day for 10 days; maintenance dose was 0.5–4.0 mg daily. Although there were some positive effects on laboratory data (especially on the prognostic parameters bilirubin and albumin) and liver histology, the drug should not be considered for further studies, since bone marrow suppression occurred in 30% and untreatable acute non-lymphocytic leukaemia was observed.

Cyclosporine is a potent immunosuppressive drug successfully used after organ transplantation. In a study with 29 patients who had been treated with 4 mg/kg per day[29] symptoms had improved or stabilized compared to the placebo group; routine laboratory data and especially IgM and AMA decreased significantly (IgM $p < 0.01$; AMA $p < 0.03$). Differences between liver biopsies were significantly better in the treated group ($p < 0.003$). However, hypertension developed in more than 50% of the patients and depression of renal function was seen in 47%[29,30]. In the largest controlled trial of Lombard *et al.*[31] renal suppression and hypertension occurred in only 10%, which might be due to the lower dosage used. Nevertheless side-effects of cyclosporine cause the drug to be of uncertain long-term value (Tables 3 and 4). Whether other immunosuppressive drugs with modes of action similar to cyclosporine, such as FK-506, will be helpful, remains to be seen.

Studies with combination therapy

The question of whether, using the combination of UDCA with one of the already mentioned drugs, the beneficial effect of UDCA is enhanced by the added second drug, or whether UDCA enhances the effects of the other compounds, is difficult to answer. From eight controlled trials (Table 5), in which different combinations had been tested, one can conclude that MTX may be useful in those patients in whom UDCA alone did not improve the laboratory data sufficiently. On the other hand one has to consider that MTX is a toxic substance, which probably has to be given lifelong in a slowly progressing disease with a relatively long spontaneous life expectancy[2,32–38].

Table 5 Combination therapy of primary biliary cirrhosis: controlled trials

Reference	*Drug*	*Dosage*	*Patients*	*Symptoms*	*Laboratory*	*Histology*	*Toxicity*
32	UDC followed by UDC/MTX	UDC 15 mg/kg MTX 2.5 mg/day	8	–	+	0	+
33	UDC/MTX vs no therapy	UDC 500 mg MTX 15 mg/week	14	–	+	–	
34	UDC/MTX vs UDC	UDC 13–15 mg MTX 0.25 mg/kg/week	32	–	–	–	+
35	UDC/Colchicine vs UDC	UDC 600 mg Colchicine 1 mg	22	+	+	0	–
36	UDC/Colchicine vs UDC/placebo	UDC 10 mg/kg Colchicine 1 mg	22	–	–	–	–
37	UDC/Colchicine vs UDC/placebo	UDC 500 mg Colchicine 1 mg	88	–	–	0	
38	Colchicine followed by UDC/Colchicine		45	0	+	0	
2	UDC/prednisolone vs UDC/placebo	UDC 10 mg/kg Prednisolone 10 mg	30	–	–	+	–

–, Not changed vs control; +, improved vs control; Tox +, present; 0, not investigated

Glucocorticoids given in the low dose of 10 mg/day obviously do not increase bone loss in PBC patients[2]. Additionally, UDCA could prevent deterioration of pre-existing osteoporosis, decreasing S-PIP concentrations in the serum[16], or stimulating the activity of osteoblasts[39]. Since it has been shown that UDCA also activates latent glucocorticoid receptors[40], the combination of prednisolone with UDCA could possibly be beneficial[40]. Glucocorticoids do not negatively influence UDCA concentrations in the serum, as shown during a 9-month treatment period[2] with prednisolone (10 mg/day) compared to UDCA alone (10 mg/kg per day), while MTX (0.25 mg/kg per week, for a period of 2 years) increased biliary UDCA concentrations (52%) significantly compared to UDCA alone (41%) (13–15 mg/kg per day; *p*-value in the reprint not given)[34].

MEDICAL THERAPY OF PSC

Therapy of PSC is rather difficult, since intra- and extrahepatic bile duct strictures, sacculations, sludge and gallstones may develop. Besides medical therapy there are some endoscopic and surgical options (Table 6), which will not be discussed here.

There are only two controlled medical studies in patients with PSC. In one penicillamine has been tested versus placebo[41]; the second one used a combination of UDCA/MTX versus UDCA alone[42]. In both studies there were no positive effects (Table 7) concerning symptoms, liver enzymes, histological progress or survival. In the study with penicillamine the majority of patients had stage III or IV of the disease, which may have biased the results. Twenty-one per cent of the patients were lost due to side-effects. In the study with UDCA/MTX combination, five patients discontinued combination therapy because of hair loss and pulmonary problems, and three were referred for transplantation[42]. Therefore there is low support for the MTX/UDCA combination.

Table 6 Endoscopic and surgical options in the management of PSC

Endoscopy	
Cholangioplasty, stent insertion, stone removal or sphincterotomy	Improve biochemistry, symptoms. Recurrence rate 20–50% Complications
Surgery	
T-tube placement	Historical
Choledochojejunal cutaneous fistulas	Temporary transhepatic stents
Procto/colectomy	No change
OLT (6% of all transplantations)	1 year survival: 90% 3 years: 87% Second transplantation: 16% (PBC: 2%) PSC recurrence not known, but non-anastomotic strictures increased compared to other OLT
OLT plus immunosuppression	Risk factor for colon cancer?

OLT = liver transplantation

A controlled study with corticosteroids and colchicine[43] has been published only in abstract form. In 12 patients corticosteroids and colchicine were superior to a control group, but improvement was not sustained at 2 years.

CONCLUSIONS

Most data suggest that the aetiology of PBC and PSC is based on some abnormalities of immunoregulation; yet it is of interest that immunosuppressives do not improve, only marginally improve, the diseases, although PBC resembles rejection of a transplanted liver, which can be successfully treated with immunosuppressives such as glucocorticoids, cyclosporine and azathioprine. Therefore something else, bacteria or viruses from the intestinal or lymphatic system, should be investigated.

On the other hand, the widely used UDCA is also unable to cure the disease. UDCA shifts the hydrophobic to a hydrophilic bile acid pool, and thus reduces cytotoxic reactions between apolar bile salts and liver cells, which may be followed by some immunological improvement. A combination of UDCA with immunosuppressives could be superior to each monotherapy, since bile salts interact with cholestasis, and immunosuppressives with the inflammation. Glucocorticoids, already used in long-term treatment of chronic liver diseases,

Table 7 Medical therapy of primary sclerosing cholangitis: controlled trials

Reference	*Drug*	*Dosage*	*Patients*	*Symptoms*	*Laboratory*	*Histology*	*Toxicity*	*Survival*
41	D-penicillamine vs placebo	3 × 250 mg	70	–	–	–	+	–
42	UDC/MTX vs UDC	UDC 13–15 mg/kg MTX 0.25 mg/kg per week	29	–	–	0	MTX+	0

+, present; –, no effect; 0, not investigated

Table 8 Definitive medical therapy for primary biliary cirrhosis

Promising medical therapies	*Uncertain efficacy*	*Not recommended*
Ursodeoxycholic acid or combination therapies	Azathioprine, colchicine	D-penicillamine, glucocorticoids, cyclosporine, chlorambucil, thalidomide

and having few and well-known side-effects, should be preferred in combination with UDCA. The other drugs discussed in this chapter are less suitable, mainly because of their unpredictable and sometimes life-threatening side effects (Table 8), as seen during monotherapy.

References

1. Portmann BC. Pathology of ductopenia with a particular reference to primary biliary cirrhosis and liver allograft rejection. In: van Berge Henegouwen GP, van Hoek B, de Groote J, Matern S, Stockbrügger RW, editors. Cholestatic liver diseases. New strategies for prevention and treatment of hepatobiliary and cholestatic liver diseases. Dordrecht: Kluwer; 1994:171–84.
2. Leuschner M, Güldütuna S, You T, Hübner K, Bhatti S, Leuschner U. Ursodeoxycholic acid and prednisolone versus ursodeoxycholic acid and placebo in the treatment of early stages of primary biliary cirrhosis. J Hepatol. 1996;25:48–57.
3. Desmukh K, Nimms ME. A defect in the intramolecular and intermolecular cross linking of collagen caused by D-penicillamine. J Biol Chem. 1969;244:1787–93.
4. Nimms ME, Desmukh K, Gerth N. Collagen defect induced by D-penicillamine. Nature. 1992;240:220–1.
5. Harris Ed, Krane SM. The effects of colchicine on collagenase in cultures of rheumatoid synovium. Arthritis Rheum. 1971;14:668–84.
6. Diegelmann RF, Peterkofsky B. Inhibition of collagen secretion from bone and cultured fibroblasts by microtubular disruptive drugs. Proc Natl Acad Sci USA. 1972;69:892–6.
7. Robson SC, Neuberger JM, Williams R. The influence of cyclosporine A therapy on sex hormone levels in pre- and post-menopausal women with primary biliary cirrhosis. J Hepatol. 1994;21:412–16.
8. McCormick PA, Scott F, Epstein O, Burroughs AK, Scheuer PJ, McIntyre N. Thalidomide as therapy for primary biliary cirrhosis: a double-blind placebo controlled pilot study. J Hepatol. 1994;21:496–9.
9. Vogelsang GB, Farmer ER, Hess AD *et al.* Thalidomide for the treatment of chronic graft-versus-host disease. N Engl J Med. 1992;326:1055–8.
10. Youle M, Hawkins D, Gazzard B. Thalidomide in hyperalgic pharyngeal ulceration of AIDS. Lancet. 1990;335:1591.
11. Heathcote J, Ross A, Sherlock S. A prospective controlled trial of azathioprine in primary biliary cirrhosis. Gastroenterology. 1976;70:656–60.
12. Christensen E, Neuberger J, Crowe J *et al.* Beneficial effect of azathioprine and prediction of prognosis in primary biliary cirrhosis. Final results of an international trial. Gastroenterology. 1985;89:1084–91.
13. Warnes TW, Smith A, Lee FI, Haboubi NY, Johnson PJ, Hunt L. A controlled trial of colchicine in primary biliary cirrhosis. J Hepatol. 1987;5:1–7.
14. Kaplan MM, Alling DW, Zimmermann HJ *et al.* A prospective trial of colchicine for primary biliary cirrhosis. N Engl J Med. 1986;315:1448–54.
15. Bodenheimer H, Schaffner F, Pezzullo J. Evaluation of colchicine therapy in primary biliary cirrhosis. Gastroenterology. 1988;95:124–9.
16. Vuoristo M, Färkkilä M, Karvonen A-L *et al.* A placebo-controlled trial of primary biliary cirrhosis treatment with colchicine and ursodeoxycholic acid. Gastroenterology. 1995;108:1470–8.
17. Kaplan MM. Medical treatment of primary biliary cirrhosis. Sem Liver Dis. 1989;9:138–43.
18. Mitchison HC, Palmer JM, Bassendine MF, Watson AJ, Record CO, James OFW. A controlled trial of prednisolone treatment in primary biliary cirrhosis. J Hepatol. 1992;15:336–44.

19. Triger D, Manifold IN, Cloke P, Wunderwood JB. D-penicillamine in primary biliary cirrhosis. Two year results. Gut. 1980;21:919–20.
20. Epstein O, Jain S, Lee RG *et al.* D-penicillamine treatment improves survival in primary biliary cirrhosis. Lancet. 1981;1:1275–7.
21. Bassendine MF, Macklon AF, Mulcaly R, James OFW. Controlled trial of high and low dose D-penicillamine in primary biliary cirrhosis. Gut. 1982;23:909–13.
22. Matloff DS, Alpert E, Resnick RH, Kaplan MM. A prospective trial of D-penicillamine in primary biliary cirrhosis. N Engl J Med. 1982;306:319–26.
23. Taal BG, Schalm SW, Tenkate FW, van Berge Henegouwen GP, Brandt KH. Low therapeutic value of D-penicillamine in short-term prospective trial in primary biliary cirrhosis. Liver. 1983;3:345–52.
24. Bodenheimer HC, Schaffner F, Sternlieb I, Klion FM, Salvatore V, Pezullo J. A prospective trial of D-penicillamine in the treatment of primary biliary cirrhosis. Hepatology. 1985;5:1139–42.
25. Dickson ER, Fleming TR, Wiesner RH *et al.* Trial of penicillamine in advanced primary biliary cirrhosis. N Engl J Med. 1985;312:1011–15.
26. Neuberger J, Christensen E, Portman B *et al.* Double blind controlled trial of D-penicillamine in patients with primary biliary cirrhosis. Gut. 1985;26:114–19.
27. Kaplan MM, Knox TA. Treatment of primary biliary cirrhosis with low-dose weekly methotrexate. Gastroenterology. 1991;101:1332–8.
28. Hoofnagle JH, Davis GL, Shafer DF *et al.* Randomized trial of chlorambucil for primary biliary cirrhosis. Gastroenterology. 1986;91:1327–34.
29. Wiesner RH, Ludwig J, Lindor KD *et al.* A controlled trial of cyclosporine in the treatment of primary biliary cirrhosis. N Engl J Med. 1990;322:1419–24.
30. Minuk GY, Bohme C, Burgess E *et al.* Pilot study of cyclosporin A in patients with symptomatic primary biliary cirrhosis. Gastroenterology. 1988;95:1356–9.
31. Lombard M, Portmann PB, Neuberger J *et al.* Cyclosporine A treatment in primary biliary cirrhosis: results of a long-term placebo controlled trial and effect on survival. Gastroenterology. 1993;104:519–26.
32. Buscher H-P, Zietschmann Y, Gerok W. Positive responses to methotrexate and ursodeoxycholic acid in patients with primary biliary cirrhosis responding insufficiently to ursodeoxycholic acid alone. J Hepatol. 1993;18:9–14.
33. Van Steenbergen W, Sciot R, Van Eyken P, Desmet V, Fevery J. Methotrexate alone or in combination with ursodeoxycholic acid as possible treatment in primary biliary cirrhosis. In: Van Berge Henegouwen GP, Van Hoek B, de Groote J, Matern S, Stockbrügger RW, editors. Cholestatic liver diseases. New strategies for prevention and treatment of hepatobiliary and cholestatic liver diseases. Dordrecht: Kluwer; 1994:246–54.
34. Lindor KD, Dickson ER, Jorgensen RA *et al.* The combination of ursodeoxycholic acid and methotrexate for patients with primary biliary cirrhosis: the results of a pilot study. Hepatology. 1995;22:1158–62.
35. Ikeda T, Tozuka S, Noguchi O *et al.* Effects of additional administration of colchicine in ursodeoxycholic acid-treated patients with primary biliary cirrhosis: a prospective randomized study. J Hepatol. 1996;24:88–94.
36. Raedsch R, Stiehl A, Walker S, Scherrmann JM, Kommerell B. Kombinierte Ursodeoxycholsäure plus Colchicin-Behandlung bei primär biliärer Zirrhose: Ergebnisse einer placebokontrollierten Doppelblindstudie. Z Gastroenterol. 1992;30:55–7.
37. Podda M, Almasso P, Battezzatti PM, Crosignani A and the Italian multicenter group for the study of UDCA in PBC. Long-term effect of the administration of ursodeoxycholic acid alone or with colchicine in patients with primary biliary cirrhosis: a double-blind multicenter study. In: Paumgartner G, Stiehl A, Gerok W, editors. Bile acids and the hepatobiliary system. Dordrecht: Kluwer; 1993:310–15.
38. Schaffner F. Ursodeoxycholic acid (U) + colchicine (C) for treatment of primary biliary cirrhosis (PBC). Hepatology. 1991;14: abstract 62.
39. Palamorou-Vogiatzi C, Georgiou E, Proukakis C *et al.* Osteocalcin levels before and after ursodeoxycholic acid (UDCA) therapy in primary biliary cirrhosis (PBC). Hepatology. 1990;12:841 (abstract).
40. Tanaka H, Makino I. Ursodeoxycholic acid-dependent activation of the glucocorticoid receptor. Biochem Biophys Res Commun. 1992;188:942–8.
41. LaRusso NF, Wiesner RH, Ludwig J, MacCarty RL, Beaver SJ, Zinsmeister AR. Prospective trial of penicillamine in primary sclerosing cholangitis. Gastroenterology. 1988;95:1036–42.

42. Lindor KD, Jorgensen RA, Anderson ML, Gores GJ, Hofmann AF, LaRusso NF. Ursodeoxycholic acid and methotrexate for primary sclerosing cholangitis: a pilot study. Am J Gastroenterol. 1996;91:511–15.
43. Lindor KD, LaRusso NF, Wiesner RH. Prednisolone and colchicine are not of benefit after two years in patients with primary sclerosing cholangitis. Hepatology. 1989;10:638 (abstract).

21
Treatment of vanishing bile duct syndrome with ursodeoxycholic acid

M. PODDA, A. CROSIGNANI, A. LARGHI, P. M. BATTEZZATI, P. INVERNIZZI, M. ALLOCCA and M. ZUIN

INTRODUCTION

Progressive destruction of bile ducts characterizing the vanishing bile duct syndrome (VBDS) may be due to different aetiological agents. Whatever the aetiological agent, the retention of endogenous, detergent hepatotoxic bile acids may initiate and/or aggravate liver cell injury, which may lead to liver cirrhosis and impairment of liver function. Ursodeoxycholic acid (UDCA) was shown to improve biochemical and clinical expression of different cholestatic conditions[1] and its mechanism of action was suggested to be related, at least in part, to the dilution and/or displacement of endogenous bile acids[2–4]. Therefore, this drug may improve the clinical outcome of different diseases which are responsible for VBDS, even if it has no effect on the underlying aetiological agents.

The clinical experience on the treatment of VBDS with UDCA is limited in the adult to primary biliary cirrhosis (PBC), primary sclerosing cholangitis (PSC) and graft-versus-host disease (GVHD). However, it is only for PBC that data coming from randomized controlled trials with meaningful numbers of patients are presently available (Table 1).

Table 1 Available studies on UDCA treatment for VBDS of the adult

	Open studies	*RCT*
PBC		
No.	12	10
Patients	219	969
PSC		
No.	5	2
Patients	56	34
GVHD		
No.	1	–
Patients	12	–

URSODEOXYCHOLIC ACID FOR GRAFT-VERSUS-HOST DISEASE

Only data coming from a pilot study are available for the treatment of GVHD with UDCA[5]. A substantial improvement of serum liver enzymes related to cholestasis and cytolysis was described, but the clinical experience is limited to a small number of patients (n=12). Further studies on clinically relevant end-points are warranted.

URSODEOXYCHOLIC ACID FOR PRIMARY SCLEROSING CHOLANGITIS

For PSC, data are available from two double-blind, randomized controlled trials (RCT) (Table 1)[6,7]. In both studies the biochemical expression of the disease was shown to improve, whereas no effect on symptoms was found. In one study[6] also, a slight but significant improvement of histology was observed, compared to placebo. Overall, results from these two RCT are encouraging but require confirmation in larger series, since the number of patients enrolled is limited.

On the other hand, results from a long-term open trial performed in 43 patients treated with UDCA and endoscopic dilatation, whenever the latter was necessary, for a period longer than 3 years, indicate a significant improvement of transplantation-free survival, as compared with that predicted from survival models[8]. In addition, transplantation rate was found to be significantly lower compared to that of a group of 10 patients who had dropped out[8]. However, it is questionable if such a control group is appropriate in order to draw a definitive conclusion on the ability of UDCA to improve survival in patients with PSC.

Quite recently, at the 1996 AGA meeting, data were reported of a RCT in which 105 patients were enrolled and randomly assigned to receive UDCA (13–15 mg/kg per day) or placebo[9]. After a mean follow-up of 2.9 years a significant improvement of liver biochemistries was confirmed, but neither histology nor time until treatment failure was significantly affected by treatment.

In conclusion, to clarify the issue of the effectiveness of UDCA for the treatment of PSC, availability, as a full paper, of the results of this latter study is needed. In addition, the beneficial effects of UDCA in patients treated with endoscopic dilatation, as already suggested by Stiehl *et al.*[8], should be confirmed in a randomized controlled study.

URSODEOXYCHOLIC ACID FOR PRIMARY BILIARY CIRRHOSIS

Summary of the available data

In PBC 10 RCT have been performed in which a large number of patients were enrolled (Table 2)[10–19]. Marked improvement of serum liver enzymes, a slight decrease in serum bilirubin concentrations and a decrease in serum IgM levels were consistently found, whereas no consistent effect on pruritus was reported, as compared with placebo. In addition, UDCA was shown to be remarkably safe, since only few minimal side-effects were observed.

In the four long-term multicentre RCT[11,15,16,18], the effects of UDCA administration on histology and on survival have also been assessed. To test the effects

Table 2 Randomized controlled trials on UDCA treatment for PBC

Reference	*No. of patients*	*Duration (months)*
Leuschner *et al.*, 1989[10]	18	9
Poupon *et al.*, 1991[11]	146	24
Oka *et al.*, 1991[12]	45	6
Battezzati *et al.*, 1993[13]	88	6–12
Hwang *et al.*, 1993[14]	12	3
Heathcote *et al.*, 1994[15]	222	24
Lindor *et al.*, 1994[16]	180	24
Turner *et al.*, 1994[17]	46	24
Combes *et al.*, 1995[18]	151	24
Vuoristo *et al.*, 1995[19]	61	24

of UDCA on histology, different parameters have been evaluated in different studies. In particular, Poupon and colleagues[11] found a significant improvement for piecemeal necrosis, parenchymal necrosis, portal and lobular inflammation, cholestasis, bile duct paucity and proliferation. Conversely, only minimal improvement in terms of bile duct paucity and periportal ballooning was reported by the Canadian study[15], In the study performed at the Mayo Clinic[16], the progression of the histological stage of the disease was not affected by UDCA administration. Interestingly, Combes *et al.*[18] found a significant histological improvement in terms of piecemeal necrosis, portal inflammation, cholestasis and fibrosis, but only in patients with less severe disease (i.e. serum bilirubin < 2 mg/dl).

In none of these studies was survival shown to improve significantly. However, by the prolongation of follow-up after the completion of the study, when all patients were receiving open-label UDCA, Poupon and colleagues found a significant improvement of OLT-free survival compared to placebo for those patients who had been assigned to UDCA treatment at enrolment[20] (Figure 1). More recently, this observation was confirmed by the Mayo Clinic group when the patients enrolled in the RCT were followed up for 3 additional years after the completion of the study[21]. Furthermore, a significant improvement of

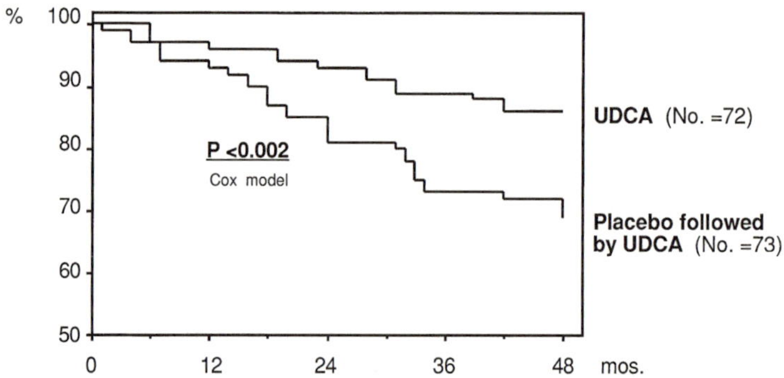

Figure 1 Probability of survival free from OLT and from major complications of liver cirrhosis in patients with PBC during long-term treatment with UDCA (modified from ref. 20)

OLT-free survival was demonstrated by a combined analysis of three RCT[22] in which 553 patients had been enrolled. Only 47 patients in the UDCA group did not survive free of OLT, as compared with 68 in the placebo group, thus indicating that the risk was reduced by 32% (p=0.014).

Which patients should be treated?

There are many open questions regarding UDCA treatment for PBC. One of the most relevant issues is the selection of the patients who may most benefit from UDCA administration. Since treatment should be prescribed life-long, problems of cost-effectiveness, if not of safety, are of great interest.

Overall, the available studies indicate that UDCA is more beneficial in patients with less advanced disease, whereas in patients with most severe PBC, when the large majority of bile ducts have been lost, treatment is unlikely to be beneficial and liver transplantation remains the only effective therapeutic tool.

As already indicated, in a multicentre study from USA[18], histology was favourably affected by UDCA in anicteric patients, but not in patients with serum bilirubin concentrations higher than 2 mg/dl at enrolment. In addition, treatment failure occurred sooner during placebo than during UDCA administration in patients with anicteric PBC, but at the same rate in similarly treated icteric patients. Our own experience on a large cohort of Italian symptomatic PBC patients is consistent with this finding since we observed, after a median time of 35 months of UDCA administration at the daily dose of 500 mg, a significantly higher rate of treatment failures (death, OLT, major complications of liver cirrhosis and doubling of bilirubin serum values to levels higher than 4 mg/dl) in patients with serum bilirubin higher than 2 mg/dl, compared to patients with values lower than 2 mg/dl[23].

On the other hand, it is still questionable if patients with very early stage of the disease may benefit from UDCA treatment, and this may be relevant for the relatively high cost of this drug, which should be taken for several decades. From the literature, and from our own experience, there is evidence that several patients presenting without symptoms may never progress to end-stage disease (Figure 2). Therefore, the most difficult decision is how to manage asymptomatic patients, since there is still no reliable way to distinguish patients whose disease is likely to progress rapidly from those with slowly progressive disease who may require no treatment.

CONCLUSIONS

Definitive data on the efficacy of UDCA treatment for vanishing bile duct syndrome are available only for PBC. In patients with PBC, UDCA was shown to delay but not to halt the progression of the disease. To improve the efficacy, association therapies with immunosuppressive or anti-fibrotic agents and the use of UDCA derivatives have been suggested[24–28]. In patients with more advanced PBC UDCA is unlikely to be effective, and high serum bilirubin concentrations are associated with lower response to treatment. On the opposite side of the spectrum of the disease, the cost-effectiveness of treating asymptomatic patients remains to be established.

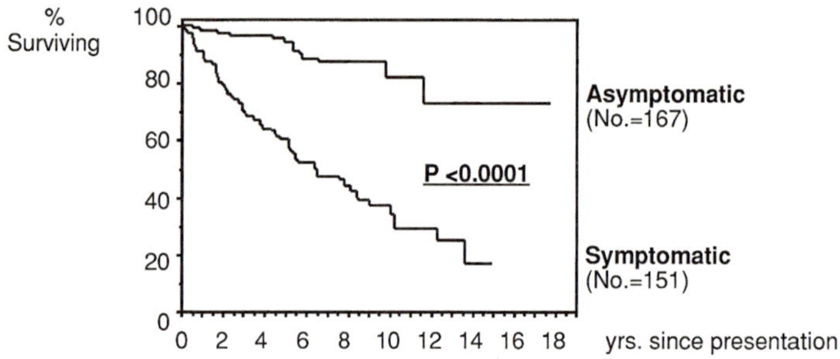

Asymptomatic	167	124	94	64	33	17	9	4	2	1	No. of patients at risk
Symptomatic	151	98	65	42	24	15	8	2	0		

Figure 2 Survival of patients with PBC presenting with or without symptoms (pruritus and/or jaundice): the clinical experience at our centre

References

1. Rubin RA, Kowalski TE, Khandelwal, Malet PF. Ursodiol for hepatobiliary disorders. Ann Intern Med. 1994;121:207–18.
2. Armstrong MJ, Carey MC. The hydrophobic–hydrophilic balance of bile salts. Inverse correlation between reverse-phase high performance liquid chromatographic mobilities and micellar cholesterol-solubilizing capacities. J Lipid Res. 1982;23:70–80.
3. Hofmann AF, Popper H. Ursodeoxycholic acid for primary biliary cirrhosis. Lancet. 1987;11:398–9.
4. Attili AF, Angelico M, Cantafora A, Alvaro D, Capocaccia L. Bile acid induced liver toxicity: relation to the hydrophobic–hydrophylic balance of bile acids. Med Hypotheses. 1986;19:57–69.
5. Fried RH, Murakami CS, Fisher LD, Willson LA, Sullivan KM, McDonald GB. Ursodeoxycholic acid treatment of refractory chronic graft-versus-host disease of the liver. Ann Intern Med. 1992;116:624–9.
6. Beuers U, Spengler U, Kruis W *et al.* Ursodeoxycholic acid for treatment of primary sclerosing cholangitis: a placebo-controlled trial. Hepatology. 1992;16:707–14.
7. Stiehl A, Walker S, Stiehl L, Rudolph G, Hofmann WJ, Theilmann L. Effect of ursodeoxycholic acid on liver and bile duct disease in primary sclerosing cholangitis. A 3-year pilot study with a placebo-controlled study period. J Hepatol. 1994;20:57–64.
8. Stiehl A. Ursodeoxycholic acid therapy in treatment of primary sclerosing cholangitis. Scand J Gastroenterol. 1994;29(Suppl. 204):59–61.
9. Lindor KD and the Mayo PSC/UDCA Study Group. A randomized trial of ursodeoxycholic acid in the treatment of primary sclerosing cholangitis. Gastroenterology. 1996;110:844A.
10. Leuschner U, Fischer H, Kurtz W *et al.* Ursodeoxycholic acid and primary biliary cirrhosis: results from a controlled double-blind trial. Gastroenterology. 1989;97:1268–74.
11. Poupon RE, Balkau B, Eschwege E, Poupon R, UDCA–PBC Study Group. A multicenter, controlled trial of ursodiol for the treatment of primary biliary cirrhosis. N Engl J Med. 1991;324:1548–54.
12. Oka K, Toda G, Ikeda Y *et al.* A multi-center double-blind controlled trial of ursodeoxycholic acid for primary biliary cirrhosis. Gastroenterol Jpn. 1991;25:774–80.
13. Battezzati PM, Podda M, Bianchi FB *et al.* Ursodeoxycholic acid for symptomatic primary biliary cirrhosis: preliminary analysis of a double-blind multicenter trial. J Hepatol. 1993;17:332–8.
14. Hwang S-J, Chan C-Y, Lee S-D, Wu J-C, Tsay S-H, Lo K-J. Ursodeoxycholic acid in the treatment of primary biliary cirrhosis: a short-term, randomized, double-blind controlled cross-over study with long-term follow up. J Gastroenterol Hepatol. 1993;8:217–23.

15. Heathcote EJ, Cauch-Dudek K, Walker V, Bailey RJ *et al.* The Canadian multicenter double-blind randomized controlled trial of ursodeoxycholic acid in primary biliary cirrhosis. Hepatology. 1994;19:1149–56.
16. Lindor KD, Dickson ER, Baldus WP, Jorgensen RA *et al.* Ursodeoxycholic acid in the treatment of primary biliary cirrhosis. Gastroenterology. 1994;106:1284–90.
17. Turner IB, Myszor M, Mitchison HC, Bennet MK, Burt AD, James OFW. A two year controlled trial examining the effectiveness of ursodeoxycholic acid in primary biliary cirrhosis. J Gastroenterol Hepatol. 1994;9:162–8.
18. Combes B, Carithers RL Jr, Maddrey WC *et al.* A randomized, double-blind, placebo-controlled trial of ursodeoxycholic acid in primary biliary cirrhosis. Hepatology. 1995;22:759–66.
19. Vuoristo M, Farkkila M, Karvonen A-L *et al.* A placebo-controlled trial of primary biliary cirrhosis treatment with colchicine and ursodeoxycholic acid. Gastroenterology. 1995;108:1470–8.
20. Poupon RR, Poupon R, Balkau B and the UDCA–PBC study group. Ursodiol for long-term treatment of primary biliary cirrhosis. N Engl J Med. 1994;330:1342–7.
21. Lindor KD, Therneau TM, Jorgensen RA, Malinchoc M, Dickson R. Effects of ursodeoxycholic acid on survival in patients with primary biliary cirrhosis. Gastroenterology. 1996;110:1515–18.
22. Heathcote EJ, Lindor KD, Poupon R, Cauch-Dudek K, Dickson ER, Trout R, Poupon RE. Combined analysis of French, American and Canadian randomized controlled trials of ursodeoxycholic acid therapy in primary biliary cirrhosis. Gastroenterology. 1995;108:1082A.
23. Podda M, Almasio P, Battezzati PM, Crosignani A and the Italian multicenter group for the study of UDCA in PBC. Long-term effect of the administration of ursodeoxycholic acid alone or with colchicine in patients with primary biliary cirrhosis. in: Paumgartner G, Stiehl A, Gerok W editors. Bile acids and the hepatobiliary system. From basic science to clinical practice. Lancaster: Kluwer; 1993:310–15.
24. Podda M, Crosignani A, Battezzati PM *et al.* Ursodeoxycholic acid for the therapy of chronic cholestatic liver disease. In: Hofmann AF, Paumgartner G, Stiehl A, editors. Bile acids in gastroenterology: basic and clinical advances. Lancaster: Kluwer; 1995;364–71.
25. Lim AG, Jazrawi RP, Northfield TC. The ursodeoxycholic acid story in primary biliary cirrhosis. Gut. 1995;35:301–4.
26. Lindor KD. Colchicine and ursodeoxycholic acid for primary biliary cirrhosis: emerging results. Gastroenterology. 1995;108:1592–4.
27. Crosignani A, Battezzati PM, Setchell KDR *et al.* Tauroursodeoxycholic acid for the treatment of primary biliary cirrhosis: a dose-response study. Dig Dis Sci. 1996;41:809–15.
28. Setchell KDR, Rodrigues CPM, Podda M, Crosignani A. Metabolism of orally administered tauroursodeoxycholic acid in patients with primary biliary cirrhosis. Gut. 1995;38:439–46.

22
Mechanism of action of UDCA in cholestatic syndromes

U. BEUERS, G.-A. KULLAK-UBLICK and G. PAUMGARTNER

INTRODUCTION

The dihydroxy bile acid ursodeoxycholic acid (UDCA) improves liver structure and function in chronic cholestatic liver diseases such as primary biliary cirrhosis (PBC) or primary sclerosing cholangitis (PSC)[1–8]. In addition, UDCA has been shown to prolong transplant-free survival in patients with PBC[9–11]. The anticholestatic effect of UDCA is not only observed in patients with autoimmune diseases of the biliary tract such as PBC or PSC, but has also been demonstrated in a number of cholestatic disorders of other origins[8]. So far the mechanism of action of UDCA in cholestatic syndromes has not been resolved[12–15].

PHYSICOCHEMICAL AND PHARMACOLOGICAL PROPERTIES OF UDCA

UDCA ($3\alpha,7\beta$-dihydroxy-5β-cholanoic acid) is a relatively hydrophilic bile acid which occurs naturally in many mammals. In humans, UDCA represents up to 3% of the total bile acid pool. UDCA is more hydrophilic than the other common dihydroxy bile acids, chenodeoxycholic acid (CDCA) and deoxycholic acid (DCA). Depending on the method used, comparison of UDCA and the trihydroxy bile acid cholic acid (CA) with regard to their hydrophilicity reveals differing results. By the criteria of critical micellar concentration, octanol–water partition coefficient, passive membrane permeation, contiguous hydrophobic area, or partition chromatography using octyl silane as the stationary phase, CA is more hydrophilic than UDCA. In contrast, UDCA is more hydrophilic than CA when partition chromatography is performed with octadecyl silane as the stationary phase[13,16–18].

After oral administration, UDCA is passively absorbed in the small intestine and is transported to the liver via the portal vein bound to albumin. After effective extraction (> 50% during first pass) by the hepatocytes, UDCA is mainly conjugated with glycine and taurine in the human liver and secreted into bile, undergoing an effective enterohepatic circulation due to active reabsorption of the UDCA amides in the terminal ileum. Thus, the glycine and taurine conjugates represent the predominant forms of UDCA in the enterohepatic and systemic circulation[13]. Glucuronidation, sulphation, glucosidation and *N*-acetylglucosaminidation of UDCA have also been described[19–21].

HEPATOTOXICITY OF BILE ACIDS

Cholestasis is a uniform reaction of the liver in response to a wide range of abnormalities at the level of the liver cell, or to mechanical obstruction of the bile ducts[22]. More than two decades ago it was proposed that retention of hepatotoxic cholephils within the liver cell might be the common feature of different forms of cholestasis, and the accumulation of hydrophobic bile acids was soon regarded as a major culprit in cholestatic liver damage. It was demonstrated that lithocholic acid (LCA) induces liver cirrhosis[23] and that its taurine conjugate (TLCA) causes cholestasis in experimental animals[24]. The hepatic levels of hydrophobic dihydroxy bile acids correlate with the degree of liver damage[25,26]. However, the molecular mechanism of bile acid-induced liver cell damage is not exactly known, and a number of pathomechanisms have been proposed[8,12–14,22,27–29].

The hydrophilic bile acid TUDCA prevents liver damage and cholestasis caused by TCA[30] and the more hydrophobic bile acids TCDCA[31,32], TDCA[32], or TLCA[33] in both experimental animals and in the isolated perfused liver. Taurine conjugation of UDCA seems to be a prerequisite for the protective effect of this bile acid[34–36].

PUTATIVE MECHANISMS OF ACTION OF UDCA IN CHRONIC CHOLESTATIC LIVER DISEASE

During the past decade a number of mechanisms have been discussed to explain the beneficial effect of UDCA in cholestatic syndromes. Among these mechanisms the following have attracted major interest:

1. Displacement of hydrophobic bile acids from the enterohepatic circulation.
2. Hypercholeresis.
3. Membrane stabilization and protection against more hydrophobic bile acids.
4. Immunomodulation.
5. Stimulation of hepatocellular secretion.

These will now be discussed in more detail.

Displacement of hydrophobic bile acids from the enterohepatic circulation

The effects of UDCA administration on endogenous bile acid kinetics and bile acid levels in serum, bile, and urine of patients with cholestatic liver disease have been studied intensively. During the first month of treatment, UDCA becomes the predominant bile acid in serum and reaches levels up to 60% of total serum bile acids when administered at doses of 13–15 mg/kg per day. Serum levels of the primary bile acid CA tended to decrease during the first weeks[37,38] and months[39–43], whereas those of the primary bile acid CDCA remained unchanged for at least 3–6 months[37,38,41,42,44] before decreasing[39,43]. Serum levels of DCA were not affected by UDCA treatment in patients with chronic cholestasis, in whom they usually are low[37,39–41,43,44]. DCA decreased only in one group of patients with predominantly early-stage PBC and normal pretreatment serum levels during UDCA treatment[38]. Serum levels of LCA increased significantly in patients with PBC during UDCA treatment[43].

In bile of patients with PBC, UDCA became the predominant biliary bile acid, almost exclusively in the conjugated form. Levels of cholic acid decreased, whereas those of CDCA and DCA were not affected, and those of LCA increased significantly after 6 months of UDCA treatment[41].

The pool sizes of CA and CDCA were not significantly affected by UDCA treatment over a period of 1–3 months[38,39,43]. Pool sizes of DCA are low in patients with chronic cholestasis, most probably due to an impairment of the enterohepatic circulation of bile acids with diminished amounts of CA reaching the colon for bacterial conversion to DCA[38], and were not significantly affected in one study[38]. In another study, in which patients mostly with early-stage PBC had DCA pool sizes within the normal range before treatment, UDCA administration led to a reduction of the DCA pool size[39] comparable to its effect in healthy subjects[38].

Reabsorption of endogenous bile acids in the small intestine is impaired by UDCA administration, as shown in patients with ileostomy[45] or by use of the SeHCAT test[46,47]. The impact of this phenomenon on the beneficial effect of UDCA in cholestasis is unclear, since impairment of bile acid absorption and reduced bile acid flow to the liver might induce an increase of hepatocellular synthesis and fractional turnover of primary bile acids. Indeed, fractional turnover and synthesis of CA increased significantly in patients with PSC under UDCA treatment[43]. In addition, fractional turnover and synthesis of CDCA tended to increase in patients with PBC and PSC[38,39,43]. CA kinetics are more strongly affected by UDCA administration than CDCA kinetics, probably for two reasons: (a) CDCA, but not CA, is reabsorbed in the proximal small intestine at a reasonable rate by non-ionic passive diffusion due to its lipophilicity[48]; (b) UDCA is partly converted to CDCA by intestinal bacteria[49–51] and the liver[52,53]. In conclusion, these data indicate that, during the first months of UDCA treatment when serum liver tests show marked improvement in patients with cholestatic liver disease, endogenous bile acids, particularly the hydrophobic bile acids, are not replaced by UDCA but are redistributed within the enterohepatic circulation, probably due to an improved hepatic clearance suggesting stimulation of hepatocellular bile acid secretion by UDCA (see below).

Hypercholeresis

In experimental studies, unconjugated, but not conjugated UDCA given to rats at high pharmacological doses induces a greater choleresis than expected from the amount of bile acids secreted into bile, a phenomenon called 'hypercholeresis'[54]. The 'cholehepatic shunt hypothesis' proposed by Hofmann and associates 10 years ago[55] still remains the best explanation for hypercholeresis[56]. According to this hypothesis, protonation of unconjugated UDC in the bile duct lumen leads to generation of a HCO_3^- anion ($UDC^- + H_2CO_3 \rightarrow UDCA + HCO_3^-$). While UDCA is taken up by the bile duct endothelium via passive non-ionic absorption and undergoes cholehepatic shunting via the peribiliary plexus, the HCO_3^- anion is secreted into the intestine. Thus, each cholehepatic cycle of a UDCA molecule may generate one HCO_3^- anion in bile. During the past decade a number of sophisticated studies have provided additional evidence for the 'cholehepatic shunt' of UDCA under experimental conditions[57–61].

Might hypercholeresis explain the beneficial effect of UDCA in patients with cholestatic syndromes? Knyrim and associates administered UDCA or CA intraduodenally at a therapeutic dose of 15 mg/kg to patients with cholelithiasis after depletion of the bile acid pool overnight. They observed a similar correlation of bile flow and bile acid secretion for either bile acid, but no hypercholeresis[62]. In addition, Crosignani and associates observed an increase of unconjugated UDCA in bile of patients with PBC from 0.4 to only 0.7% during UDCA treatment[42]. Only unconjugated, but not conjugated, UDCA has been shown to induce hypercholeresis in experimental animals[63]. Thus, hypercholeresis is unlikely to occur at considerable rates during UDCA treatment of patients with cholestatic syndromes. Therefore, the beneficial effect of UDCA in cholestasis can not be explained by hypercholeresis.

Membrane stabilization and protection against more hydrophobic bile acids

A number of *in-vitro* studies have provided evidence that UDCA exerts a membrane-stabilizing effect when artificial or biomembranes are exposed to high levels of hydrophobic bile acids.

Exposure of erythrocyte membranes to bile acids at 20 mmol/L concentrations revealed that UDCA and its conjugates were less damaging than DCA and CDCA and, at 40 mmol/L, virtually abolished the membrane-damaging effects of the latter bile acids, as demonstrated by electron paramagnetic resonance spectroscopy[64]. UDCA antagonized the increases in membrane polarity and the release of membrane cholesterol and phospholipid observed after incubation with 1–10 mmol/L CDCA[65]. UDCA conjugates also protect against membrane damage in rat and human hepatocytes induced by more hydrophobic bile acids *in vitro*[34,66], and against disruption of model membranes composed of egg lecithin and cholesterol (molar ratio $< 2 : 1$)[67]. At millimolar concentrations TUDCA inhibits protein release induced by TDCA in canalicular membranes[68]. A recent study, however, indicates that reduction of bile acid-induced permeabilization and dissolution of cholesterol-rich membranes after addition of TUDCA may result from effects on the formation and structure of simple and mixed micelles rather than a direct membrane-stabilizing effect of TUDCA[69].

In conclusion, UDCA conjugates at millimolar concentrations exert a membrane-stabilizing effect *in vitro* against membrane damage induced by hydrophobic bile acids. If these effects are of physiological importance *in vivo* the site of action of UDCA conjugates would be the bile ducts, where millimolar bile acid concentrations are found, but not the systemic circulation or the liver cell. Thus, the relevance of these findings with regard to the anticholestatic effect of UDCA *in vivo* remains unclear.

Immunomodulation

In patients with PBC and PSC, treatment with UDCA led to a reduction of aberrant major histocompatibility complex (MHC) Class I expression on hepatocellular membranes[6,70]. MHC Class I molecules are key structures for antigen recognition by cytotoxic T lymphocytes[71]. Aberrant expression of MHC Class I molecules on hepatocellular membranes can be induced by experimental cholestasis[72,73], and by exposure of hepatocytes *in vitro* to high levels of hydrophobic bile acids[74].

Thus, the reduction of MHC Class I display on liver cells, which renders these cells less vulnerable to attack by cytolytic T-cells, may be a consequence of UDCA's anticholestatic effect rather than an intrinsic immunomodulating property of this bile acid.

In vitro, UDCA modulates secretion of cytokines and immunoglobulins by immunocompetent cells[75,76]. Although these studies were partly performed using reasonable micromolar concentrations of bile acids[75] it remains uncertain whether the effects observed play a role *in vivo* when effects of bile acids on cells other than hepatocytes may be much less pronounced due to protein binding within the circulation.

In summary, immunomodulating effects of UDCA in cholestatic liver disease may be regarded as secondary phenomena and might be explained by the anticholestatic effect of UDCA.

Stimulation of hepatocellular secretion

Accumulation of potential hepatotoxins such as hydrophobic bile acids within the liver cell has been assumed to play a pivotal role in cholestasis-associated liver damage. Kitani and co-workers demonstrated that TUDCA stimulates biliary bile acid secretion in the bile fistula rat[31] and suggested that 'the cytoprotective effect is most probably exerted in the excretory pathway from the hepatocyte to the biliary canaliculus'[15]. Today, increasing experimental and clinical evidence supports this early suggestion by Kitani. TUDCA reduces intrahepatocyte content of its hydrophobic 7α-epimer, TCDCA *in vitro*[77]. In patients with PBC and PSC, biliary secretion of bile acids is markedly stimulated by UDCA treatment[78,79], and in patients with cystic fibrosis a stimulation of the biliary secretory capacity by UDCA treatment has been demonstrated[80].

What is the molecular mechanism of UDCA-induced stimulation of biliary bile acid secretion? ATP-dependent carrier-mediated transport across the canalicular membrane is the rate-limiting step in hepatocellular bile acid secretion[81]. The canalicular bile acid transport protein has not yet been identified. It has, however, been shown that canalicular membrane transport activity is highly regulated by the insertion of transport protein-carrying vesicles into this domain[82,83]. Vesicle fusion or exocytosis is regulated by a complex network of signals in secretory cells including hepatocytes, among which cytosolic free calcium $[Ca^{2+}]_i$, protein kinase C (PKC) and protein kinase A (PKA) play a key role[84–86].

TUDCA was shown to induce a sustained elevation of $[Ca^{2+}]_i$ in isolated hepatocytes at physiological bile acid levels via depletion of inositol-1,4,5-trisphosphate (IP_3)-sensitive endoplasmic Ca^{2+} stores and stimulation of Ca^{2+} inflow across the plasma membrane[87–89]. In the perfused rat liver, TUDCA, but not the primary bile acids TCA and TCDCA, induce a sustained stimulation of hepatocellular exocytosis by Ca^{2+}-dependent mechanisms[89]. In addition, TUDCA induces translocation to the hepatocellular membranes of the α-isoform of PKC[90,91], which has been functionally related to stimulation of exocytosis[92], and activates membrane-associated PKC in isolated hepatocytes[91]. TUDCA induces accumulation of s,n-1,2-diacylglycerol (DAG), the intracellular activator of PKC[91], but does not affect hepatocellular IP_3 levels[87,88], suggesting that phospholipase D, but not phosphoinositol bisphosphate (PIP_2)-dependent phospholipase C, is affected by TUDCA in hepatocytes. Thus, TUDCA stimulates Ca^{2+}- and putatively α-PKC-dependent hepatocellular exocytosis, and might thereby enhance the excretory capacitiy of the liver cell[87,89,91].

Cell swelling has also been shown to stimulate bile acid secretion in the perfused liver[93], and TUDCA induces cell swelling at physiological concentrations[93]. A comparison of the effect of TUDCA with those of other bile acids on cell volume changes could help to assess whether cell swelling contributes to the beneficial effect of TUDCA in cholestasis.

SUMMARY

A number of potential mechanisms and sites of action of UDCA in cholestatic syndromes have been discussed during the past decade. Increasing evidence suggests that stimulation of hepatocellular secretion by UDCA conjugates is of key importance for the beneficial effect of UDCA in cholestasis. The exact molecular mechanism of UDCA-induced stimulation of biliary secretion remains to be established.

References

1. Poupon RE, Balkau B, Eschwege B, Poupon R, and the PBC–UDCA study group. A multicenter, controlled trial of ursodiol for the treatment of primary biliary cirrhosis. N Engl J Med. 1991;324:1548–54.
2. Leuschner U, Fischer H, Kurtz W *et al.* Ursodeoxycholic acid in primary biliary cirrhosis: results of a controlled double-blind trial. Gastroenterology. 1989;97:1268–74.
3. Heathcote EJ, Cauch-Dudek K, Walker V *et al.* The Canadian multicenter double-blind randomized controlled trial of ursodeoxycholic acid in primary biliary cirrhosis. Hepatology. 1994;19:1149–56.
4. Lindor KD, Dickson ER, Baldus WP *et al.* Ursodeoxycholic acid in the treatment of primary biliary cirrhosis. Gastroenterology. 1994;106:1284–90.
5. Combes B, Carithers RL, Maddrey WC *et al.* A randomized, double-blind, placebo-controlled trial of ursodeoxycholic acid in primary biliary cirrhosis. Hepatology. 1995;22:759–66.
6. Beuers U, Spengler U, Kruis W *et al.* Ursodeoxycholic acid for treatment of primary sclerosing cholangitis: a placebo-controlled trial. Hepatology. 1992;16:707–14.
7. Stiehl A, Walker S, Stiehl S, Rudolph G, Hofmann WJ, Theilmann L. Effect of ursodeoxycholic acid on liver and bile duct disease in primary sclerosing cholangitis. A 3-year pilot study with a placebo-controlled study period. J Hepatol. 1994;20:57–64.

8. Reichen J. Pharmacologic treatment of cholestasis. Semin Liver Dis. 1993;13:302–15.
9. Poupon RE, Poupon R, Balkau B. Ursodiol for the long-term treatment of primary biliary cirrhosis. N Engl J Med. 1994;330:1342–7.
10. Heathcote EJ, Lindor KD, Poupon R *et al.* Combined analysis of French, American and Canadian randomized controlled trials of ursodeoxycholic acid therapy in primary biliary cirrhosis. Gastroenterology. 1995;108:A1082.
11. Lindor KD, Therneau TM, Jorgensen RA, Malinchoc M, Dickson ER. Effects of ursodeoxycholic acid on survival in patients with primary biliary cirrhosis. Gastroenterology. 1996;110:1515–18.
12. Poupon RE, Poupon R. Ursodeoxycholic acid therapy of chronic cholestatic conditions in adults and children. Pharmacol Ther. 1995;66:1–15.
13. Hofmann AF. Bile acids. In: Arias IM, Boyer JL, Fausto N, Jakoby WB, Schachter DA, Shafritz DA, editors. The liver. Biology and pathobiology. New York: Raven Press. 1994:677–718.
14. Heuman DM. Hepatoprotective properties of ursodeoxycholic acid. Gastroenterology. 1993;104:1865–70.
15. Kitani K. Hepatoprotective effect of ursodeoxycholate in experimental animals. In: Paumgartner G, Stiehl A, Barbara L, Roda E, editors. Strategies for the treatment of hepatobiliary diseases. Lancaster: Kluwer. 1990:43–56.
16. Hofmann AF. Bile acid hepatotoxicity and the rationale of UDCA therapy in chronic cholestatic liver disease: some hypotheses. In: Paumgartner G, Stiehl A, Barbara L, Roda E, editors. Strategies for the treatment of hepatobiliary diseases. Lancaster: Kluwer. 1990:13–33.
17. Armstrong MJ, Carey MC. The hydrophobic–hydrophilic balance of bile salts. Inverse correlation between reverse high performance liquid chromatographic mobilities and micellar cholesterol-solubilizing capacities. J Lipid Res. 1982;23:70–80.
18. Heuman DM. Quantitative estimation of the hydrophobic–hydrophilic balance of mixed bile salt solutions. J Lipid Res. 1989;30:719–30.
19. Stiehl A, Rudolph G, Raedsch R *et al.* Ursodeoxycholic acid-induced changes of plasma and urinary bile acids in patients with primary biliary cirrhosis. Hepatology. 1990;12:492–7.
20. Marschall HU, Matern H, Wietholtz, Egestad B, Matern S, Sjövall J. Bile acid *N*-acetylglucosaminidation. J Clin Invest. 1992;89:1981–7.
21. Marschall HU, Griffiths WJ, Götze U *et al.* The major metabolites of ursodeoxycholic acid in human urine are conjugated with *N*-acetylglucosamine. Hepatology. 1994;20:845–53.
22. Reichen J, Simon R. Cholestasis. In: Arias IM, Boyer JL, Fausto N, Jakoby WB, Schachter DA, Shafritz DA, editors. The liver. Biology and pathobiology. New York: Raven Press. 1994:1291–326.
23. Holsti P. Cirrhosis of the liver induced in rabbits by gastric instillation of 3-monohydroxycholynic acid. Nature. 1960;186:250.
24. Javitt JB. Cholestasis in rats induced by taurolithocholate. Nature. 1966;210:1262–3.
25. Greim H, Trulzsch D, Roboz J *et al.* Mechanism of cholestasis. 5. Bile acids in normal rat livers and in those after bile duct ligation. Gastroenterology. 1972;63:837–45.
26. Greim H, Trulzsch D, Czygan P *et al.* Mechanism of cholestasis. 6. Bile acids in human livers with or without biliary obstruction. Gastroenterology. 1972;63:846–50.
27. Attili AF, Angelico M, Cantafora A, Alvaro D, Capocaccia L. Bile acid-induced liver toxicity: relation to the hydrophobic-hydrophilic balance of bile acids. Med Hypotheses. 1986;19:57–69.
28. Spivey JR, Bronk SF, Gores GJ. Glycochenodeoxycholate-induced lethal hepatocellular injury in rat hepatocytes. J Clin Invest. 1993;92:17–24.
29. Patel T, Spivey J, Vadakekalam J, Gores GJ. Apoptosis – an alternative mechanism of bile salt hepatotoxicity. In: Paumgartner G, Beuers U, editors. Bile acids in liver diseases. Lancaster: Kluwer. 1995:88–95.
30. Kitani K, Kanai S. Tauroursodeoxycholate prevents taurocholate-induced cholestasis. Life Sci. 1982;30:515–23.
31. Kitani K, Ohta M, Kanai S. Tauroursodeoxycholate prevents the hepatocellular damage caused by other bile salts in the rat. Am J Physiol. 1985;248:G407–17.
32. Heuman DM, Mills AS, McCall J, Hylemon PB, Pandak WM, Vlahcevic ZR. Conjugates of ursodeoxycholate protect against cholestasis and hepatocellular necrosis caused by more hydrophobic bile salts. Gastroenterology. 1991;100:203–11.
33. Schoelmerich J, Baumgartner U, Miyai K, Gerok W. Tauroursodeoxycholate prevents taurolithocholate-induced cholestasis and toxicity in rat liver. J Hepatol. 1990;10:280–3.

34. Heuman DM, Pandak WM, Hylemon PB, Vlahcevic ZR. Conjugates of ursodeoxycholate protect against toxicity of more hydrophobic bile salts: *in vitro* studies in rat hepatocytes and human erythrocytes. Hepatology. 1991;14:920–6.
35. Tsukahara K, Kanai S, Ohta M, Kitani K. Taurine conjugate of ursodeoxycholate plays a major role in the hepatoprotective effect against cholestasis induced by taurochenodeoxycholate in rats. Liver. 1993;13:262–9.
36. Baumgartner U, Schoelmerich J, Sellinger M, Reinhardt M, Ruf G, Farthmann EH. Different protective effects of tauroursodeoxycholate, ursodeoxycholate, and 23-methyl-ursodeoxycholate against taurolithocholate-induced cholestasis. Dig Dis Sci. 1996;41:250–5.
37. Beuers U, Fischer S, Spengler U, Paumgartner G. Formation of iso-ursodeoxycholic acid during administration of ursodeoxycholic acid in man. J Hepatol. 1991;13:97–103.
38. Beuers U, Spengler U, Zwiebel FM, Pauletzki J, Fischer S, Paumgartner G. Effect of ursodeoxycholic acid on the kinetics of the major hydrophobic bile acids in health and in chronic cholestatic liver disease. Hepatology. 1992;15:603–8.
39. Mazzella G, Parini P, Bazzoli F *et al.* Ursodeoxycholic acid administration on bile acid metabolism in patients with early stages of primary biliary cirrhosis. Dig Dis Sci. 1993;38:896–902.
40. Batta AK, Arora R, Salen G, Tint S, Eskreis D, Katz S. Characterization of serum and urinary bile acids in patients with primary biliary cirrhosis by gas–liquid chromatography–mass spectrometry: effect of ursodeoxycholic acid treatment. J Lipid Res. 1989;30:1953–62.
41. Stiehl A, Rudolph G, Raedsch R *et al.* Ursodeoxycholic acid-induced changes of plasma and urinary bile acids in patients with primary biliary cirrhosis. Hepatology. 1990;12:492–7.
42. Crosignani A, Podda M, Battezzati PM *et al.* Changes in bile acid composition in patients with primary biliary cirrhosis induced by ursodeoxycholic acid administration. Hepatology. 1991;14:1000–7.
43. Rudolph G, Endele R, Senn M, Stiehl A. Effect of ursodeoxycholic acid on the kinetics of cholic acid and chenodeoxycholic acid in patients with primary sclerosing cholangitis. Hepatology. 1993;17:1028–32.
44. Poupon RE, Chrétien Y, Poupon R, Paumgartner G. Serum bile acids in primary biliary cirrhosis: effect of ursodeoxycholic acid therapy. Hepatology. 1993;17:599–604.
45. Stiehl A, Raedsch R, Rudolph G. Acute effects of ursodeoxycholic and chenodeoxycholic acid on the small intestinal absorption of bile acids. Gastroenterology. 1990;98:424–8.
46. Marteau P, Chazouilleres O, Myara A, Jian R, Rambaud JC, Poupon R. Effect of chronic administration of ursodeoxycholic acid on the ileal absorption of endogenous bile acids in man. Hepatology. 1990;12:1206–8.
47. Eusufzai S, Ericsson S, Cederlund T, Einarsson K, Angelin B. Effect of ursodeoxycholic acid treatment on ileal absorption of bile acids in man as determined by the SeHCAT test. Gut. 1991;32:1044–8.
48. van Berge Henegouwen GP, Hofmann AF. Pharmacology of chenodeoxycholic acid. II. Absorption and metabolism. Gastroenterology. 1977;73:300–9.
49. Fedorowski T, Salen G, Tint GS, Mosbach EH. Transformation of chenodeoxycholic and ursodeoxycholic acid by human intestinal bacteria. Gastroenterology. 1979;77:1068–73.
50. Fromm H, Sarva RP, Bazzoli F. Formation of ursodeoxycholic acid from chenodeoxycholic acid in the human colon: studies of the role of 7-ketolithocholic acid as an intermediate. J Lipid Res. 1983;24:841–53.
51. Macdonald IA, Bokkenheuser VD, Winter J, McLernon AM, Mosbach EH. Degradation of steroids in the human gut. J Lipid Res. 1983;24:675–700.
52. Fromm H, Carlson GL, Hofmann AF, Farivar S, Amin P. Metabolism in man of 7-ketolithocholic acid: a precursor of cheno- and ursodeoxycholic acids. Am J Physiol. 1980;239:G161–6.
53. Salen G, Verga D, Batta AK, Tint GS, Shefer S. Effect of 7-ketolithocholic acid on bile acid metabolism in humans. Gastroenterology. 1982;83:341–7.
54. Dumont M, Erlinger S, Uchman S. Hypercholeresis induced by ursodeoxycholic acid and 7-ketolithocholic acid in the rat: possible role of bicarbonate transport. Gastroenterology. 1980;79:82–9.
55. Yoon YB, Hagey LR, Hofmann AF, Gurantz D, Michelotti EL, Steinbach JH. Effect of side-chain shortening on the physiological properties of bile acids: hepatic transport and effect on biliary secretion of 23-norursodeoxycholate in rodents. Gastroenterology. 1986;90:837–52.
56. Erlinger S. Hypercholeretic bile acids: a clue to the mechanism? Hepatology. 1990;11;888–90.

57. Lake JR, Renner EL, Scharschmidt BF *et al.* Inhibition of Na^+/H^+ exchange in the rat is associated with decreased ursodeoxycholate hypercholeresis, decreased secretion of unconjugated ursodeoxycholate, and increased ursodeoxycholate glucuronidation. Gastroenterology. 1988;95:454–63.
58. Gautam A, Ng OC, Strazzabosco M, Boyer JL. Quantitative assessment of canalicular bile formation in isolated rat hepatocyte couplets using microscopic optical planimetry. J Clin Invest. 1989;83:565–73.
59. Farges O, Corbic M, Dumont M, Maurice M, Erlinger S. Permeability of the rat biliary tree to ursodeoxycholic acid. Am J Physiol. 1989;256:G653–60.
60. Alvaro D, Mennone A, Boyer JL. Effect of ursodeoxycholic acid on intracellular pH regulation in isolated rat bile duct epithelial cells. Am J Physiol. 1993;265:G783–91.
61. Strazzabosco M, Poci C, Spirlí C, Sartori L, Knuth A, Crepaldi G. Effect of ursodeoxycholic acid on intracellular pH in a bile duct epithelium-like cell line. Hepatology. 1994;19:145–54.
62. Knyrim K, Vakil N, Pfab R, Classen M. The effects of intraduodenal bile acid administration on biliary secretion of ionized calcium and carbonate in man. Hepatology. 1989;10:134–42.
63. Gurantz D, Schteingart CD, Hagey LR, Steinbach JH, Grotmol T, Hofmann AF. Hypercholeresis induced by unconjugated bile acid infusion correlates with recovery in bile of unconjugated bile acids. Hepatology. 1991;13:540–50.
64. Leuschner U, Fischer H, Kurtz W *et al.* Ursodeoxycholic acid in primary biliary cirrhosis: results of a controlled double-blind trial. Gastroenterology. 1989;97:1268–74.
65. Güldütuna S, Zimmer G, Imhof M, Bhatti S, You T, Leuschner U. Molecular aspects of membrane stabilization by ursodeoxycholate. Gastroenterology. 1993;104:1736–44.
66. Galle PR, Theilmann L, Raedsch R, Otto G, Stiehl A. Ursodeoxycholate reduces hepatotoxicity of bile salts in primary human hepatocytes. Hepatology. 1990;12:486–91.
67. Heuman DM, Bajaj R. Ursodeoxycholate conjugates protect against disruption of cholesterol-rich membranes by bile salts. Gastroenterology. 1994;106:1333–41.
68. Heuman DM. Disruptive and protective interactions of bile salts, cholesterol : lecithin vesicles, and canalicular membranes. In: Hofmann AF, Paumgartner G, Stiehl A, editors. Bile acids in gastroenterology. Lancaster: Kluwer; 1995:283–9.
69. Heuman DM, Bajaj RS, Lin Q. Adsorption of mixtures of bile salt taurine conjugates to lecithin-cholesterol membranes: implications for bile salt toxicity and cytoprotection. J Lipid Res. 1996;37:562–73.
70. Calmus Y, Gane P, Pouger P, Poupon R. Hepatic expression of class I and class II major histocompatibility complex molecules in primary biliary cirrhosis: effect of ursodeoxycholic acid. Hepatology. 1990;11:12–15
71. Benacerraf B. Role of MHC gene products in immune regulation. Science. 1981;212:1229–38.
72. Innes GK, Nagafuchi Y, Fuller BJ, Hobbs KEF. Increased expression of major histocompatibility antigens in the liver as a result of cholestasis. Transplantation. 1988;45:749–52.
73. Calmus Y, Arvieux C, Gane P *et al.* Cholestasis induces major histocompatibility complex class I expression in hepatocytes. Gastroenterology. 1992;102:1371–7.
74. Hillaire S, Boucher E, Calmus Y *et al.* Effects of bile acids and cholestasis on major histocompatibility complex class I in human and rat hepatocytes. Gastroenterology. 1994;107:781–8.
75. Yoshikawa M, Tsujii T, Matsumura K *et al.* Immunomodulatory effects of ursodeoxycholic acid on immune responses. Hepatology. 1992;16:358–64.
76. Calmus Y, Arvieux C, Gane P *et al.* Cholestasis induces major histocompatibility complex class I expression in hepatocytes. Gastroenterology. 1992;102:1371–7.
77. Ohiwa T, Katagiri K, Hoshino M, Hayakawa T, Nakai T. Tauroursodeoxycholate and tauro-β-muricholate exert cytoprotection by reducing intrahepatocyte taurochenodeoxycholate content. Hepatology. 1993;17:470–6.
78. Jazrawi RP, de Caestecker JS, Goggin PM *et al.* Kinetics of hepatic bile acid handling in cholestatic liver disease: effect of ursodeoxycholic acid. Gastroenterology. 1994;106:134–42.
79. Stiehl A, Rudolph G, Sauer P, Theilmann L. Biliary secretion of bile acids and lipids in primary sclerosing cholangitis. Influence of cholestasis and effect of ursodeoxycholic acid treatment. J Hepatol. 1995;23:283–9.
80. Colombo C, Castellani MR, Balistreri WF, Seregni E, Assaido ML, Giunta A. Scintigraphic documentation of an improvement in hepatobiliary excretory function after treatment with ursodeoxycholic acid in patients with cystic fibrosis and associated liver disease. Hepatology. 1992;15:677–84.

81. Arias IM, Che M, Gatmaitan Z, Leveille C, Nishida T, St Pierre M. The biology of the bile canaliculus, 1993. Hepatology. 1993;17:318–29.
82. Benedetti A, Strazzabosco M, Ng OC, Boyer JL. Regulation of activity and apical targeting of the Cl^-/HCO_3^- exchanger in rat hepatocytes. Proc Natl Acad Sci USA. 1994;91:792–6.
83. Boyer JL, Soroka CJ. Vesicle targeting to the apical domain regulates bile excretory function in isolated rat hepatocyte couplets. Gastroenterology. 1995;109:1600–11.
84. Burgoyne RD, Morgan A. Regulated exocytosis. Biochem J. 1993;293:305–16.
85. Nathanson MH, Boyer JL. Mechanisms and regulation of bile secretion. Hepatology. 1991;14:551–66.
86. Nathanson MH, Boyer JL. Vesicular trafficking in the hepatocyte. In: Arias IM, Boyer JL, Fausto N, Jakoby WB, Schachter DA, Shafritz DA, editors. The liver. Biology and pathobiology. New York: Raven Press; 1994:655–64.
87. Beuers U, Nathanson MH, Boyer JL. Effects of tauroursodeoxycholic acid on cytosolic Ca^{++} signals in isolated rat hepatocytes. Gastroenterology. 1993;104:604–12.
88. Bouscarel B, Fromm H, Nussbaum R. Ursodeoxycholic acid mobilizes intracellular calcium and activates phosphorylase-a in isolated hepatocytes. Am J Physiol. 1993;264:G243–51.
89. Beuers U, Nathanson MH, Isales CM, Boyer JL. Tauroursodeoxycholic acid stimulates hepatocellular exocytosis and mobilizes extracellular Ca^{++} mechanisms defective in cholestasis. J Clin Invest. 1993;92:2984–93.
90. Bouscarel B, Gettys TW, Fromm H, Dubner H. Ursodeoxycholic acid inhibits glucagon-induced cAMP formation in hamster hepatocytes: a role for PKC. Am J Physiol. 1995;268:G300–10.
91. Beuers U, Throckmorton DC, Anderson MS *et al.* Tauroursodeoxycholic acid activates protein kinase C in isolated rat hepatocytes. Gastroenterology. 1996;110:1553–63.
92. Ganesan S, Calle R, Zawalich K, Smallwood JI, Zawalich WS, Rasmussen H. Glucose-induced translocation of protein kinase C in pancreatic islets. Proc Natl Acad Sci USA. 1990;87:9893–7.
93. Häussinger D, Schliess F. Cell volume and hepatocellular function. J Hepatol. 1995;22:94–100.

23
Vanishing bile duct syndrome – from bench to bedside

J. L. BOYER

This international Falk workshop on 'The Vanishing Bile Duct Syndrome' focuses on the most recent developments in cholangiocyte biology and the pathophysiology and therapy of these disorders. In these concluding remarks it is impossible to do justice to all of the presentations and I take great risk in attempting to review the highlights. Apologies are given to those whose work has been omitted and a request is made for forbearance from authors whose work is oversimplified by the 'cartoons' that attempt to focus on some of the main points.

This symposium began with detailed anatomical descriptions of the biliary epithelium. Desmet and Jezequel remind us (Fig. 1) that this structure is composed of multiple segments of increasing diameter. Cholangiocytes are first recognized at the canal of Hering where the ducts measure less than 15 μm in cross-section and then widen progressively. At least 6 definable segments and approximately 12 branches can be identified based on the diameters of the segments as bile leaves the canaliculus of the hepatocyte and ultimately enters the common bile duct. In addition (Fig. 2), the location of isolated bile duct cells may be inferred both by their size which increases and by the ratio of nucleus to cytoplasm which decreases as one moves distally from the ductules to interlobular ducts and then to septal ducts. These studies imply that one may begin to identify the regional location of isolated duct cells, since there is also uniformity to the size and nuclear/cytoplasmic ratio within a given bile duct segment.

Work of Alpini, LeSage, LaRusso and colleagues has also begun to suggest that the structural heterogeneity of the duct segments is associated with functional differences in transport systems that line the lumen of this epithelium (Fig. 3). For example, cells isolated from bile ductules appear to lack secretin receptors and thus do not respond to this hormone with increases in cellular cyclic AMP and activation of chloride conductances, as normally observed with cholangiocytes located in interlobular and septal ducts. Interestingly, only septal ducts appear to have somatostatin receptors which inhibit the normal secretin response. Understanding the functional differences of the bile duct segments at the cellular and molecular level is a major area of future interest for this field.

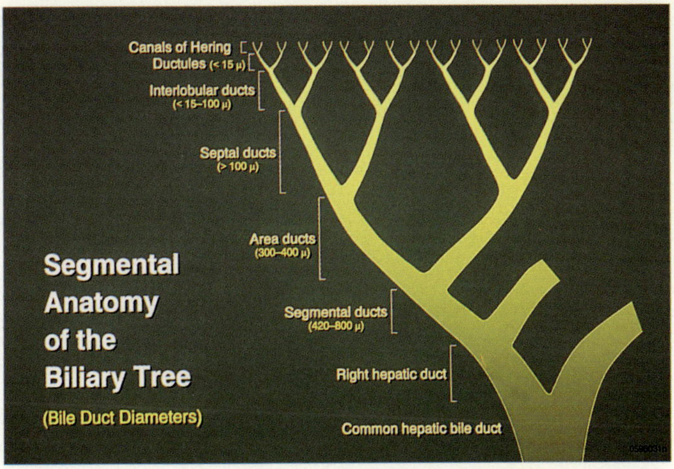

Figure 1

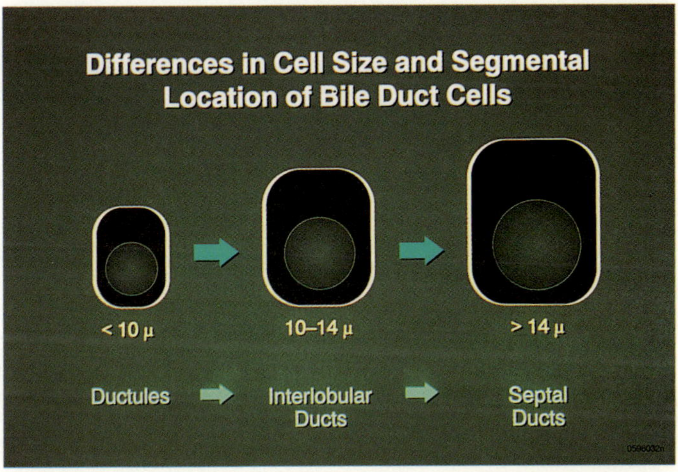

Figure 2

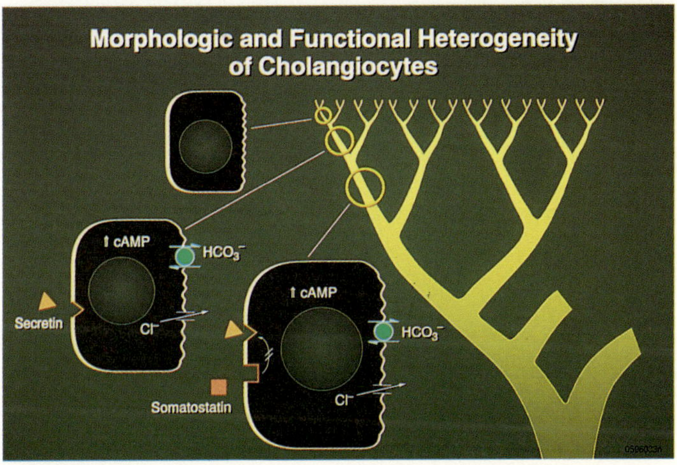

Figure 3

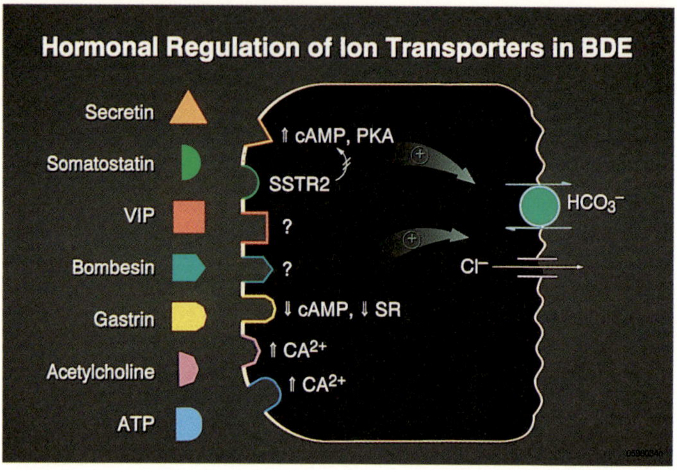

Figure 4

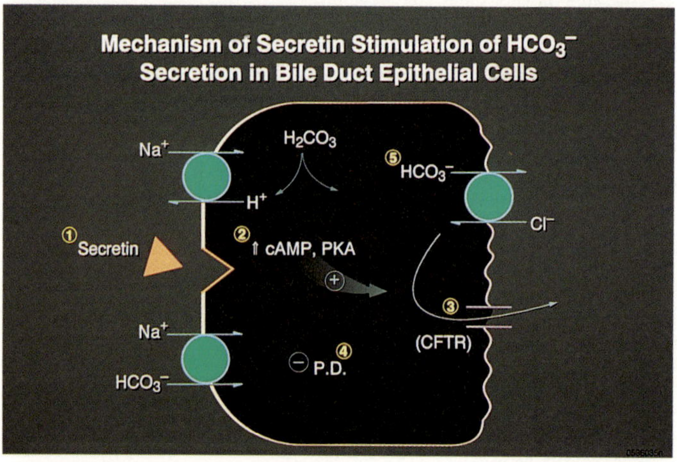

Figure 5

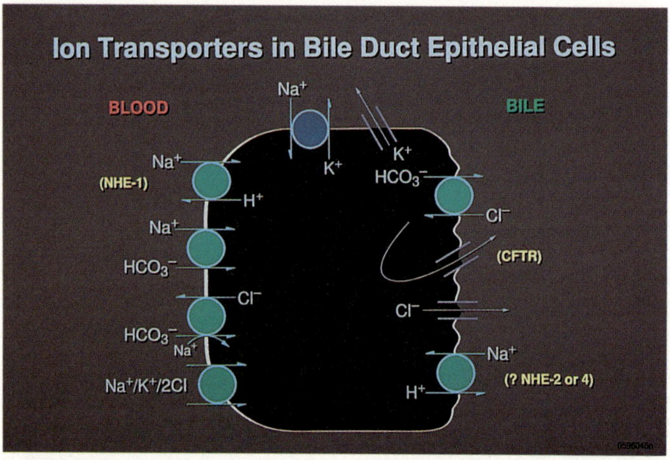

Figure 6

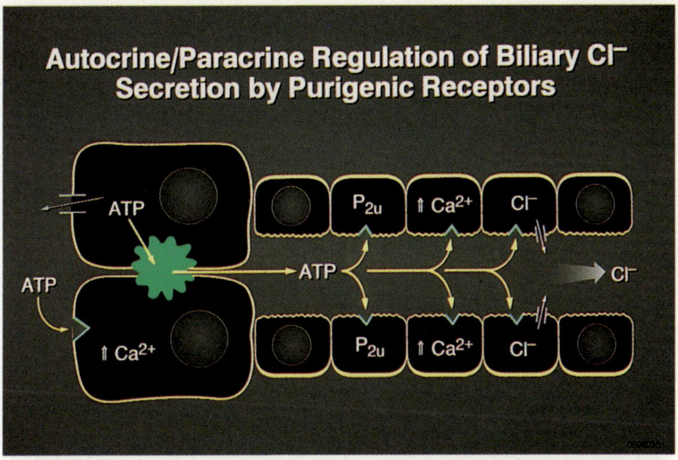

Figure 7

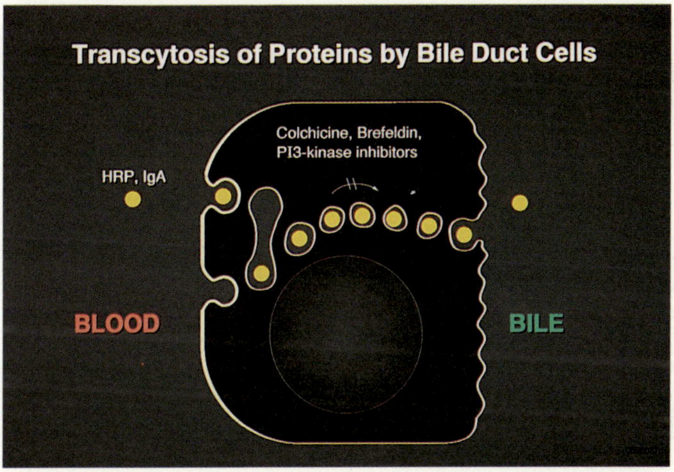

Figure 8

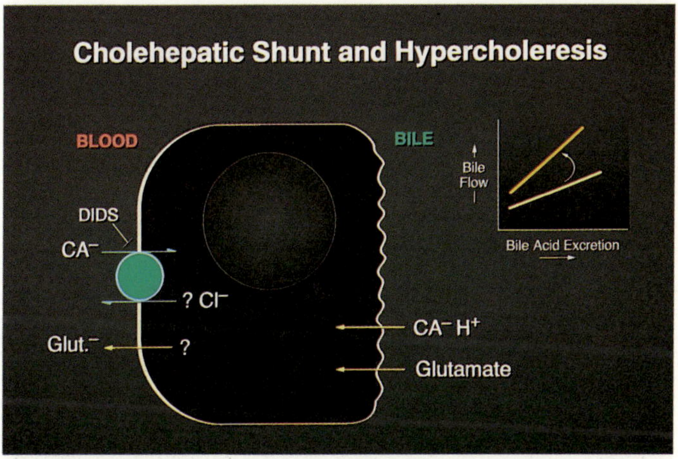

Figure 9

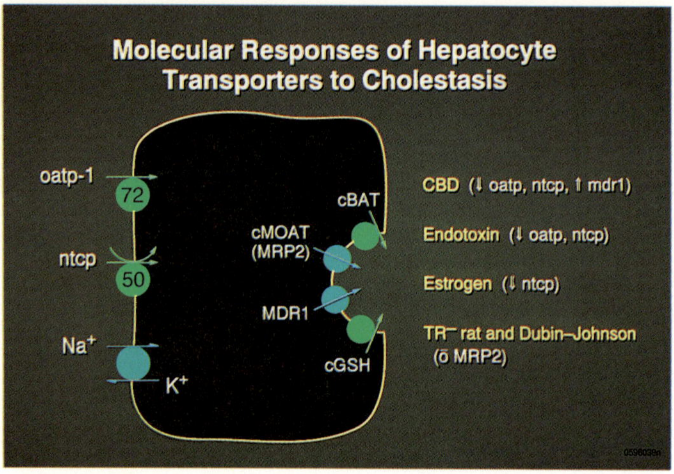

Figure 10

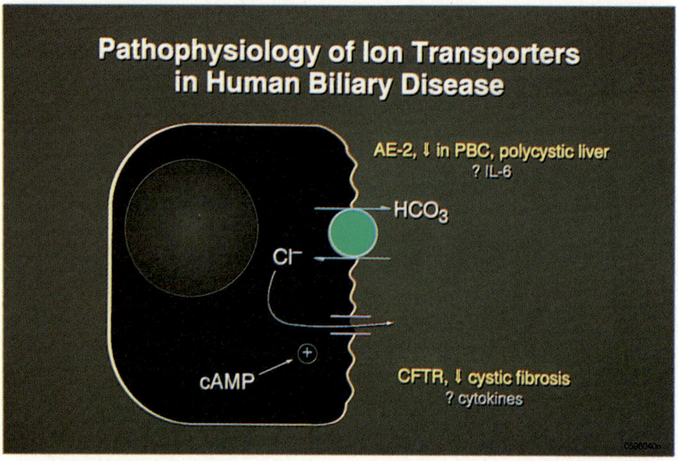

Figure 11

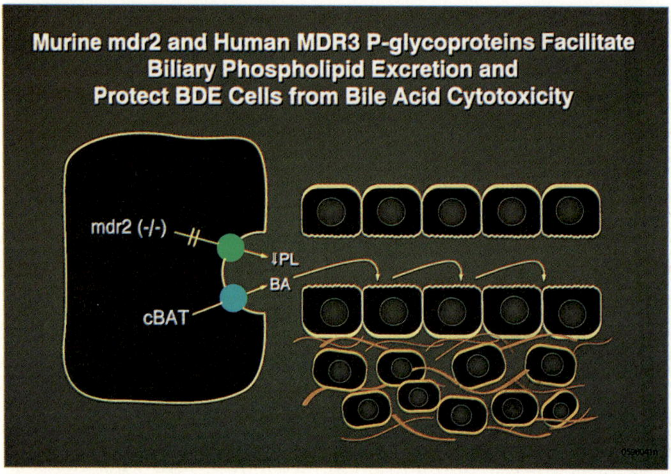

Figure 12

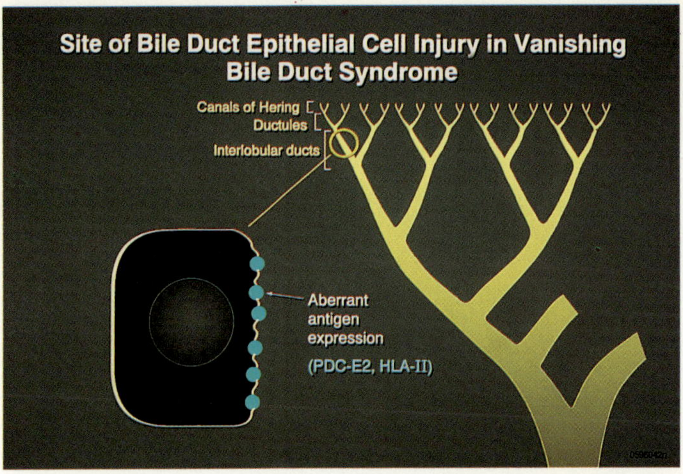

Figure 13

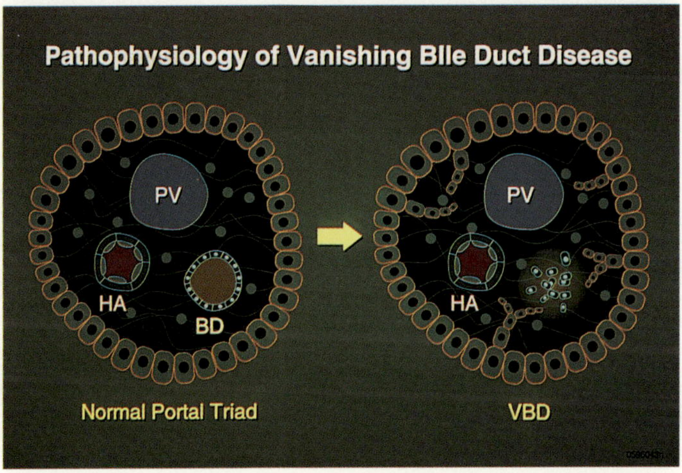

Figure 14

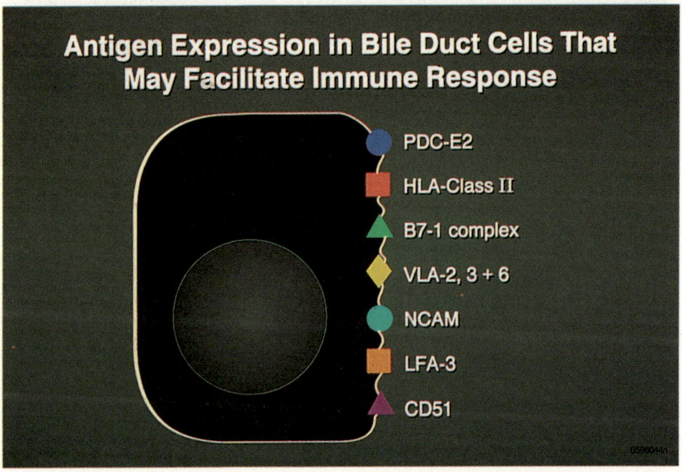

Figure 15

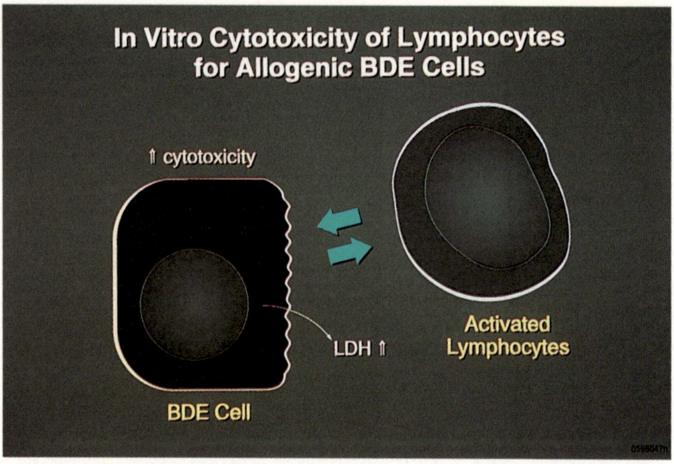

Figure 16

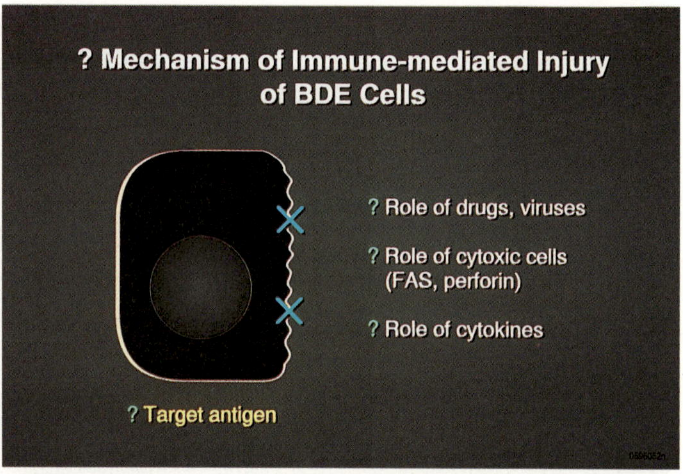

Figure 17

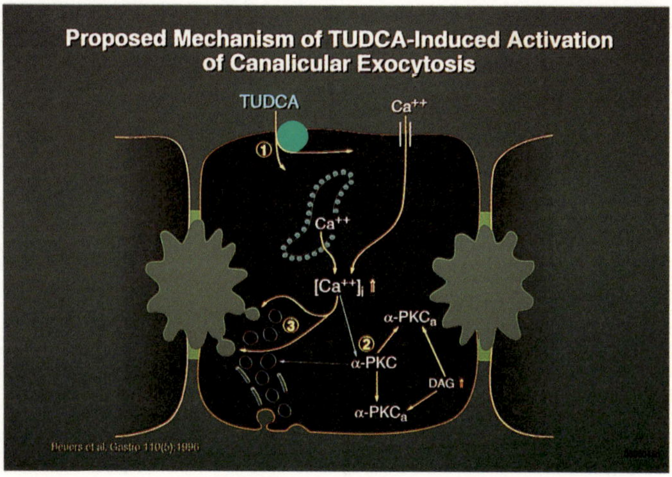

Figure 18

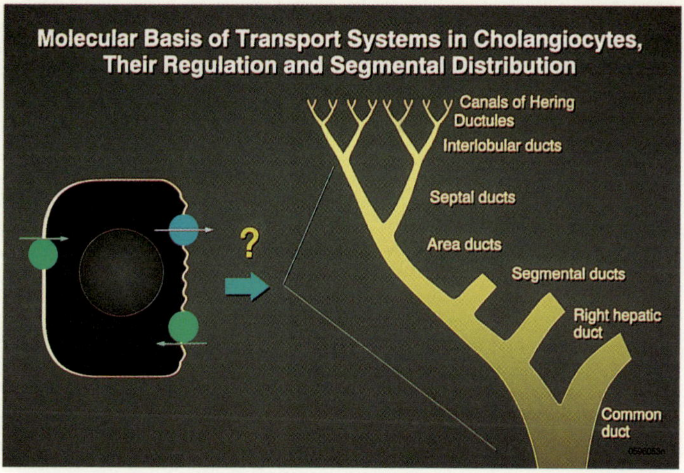

Figure 19

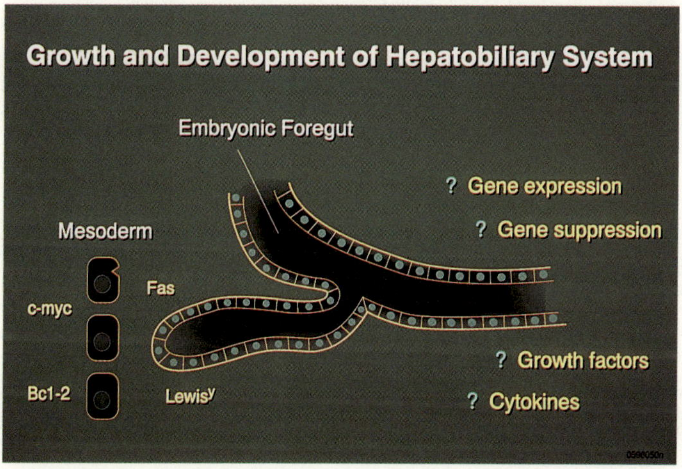

Figure 20

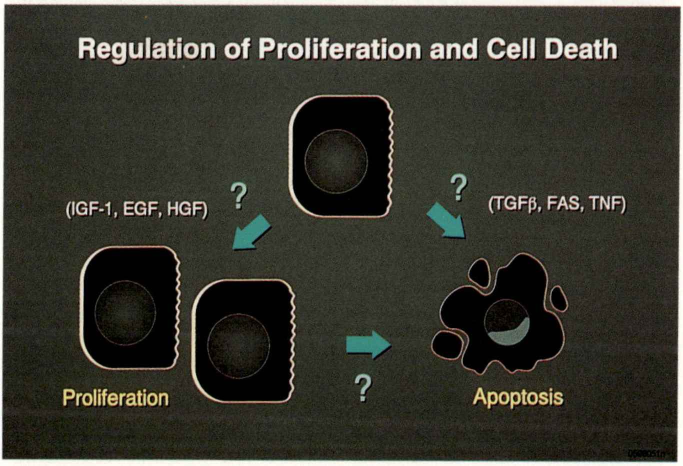

Figure 21

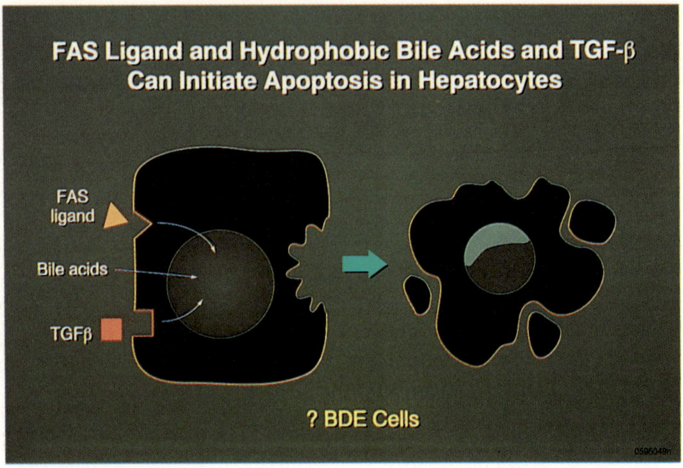

Figure 22

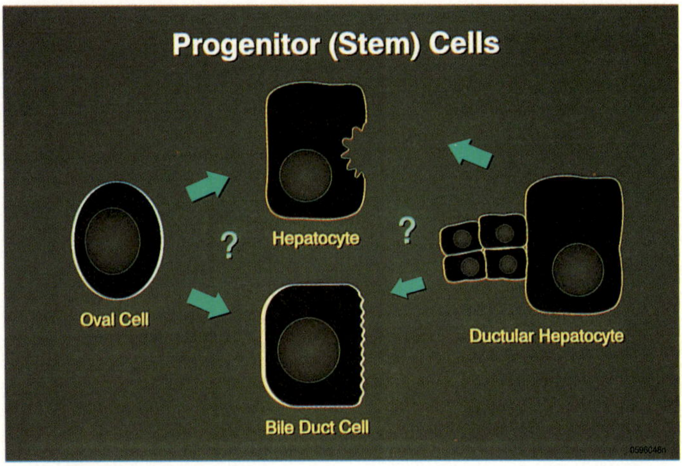

Figure 23

Bile duct epithelia generate a bicarbonate-rich fluid and much has been learned recently about the hormonal regulation of this secretion as summarized by Alvaro's and Fitz's presentations (Fig. 4). The secretin response, which is mediated by cyclic AMP, acts via protein kinase A presumably to phosphorylate a low conductance chloride channel that shares identity with the cystic fibrosis gene product. Studies by Cho in isolated bile duct units and perfused rat livers indicate that the neuropeptides, bombesin and vasointestinal peptide, can also stimulate fluid and bicarbonate excretion from the biliary epithelium, although the second messengers and signal transduction pathways have not yet been identified. Gastrin receptors also exist in biliary epithelial cells, according to Alpini, and function both to inhibit the cyclic AMP response to secretin and to down-regulate secretin receptors. Purigenic receptors (P_{2u}) have also been characterized functionally in biliary epithelium by Fitz, and extracellular ATP and UTP induce increases in intracellular calcium in human bile duct cell lines. Acetylcholine also mediates increases in intracellular calcium in isolated bile duct units, according to Nathanson, but it is not known whether these diverse agonists and receptors mediate physiological signal transduction pathways in the intact animal.

Several new techniques and experimental models which have led to progress in this field were reviewed by Levine, and others were also discussed in detail during this symposium (Table 1). Major advances are now being made in the isolation, culture and immortalization of bile duct cells from several animal species including human liver preparations. The ability to study secretory and absorptive functions in isolated bile duct units and cell monolayers is particularly important for studies of basic transport properties and should also be the source of much future work. These models have already led to the characterization of the cellular mechanism for secretin stimulated HCO_3^- secretion (Fig. 5) as well as a number of other ion transporters in bile duct epithelia. Many of these transport proteins regulate intracellular pH, cell volume, secretion and reabsorptive functions (Fig. 6). Singh has identified a Na^+/H^+ exchanger on the luminal membrane of bile duct cells that functions to extrude protons in an acid microclimate and a $Na^+/K^+/2Cl$ co-transporter on the basolateral domain whose function is to facilitate chloride secretion by the bile duct cell.

Several groups (Fitz *et al.* and Nathanson *et al.*) provide evidence that biliary epithelial cell function may be regulated in part by autocrine/paracrine phenomena (Fig. 7). ATP is released by hepatocytes and is present in bile, where it stimulates P_{2u} receptors in cholangiocytes leading to increases in cell calcium which may possibly stimulate Cl^- secretion. These observations imply that increases in metabolic activity in the hepatic parenchyma may lead to messages that have effects downstream in the bile duct epithelium.

Table 1 Experimental models for the study of bile duct epithelial cell (BDE) function

• Bile duct obstruction	• BDE cell cultures
• ANIT	• Immortalized BDE cells
• 2-acetoaminofluorine	• Cholangiocarcinoma cell lines
• Immune mediated cholangitis	• Subcellular fractionations
• Isolated BDE cells	
• Isolated BDE units	

Evidence was presented by Benedetti that proteins move across bile duct cells from basolateral to apical regions of the cell after endocytosis and transcytosis in intracellular vesicles. The process is dependent on the function of microtubules and can be inhibited by colchicine, brefeldin-A and by the phosphoinositol-3 kinase inhibitor, wortmannin (Fig. 8). In human cholangiocytes, secretory IgA enters bile via this pathway. Transport of biliary constituents in the reverse direction from the biliary lumen to the blood side of the bile duct epithelium has been proposed by Hofmann's group and termed 'the cholehepatic shunt' (Fig. 9). This process helps to explain the hypercholeretic effect of certain bile acids such as ursodeoxycholic. Studies by Benedetti demonstrate a carrier-mediated saturable, sodium-independent, chloride-dependent transport system for cholic acid on the basolateral membrane which could function as an anion exchanger for weak acids that accumulate in cholangiocytes from the biliary lumen. Gebhardt provided additional evidence for cholehepatic shunting using glutamic acid in a monolayer co-culture using Transwell technology.

Considerable information has accumulated on the effects of bile duct obstruction and other models of cholestasis on the molecular regulation of cloned transporters in hepatocytes. This important area was reviewed by Meier. In general, cholestasis results in the down-regulation of the mRNA and protein of the sinusoidal transporters for sodium dependent bile acids (ntcp) and the multi-specific organic anion transporter (oatp), which facilitates uptake of bilirubin and other organic anions into hepatocytes by sodium-independent mechanisms (Fig. 10). In contrast, some canalicular transporters may be unaffected and in some cases are actually up-regulated at both transcriptional and translational levels, as demonstrated for the multi-drug resistant P-glycoprotein, MDR-1. A second multi-drug resistant protein, MRP-2 (identical to the multi-specific organic anion transporter cMOAT), and the canalicular bile acid transporter (not yet cloned) are functionally impaired in cholestatic animal models. MRP is also absent in the Dubin–Johnson syndrome and the TR–, Groningen and EBHR mutant rats, accounting for the defect in biliary organic anion excretion in these genetic disorders.

Defects in transport systems in bile duct epithelium are beginning to be recognized in human disorders that affect this epithelium, as reviewed by Strazzabosco (Fig. 11). Biliary fibrosis and cirrhosis are well-known complications of cystic fibrosis, a genetic disorder with multiple gene defects that lead to alterations or reductions in a low conductance chloride channel in the luminal membrane of cholangiocytes. The anion exchanger for Cl^-/HCO_3^- (the AE-2 isoform) is also present on the luminal membrane of cholangiocytes and is involved in the secretion of HCO_3^-. Some studies have demonstrated a reduction in the message for AE-2 in biliary and peripheral blood cells from patients with primary biliary cirrhosis. Similar deficiencies have also been demonstrated in cells from polycystic diseases of the liver.

Remarkable advances have been made on the role of the mdr-2 P-glycoprotein in lipid secretion into bile and its protective effect for the biliary epithelium, as reviewed by Oude-Elferink. Knock-out mice, which lack this canalicular protein, are unable to excrete phospholipids into bile yet maintain normal bile acid excretion. Bile acids which normally aggregate in lipid micelles in bile now exert detergent effects on cholangiocytes, leading to progressive injury which induces bile duct proliferation and fibrosis, resulting ultimately in a biliary-type cirrhosis (Fig. 12). These studies emphasize the power of molecular biology in elucidating hitherto unsuspected functions of membrane transporters and demonstrate the close interrelationships between hepatocyte and cholangiocyte functions.

Clinical studies have clearly demonstrated the primary site of injury in vanishing bile duct syndromes that are mediated by immunological phenomena. Aberrant expression of a mitochondrial antigen (the pyruvate decarboxylase E2 antigen) is a specific defect in patients with primary biliary cirrhosis and is expressed on the luminal surface of the interlobular duct segments (Fig. 13). HLA Class-II antigens are also up-regulated in association with E2, providing a potential target for cytotoxic T-cells which lead ultimately to destruction and loss of these bile duct segments, as reviewed by both Gershwin and Vierling (Fig. 14). This immune-mediated destruction of cholangiocytes may be facilitated by the luminal surface expression of other antigens, as illustrated in Fig. 15. Studies by Joplin and colleagues demonstrate that activated lymphocytes exhibit allogeneic cytotoxicity for isolated human cholangiocytes *in vitro* (Fig. 16), suggesting that such assays might ultimately be useful in defining the pathogenesis of vanishing bile duct diseases. However as yet neither the aetiological stimulus nor the precise target antigen(s) have been identified for this disease. Thus considerable speculation exists concerning pathogenesis and the role of viruses, drugs, fas-mediated cell injury, porins and inflammatory mediators (Fig. 17).

No advances in the treatment of vanishing bile duct diseases were proposed at this symposium, although the status of past and current therapeutic approaches were reviewed by both Leuschner and Podda (Table 2). Treatment with ursodeoxycholic acid is the currently accepted therapy for primary biliary cirrhosis and may extend life, according to the results of 3 combined clinical trials. Ursodeoxycholic acid therapy may also be of benefit in sclerosing cholangitis, cholestasis of pregnancy, and cystic fibrosis, although no large double-blind trials have been undertaken in these diseases.

Speculation exists concerning the mechanism by which ursodeoxycholic acid may be beneficial in cholestatic liver diseases of this type. Immunomodulatory properties of ursodeoxycholic acid were reviewed by Calmus and suggest that ursodeoxycholic acid may moderate the cytotoxic immune response by suppressing T-cell function and by down-regulating HLA class I antigens on hepatocytes. On the basis of experimental studies in rat liver, Beuers *et al.* have proposed that the taurine conjugate of ursodeoxycholic acid (TUDCA) may stimulate biliary excretory mechanisms by acting like a calcium-stimulating hormone. Following transport into hepatocytes via the basolateral bile acid carrier, TUDCA is capable of stimulating the release of Ca^{++} from IP_3^- sensitive

Table 2 Treatment of vanishing bile duct disorders

- Corticosteroids
- Penicillamine
- Azathioprine
- Colchicine
- Methotrexate
- Ursodeoxycholic acid

intracellular stores by IP_3^- insensitive mechanisms; this leads to the translocation of the α subunit of protein kinase C from the cytoplasm to the plasma membrane and the simultaneous opening of Ca^{++} channels, which results in the sustained elevation of intracellular calcium. The combination of these events leads to increased fusion of intracellular vesicles containing canalicular membrane transporters with the canalicular membrane, which in turn leads to an increased capacity to excrete bile acids and other substances into bile (Fig. 18). Clinical studies support the view that the ursodeoxycholic acid therapy results in increased capacity of the liver to excrete bile acids, possibly leading to the diminished retention of more hydrophobic bile acids and reducing liver cell injury. These concepts remain speculative and more than one mechanism may be responsible for the therapeutic benefits of TUDCA.

Despite the remarkable advances in this field, and the comprehensiveness of the topics covered in this symposium, much remains for future study. There are compelling needs to improve the therapy of vanishing bile duct syndromes, and little was mentioned concerning new advances in therapy which to date remain largely untried (Table 3). Applications of cellular and molecular biology to the understanding of bile duct epithelial cell function and their membrane transport systems lag behind work with their counterparts in hepatocytes, and much remains to be learned about the heterogeneity of bile duct epithelial cell function throughout the various anatomical segments of the biliary tree (Fig. 19).

No mention was made in this symposium concerning mechanisms of growth and development of the biliary system, an area of substantial interest if we are to understand how neonatal cholestatic liver diseases and congenital disorders of the biliary epithelium occur. Growth factors and cytokines which influence the development of the bile ducts and mechanisms of differentiation and programmed cell death are rapidly being identified and defined with respect to their role in regulation of gene expression and suppression (Fig. 20).

Much also remains to be learned regarding how bile duct cells undergo such dramatic proliferative activity in response to cell injury and how their cell mass may be regulated by the process of apoptosis (Fig. 21). In hepatocytes, fas ligand, TGF-β and bile acids may each induce programmed cell death, as discussed by Smolarek and colleagues (Fig. 22), but less is known about these processes in cholangiocytes.

Finally, there was no time in this symposium to review the exciting work which is characterizing the oval cell as a pluri-potential cell capable of transforming into both hepatocytes or cholangiocytes under conditions of extreme injury or during malignant transformation (Fig. 23). Clearly much challenging work remains for the future. Cholangiocyte pathobiology and disease is no

Table 3 Improved treatment of vanishing bile duct syndromes

- Drugs that cycle in cholehepatic shunt
- Drugs that stimulate secretion of hydrophobic bile acids (?MDR3)
- Gene targeting
- Modulation of cytotoxic lymphocytes and inflammatory cytokines
- Modification of target antigens

longer the new frontier of hepatology but is now a main-stream interest. Symposia to follow will have much to explore.

Before closing this summary, let me express deep appreciation to the three wonderful organizers of this symposium, Drs. Domenico Alvaro (Rome), Antonio Benedetti (Ancona) and Mario Strazzabosco (Padova) for their foresight and imagination which brought us to this beautiful city of Spoleto and for their hard work and cooperation which enabled all of us to enjoy this meeting and its special hospitality. I thank them also for indulging me with the privilege of providing these concluding remarks. As always, this meeting would not have been possible without the extraordinary generosity of our sponsor, Herbert Falk, to whom the final and most important thanks must go. Arrivederci – until we meet again.

Index

Falk Symposium Series

43. Reutter W, Popper H, Arias IM, Heinrich PC, Keppler D, Landmann L, eds.: *Modulation of Liver Cell Expression*. Falk Symposium No. 43. 1987 ISBN: 0-85200-677-2*
44. Boyer JL, Bianchi L, eds.: *Liver Cirrhosis*. Falk Symposium No. 44. 1987 ISBN: 0-85200-993-3*
45. Paumgartner G, Stiehl A, Gerok W, eds.: *Bile Acids and the Liver*. Falk Symposium No. 45. 1987 ISBN: 0-85200-675-6*
46. Goebell H, Peskar BM, Malchow H, eds.: *Inflammatory Bowel Diseases – Basic Research & Clinical Implications*. Falk Symposium No. 46. 1988 ISBN: 0-7462-0067-6*
47. Bianchi L, Holt P, James OFW, Butler RN, eds.: *Aging in Liver and Gastrointestinal Tract*. Falk Symposium No. 47. 1988 ISBN: 0-7462-0066-8*
48. Heilmann C, ed.: *Calcium-Dependent Processes in the Liver*. Falk Symposium No. 48. 1988 ISBN: 0-7462-0075-7*
50. Singer MV, Goebell H, eds.: *Nerves and the Gastrointestinal Tract*. Falk Symposium No. 50. 1989 ISBN: 0-7462-0114-1
51. Bannasch P, Keppler D, Weber G, eds.: *Liver Cell Carcinoma*. Falk Symposium No. 51. 1989 ISBN: 0-7462-0111-7
52. Paumgartner G, Stiehl A, Gerok W, eds.: *Trends in Bile Acid Research*. Falk Symposium No. 52. 1989 ISBN: 0-7462-0112-5
53. Paumgartner G, Stiehl A, Barbara L, Roda E, eds.: *Strategies for the Treatment of Hepatobiliary Diseases*. Falk Symposium No. 53. 1990 ISBN: 0-7923-8903-4
54. Bianchi L, Gerok W, Maier K-P, Deinhardt F, eds.: *Infectious Diseases of the Liver*. Falk Symposium No. 54. 1990 ISBN: 0-7923-8902-6
55. Falk Symposium No. 55 not published

55B. Hadziselimovic F, Herzog B, Bürgin-Wolff A, eds.: *Inflammatory Bowel Disease and Coeliac Disease in Children*. International Falk Symposium. 1990 ISBN 0-7462-0125-7

56. Williams CN, eds.: *Trends in Inflammatory Bowel Disease Therapy*. Falk Symposium No. 56. 1990 ISBN: 0-7923-8952-2
57. Bock KW, Gerok W, Matern S, Schmid R, eds.: *Hepatic Metabolism and Disposition of Endo- and Xenobiotics*. Falk Symposium No. 57. 1991 ISBN: 0-7923-8953-0
58. Paumgartner G, Stiehl A, Gerok W, eds.: *Bile Acids as Therapeutic Agents: From Basic Science to Clinical Practice*. Falk Symposium No. 58. 1991 ISBN: 0-7923-8954-9
59. Halter F, Garner A, Tytgat GNJ, eds.: *Mechanisms of Peptic Ulcer Healing*. Falk Symposium No. 59. 1991 ISBN: 0-7923-8955-7
60. Goebell H, Ewe K, Malchow H, Koelbel Ch, eds.: *Inflammatory Bowel Diseases – Progress in Basic Research and Clinical Implications*. Falk Symposium No. 60. 1991 ISBN: 0-7923-8956-5
61. Falk Symposium No. 61 not published
62. Dowling RH, Folsch UR, Löser Ch, eds.: *Polyamines in the Gastrointestinal Tract*. Falk Symposium No. 62. 1992 ISBN: 0-7923-8976-X
63. Lentze MJ, Reichen J, eds.: *Paediatric Cholestasis: Novel Approaches to Treatment*. Falk Symposium No. 63. 1992 ISBN: 0-7923-8977-8
64. Demling L, Frühmorgen P, eds.: *Non-Neoplastic Diseases of the Anorectum*. Falk Symposium No. 64. 1992 ISBN: 0-7923-8979-4

64B. Gressner AM, Ramadori G, eds.: *Molecular and Cell Biology of Liver Fibrogenesis*. International Falk Symposium. 1992 ISBN: 0-7923-8980-8

*These titles were published under the MTP Press imprint.

65. Hadziselimovic F, Herzog B, eds.: *Inflammatory Bowel Diseases and Morbus Hirschprung*. Falk Symposium No. 65. 1992 ISBN: 0-7923-8995-6
66. Martin F, McLeod RS, Sutherland LR, Williams CN, eds.: *Trends in Inflammatory Bowel Disease Therapy*. Falk Symposium No. 66. 1993 ISBN: 0-7923-8827-5
67. Schölmerich J, Kruis W, Goebell H, Hohenberger W, Gross V, eds.: *Inflammatory Bowel Diseases – Pathophysiology as Basis of Treatment*. Falk Symposium No. 67. 1993 ISBN: 0-7923-8996-4
68. Paumgartner G, Stiehl A, Gerok W, eds.: *Bile Acids and The Hepatobiliary System: From Basic Science to Clinical Practice*. Falk Symposium No. 68. 1993 ISBN: 0-7923-8829-1
69. Schmid R, Bianchi L, Gerok W, Maier K-P, eds.: *Extrahepatic Manifestations in Liver Diseases*. Falk Symposium No. 69. 1993 ISBN: 0-7923-8821-6
70. Meyer zum Büschenfelde K-H, Hoofnagle J, Manns M, eds.: *Immunology and Liver*. Falk Symposium No. 70. 1993 ISBN: 0-7923-8830-5
71. Surrenti C, Casini A, Milani S, Pinzani M , eds.: *Fat-Storing Cells and Liver Fibrosis*. Falk Symposium No. 71. 1994 ISBN: 0-7923-8842-9
72. Rachmilewitz D, ed.: *Inflammatory Bowel Diseases – 1994*. Falk Symposium No. 72. 1994 ISBN: 0-7923-8845-3
73. Binder HJ, Cummings J, Soergel KH, eds.: *Short Chain Fatty Acids*. Falk Symposium No. 73. 1994 ISBN: 0-7923-8849-6

73B. Möllmann HW, May B, eds.: *Glucocorticoid Therapy in Chronic Inflammatory Bowel Disease: from basic principles to rational therapy*. International Falk Workshop. 1996 ISBN 0-7923-8708-2

74. Keppler D, Jungermann K, eds.: *Transport in the Liver*. Falk Symposium No. 74. 1994 ISBN: 0-7923-8858-5

74B. Stange EF, ed.: *Chronic Inflammatory Bowel Disease*. Falk Symposium. 1995 ISBN: 0-7923-8876-3

75. van Berge Henegouwen GP, van Hoek B, De Groote J, Matern S, Stockbrügger RW, eds.: *Cholestatic Liver Diseases: New Strategies for Prevention and Treatment of Hepatobiliary and Cholestatic Liver Diseases*. Falk Symposium 75. 1994. ISBN: 0-7923-8867-4
76. Monteiro E, Tavarela Veloso F, eds.: *Inflammatory Bowel Diseases: New Insights into Mechanisms of Inflammation and Challenges in Diagnosis and Treatment*. Falk Symposium 76. 1995. ISBN 0-7923-8884-4
77. Singer MV, Ziegler R, Rohr G, eds.: *Gastrointestinal Tract and Endocrine System*. Falk Symposium 77. 1995. ISBN 0-7923-8877-1
78. Decker K, Gerok W, Andus T, Gross V, eds.: *Cytokines and the Liver*. Falk Symposium 78. 1995. ISBN 0-7923-8878-X
79. Holstege A, Schölmerich J, Hahn EG, eds.: *Portal Hypertension*. Falk Symposium 79. 1995. ISBN 0-7923-8879-8
80. Hofmann AF, Paumgartner G, Stiehl A, eds.: *Bile Acids in Gastroenterology: Basic and Clinical Aspects*. Falk Symposium 80. 1995 ISBN 0-7923-8880-1
81. Riecken EO, Stallmach A, Zeitz M, Heise W, eds.: *Malignancy and Chronic Inflammation in the Gastrointestinal Tract – New Concepts*. Falk Symposium 81. 1995 ISBN 0-7923-8889-5
82. Fleig WE, ed.: *Inflammatory Bowel Diseases: New Developments and Standards*. Falk Symposium 82. 1995 ISBN 0-7923-8890-6

Falk Symposium Series

82B. Paumgartner G, Beuers U, eds.: *Bile Acids in Liver Diseases.* International Falk Workshop. 1995 ISBN 0-7923-8891-7

83. Dobrilla G, Felder M, de Pretis G, eds.: *Advances in Hepatobiliary and Pancreatic Diseases: Special Clinical Topics.* Falk Symposium 83. 1995. ISBN 0-7923-8892-5

84. Fromm H, Leuschner U, eds.: *Bile Acids – Cholestasis – Gallstones: Advances in Basic and Clinical Bile Acid Research.* Falk Symposium 84. 1995 ISBN 0-7923-8893-3

85. Tytgat GNJ, Bartelsman JFWM, van Deventer SJH, eds.: *Inflammatory Bowel Diseases.* Falk Symposium 85. 1995 ISBN 0-7923-8894-1

86. Berg PA, Leuschner U, eds.: *Bile Acids and Immunology.* Falk Symposium 86. 1996 ISBN 0-7923-8700-7

87. Schmid R, Bianchi L, Blum HE, Gerok W, Maier KP, Stalder GA, eds.: *Acute and Chronic Liver Diseases: Molecular Biology and Clinics.* Falk Symposium 87. 1996 ISBN 0-7923-8701-5

88. Blum HE, Wu GY, Wu CH, eds.: *Molecular Diagnosis and Gene Therapy.* Falk Symposium 88. 1996 ISBN 0-7923-8702-3

88B. Poupon RE, Reichen J, eds.: *Surrogate Markers to Assess Efficacy of TReatment in Chronic Liver Diseases.* International Falk Workshop. 1996 ISBN 0-7923-8705-8

89. Reyes HB, Leuschner U, Arias IM, eds.: *Pregnancy, Sex Hormones and the Liver.* Falk Symposium 89. 1996 ISBN 0-7923-8704-X

89B. Broelsch CE, Burdelski M, Rogiers X, eds.: *Cholestatic Liver Diseases in Children and Adults.* International Falk Workshop. 1996 ISBN 0-7923-8710-4

90. Lam S-K, Paumgartner P, Wang B, eds.: *Update on Hepatobiliary Diseases 1996.* Falk Symposium 90. 1996 ISBN 0-7923-8715-5

91. Hadziselimovic F, Herzog B, eds.: *Inflammatory Bowel Diseases and Chronic Recurrent Abdominal Pain.* Falk Symposium 91. 1996 ISBN 0-7923-8722-8

91B. Alvaro D, Benedetti A, Strazzabosco M, eds.: *Vanishing Bile Duct Syndrome – Pathophysiology and Treatment.* International Falk Workshop. 1996 ISBN 0-7923-8721-X